The
Rebellious Body

Reclaim Your Life from
Environmental Illness or
Chronic Fatigue Syndrome

The
Rebellious Body

Reclaim Your Life from Environmental Illness or Chronic Fatigue Syndrome

Janice Strubbe Wittenberg, R.N.

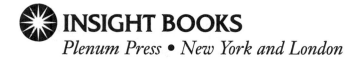 **INSIGHT BOOKS**
Plenum Press • New York and London

Library of Congress Cataloging in Publication Data

Wittenberg, Janice Strubbe
  The rebellious body: reclaim your life from environmental illness or chronic fatigue syndrome / Janice Strubbe Wittenberg.
    p.   cm.
  Includes bibliographical references and index.
  ISBN 0-306-45402-5
  1. Chronic fatigue syndrome—Popular works. 2. Environmentally induced diseases—Popular works. 3. Chronic fatigue syndrome—Alternative treatment. 4. Environmentally induced diseases—Alternative treatment. I. Title.
RB150.F37W56 1996   96-32725
616'.047—dc20   CIP

The information in this book is based on the personal experiences and research of the author. This material is for information purposes only and should not be construed as medical advice. The reader is strongly advised not to self-diagnose and is also advised to check with a qualified health professional before implementing any intervention. The author and publisher assume no responsibility for any treatments undertaken by the reader. Companies, interventions, and products are mentioned without bias to increase your knowledge only, not as a recommendation, promise of a cure, mitigation, prescription, or prevention of your medical condition. The names of individuals interviewed on these pages have been changed and composited to protect their privacy.

The cover artwork is based on the painting "Woman with Fish (#1)," © 1995, by Anna P. Oneglia. The figure on page 62 is adapted with permission from Aristo Vojdani, Ph.D., M.T., Immunosciences Laboratories, Beverly Hills, California. The illustrations on pages 73, 78, and 117 are by John Diggins.

ISBN 0-306-45402-5

© 1996 Janice Strubbe Wittenberg
Insight Books is a Division of Plenum Publishing Corporation
233 Spring Street, New York, N.Y. 10013-1578

An Insight Book

10 9 8 7 6 5 4 3 2 1

Printed in the United States of America

To John David Wittenberg, my soulmate, who helped put the eyebrows on my computer skills and who adored and angered me into health.

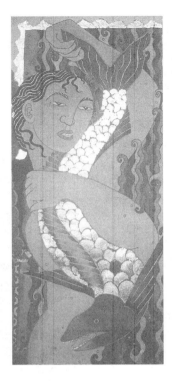

Foreword

*M*illions of Americans (and countless more worldwide) are living a nightmare of sorts. They feel bad, day after day, month after month, with a variety of distressing symptoms such as fatigue, headache, muscle and joint pains, abdominal discomfort, and problems with memory and concentration. Worse yet, when they seek help from their doctors, they are often told there is nothing really wrong with them, or the problem is all in their head. Even if they are given a diagnosis such as chronic fatigue syndrome or environmental illness, they are often told that not much can be done for them, that their illness is chronic and incurable.

If you are one of those millions of sufferers, have a friend or loved one who is chronically ill, or are a health practitioner, this is a book that can change your life for the better.

I am a family practitioner in northern California who has long had a special interest in helping patients suffering from chronic fatigue and food and chemical sensitivities. Like many physicians, I was unsatisfied with the limited approaches I was taught in medical school. While I appreciate the powers of prescription drugs and surgery, they seem of limited value in most chronic illnesses, usually serving more to treat symptoms than to actually cure the patient. To cure chronic illness it is necessary to look for the underlying causes and try to address them. This is best done using complementary therapies such as diet and life-style modification, nutritional supplements, herbs, homeopathy, and acupuncture. Each patient needs to be approached within the context of his family, social, and physical environment. With proper treatment these patients improve and eventually recover.

I can think of no one more qualified to write a book about recovering from chronic fatigue syndrome and environmental illness than a health professional who has had these illnesses and recovered. Janice Strubbe Wittenberg is such a person. I have had the honor of being part of her healthcare team and witnessing her healing over the past 7 years. She is a great example of the proactive patient, one who has taken responsibility for her health and has taken charge of her recovery. She has explored and experimented with a tremendous variety of conventional and alternative therapies, separating the wheat from the chaff, learning which were truly helpful. One of the secrets of my success as a physician is that I learn from my patients. There are many innovative therapies that I first learned about from Janice. She has been a valuable resource of information for me.

I have read many fine books about chronic fatigue syndrome and environmental illness, but I have not seen any as wide-ranging and comprehensive as this one. Because Janice addresses the underlying causes of illness, the information in this book will prove useful to *anyone* with a chronic health problem such as heart disease, arthritis, and cancer. This book also contains invaluable information for anyone interested in maintaining optimal health in today's world.

There is an amazing amount of information in this book. Janice has taken a truly holistic approach to her subject, exploring it from multiple perspectives. She explores the variety of theories as to the causes of these illnesses, provides clear and concise information about the human body and the functioning of the immune system, and explores as wide a range of treatments as I have seen assembled in one book. Her detailed discussions of diet, supplements, herbs, energy-based approaches, environmental factors, and mental and emotional aspects of health provide the comprehensive information people need for their recovery. Throughout the book she shares the experiences of real people who are fighting these illnesses, grounding the theoretical with the practical.

As a medical doctor, I feel obligated to emphasize that there is much about the causes and treatment of chronic fatigue syndrome and environmental illness that medical science does not understand. Many of the concepts and therapies Janice discusses have been scientifically validated, but many of these concepts and therapies remain unproven to the satisfaction of medical science. I am certain that many doctors will be highly skeptical about some of the concepts and treatments in this book. A certain amount of skepticism is reasonable, but one should be aware that a high percentage of the treatments commonly used in Western medicine are also unproven, and just because a treatment has not been proven to be effective does not mean it may not be helpful. Not every therapy in this book will be helpful to everyone, but everyone is likely to benefit from at least some of the treatments recommended.

Janice writes with wisdom and compassion. This book is a treasure-house of information. Anyone who takes the advice in this book to heart will find themselves on the road to better health of mind, body, and spirit. I wish the readers well on their journey.

Randy S. Baker, MD
Director, Pacific Center for Integral Health
Santa Cruz, California

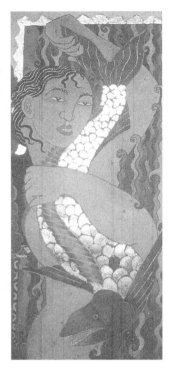

Acknowledgments

i wish to thank my husband, John Wittenberg, for his support and encouragement. I thank my mother, Jane Strubbe, and my deceased father, Jack Strubbe, for their gift of tenacity. I salute my wild, wonderful siblings, Dick, Anne, Bill, and John Strubbe, and their families, including Susan, Cristen, Jason, and Nicholas. Plus, my fine stepson, Shiloh Klepp.

I thank my healthcare team: Randy Baker, MD, Vincent Mark, MD, Mary Ellen Mark, RN, DOM, Julie Carter Hinson, DOM, Arthur Faygenholtz, DOC, Rajyo Huntley, CMT, Virginia Dixon, healer, and Grace Laurencin, MD. I also thank Michael Mamas, DOVM, founder of The School for Enlightenment and Healing, for helping to release my fear of success.

I wish to acknowledge my writing team: my dear friend Deborah Allen, for the idea of the book; Pilar Pederson, for thinking I can do anything I choose; Laurie Harper, my literary agent, for believing in the project; Frank K. Darmstadt, my editor, who was willing to take a chance; Barbara Selfridge, wonder-writer and dear friend; Barry Shepherd, PA, and Terri Frazier, for their important input; John Gillette, MD, Anna Keck, RN, NP, and John Abrams, PhD, for their technical advice. And to Joyce Robinson, friend and colleague, for her loving, ever-constant support.

Most of all, I wish to acknowledge my fellow strugglers who helped guide me with their courage and wisdom: Lari Jacqueline Doughty, Elizabeth Good, Mark Norman, Ellie Skulnick, Joanne Warobick, Terry Cleary, Gail Byrum, Louise Caraco, Sara Sanderson, Mette Hansen, Nancy Keating, Susan Van Ordstrom, Rita Mumm, and Tzivia Gover. I also wish to remember Matthew Wolf for his insights and for his courage in death. Finally, I wish to thank and express my love for Great Mother Earth.

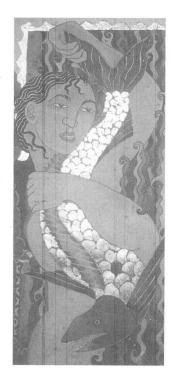

Contents

Part Two: Complementary Interventions

Part Three: What Helps

Part Four: Examining and Changing Your Beliefs

Part Five: Sustaining Your Healing

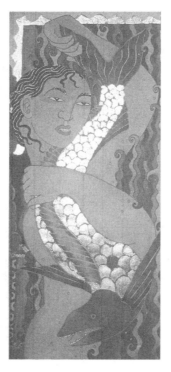

Introduction

*t*his is the book I wish someone had given me when I was ill with environmental illness (EI) and chronic fatigue syndrome (CFS). I wanted a practical book that would help me heal my unhealthy body, but also one that would go further, helping to heal my mind and spirit as well. This is such a book.

It is a book for people who are hungry to discover their path to recovery for themselves. The information and the strategies offered on these pages are meant to encourage and empower you. Other books offer a piece of the puzzle, but this one contains an entire smorgasbord of options, including feedback from sufferers regarding sources of relief. While I make no pretense at scientific mastery, hopefully this information will help you cut some corners, and prevent you from being as lost and confused as I was for such a long time.

Assuming that you already have medical support, the information on these pages will augment your recovery. If you are health-oriented and interested in taking charge of your life, this book may assist your journey. Even if you are not acutely ill, but find yourself living at half-mast with low energy and multiple, vague symptoms, this book can help you.

This book is for people of varying levels of expertise, for health practitioners, for family members, or for individuals who are ill. Some may choose to read all the way through, whereas others may seek specific information. You may use it as a resource, referring to it repeatedly. If you already know all the scientific information you care to about these illnesses or are not interested in paying attention to a lot of details, you may wish to skip the first few chapters and go directly to any other part of the book that offers specific interventions and relief. The only prerequisite to using this information is that you must believe that you can actually help yourself to become well. Without this glimmer of hope you will work against yourself.

Much of the work that awaits has to do with a multilevel approach that emphasizes boosting your immune capabilities and changing harmful attitudes. EI and CFS are tenacious, complex illnesses of the immune system that require deep and profound change on all levels. Learning to mitigate environmental factors that impact your body is one step toward healing. Cultivating healthy relationships and examining and challenging your ideas about who you are and what you are worth will also support and strengthen you.

Emotional states, habitual thought patterns, attitudes, diet, daily routines, and spiritual practices are all vital aspects of recovery. Living in harmony and internal balance will have a positive resonant effect on your ability to live in harmony with nature. Recognition that you can consciously impact all of these variables will help activate your immune system. As the helmsman of your life, you are the source of the power and the sails. Over time, in the process of healing you can determine the direction to be sailed, navigating your life toward your chosen destination.

Even if you are not able to directly impact the illness itself, there is much you can do to enhance your health. Though there is no single element that offers the magic bullet to protect you from viral, chemical, and bacterial influences, there are specific things that can accelerate your recovery. These specific interventions form the five major parts of this book and are as follows.

- *Understanding These Illnesses:* Information is *power*. This part offers information about EI and CFS, about the importance of maximizing immune function, and about the ways that the body is impacted by the disease process. It does not describe these illnesses in depth; mostly it sets a foundation for what you can do about these problems in later chapters. The more you understand both illnesses, the greater the range of choices you have toward creating your recovery.
- *Complementary Interventions:* Augmenting the medical model can be scary, but it is an important step in the process of healing. By shifting from a passive to a more proactive stance, you may find other models that suit your needs. This part explores several forms of subtle energy work as well as therapies that can help the recovery process.
- *What Helps:* You will be given tools for discovery and exploration that you can use to implement a multidimensional program that can bring about tangible relief. Recovery means taking action to protect yourself and

engaging in activities that strengthen your body. Included here are simple practical things you can do to achieve relief.

- *Examining and Changing Your Beliefs:* Exploring mental and emotional factors that influence health gives you the opportunity to influence your own perceptions and make choices that impact emotional states. As a result, you may be able to see which habits are obstructing your progress and steer your life in the direction you choose. Fearlessly examining and changing beliefs makes it possible to alter your relationship to the experience of illness. Creating a synergy with all of this information will enable you to establish a personal program of recovery.

- *Sustaining Your Healing:* The return of health does not end the work that must be done to sustain recovery. Return to the real world holds inevitable hazards that require ongoing self-protective measures. Your experience of illness may give rise to a budding consciousness that calls you into action to help the earth to recover from the same factors that have harmed you.

Experimenting with the information in these five parts, you will discover what works for you, using what is here to your best advantage. You may establish one program that works well for a time, but may eventually reach a plateau so there is no further progress. In deference to the changing needs of your body, you may need to select different interventions at different times.

These illnesses have many causes—genetic, hereditary, dietary, environmental, life-style, and personality factors all play a role. There is no one identifiable causative factor at work here. The question as to whether it is the body or the mind that caused you to become sick is unresolved. What makes sense is that emotional disharmony works synergistically with genetic frailties, as well as toxic and viral exposures, to make you sick.

While you can affect your response to what is occurring, you cannot control every curve ball these illnesses toss your way. Adhering to the notion that you should be in control of all that has happened is a sensitive issue that evokes resentment and resistance. Yet, it can be helpful to examine the mind–body conundrum. While no one factor caused you to become ill from EI and CFS, your state of mind may have had a major role in disease onset. Years of imbalance created by unhappiness, self-denial, and an overabundance of worry about the opinions of others may have helped make you sick.

There can be great freedom in accepting the idea that your state of mind has an enormous influence on the course of your health. Healing requires that a transformation of consciousness take place. This is often the pivotal point of recovery, accepting the involvement of the mind in healing and moving from there to help yourself. This is the only part of the illness you can control. Until you understand this, you may be locked into resistance; doing all you can to hate these illnesses, to hate yourself, and to hate the world that has seemingly cornered you and limited your options.

When you accept personal responsibility for your mental states, you can embark on the process of deeper healing. How you come to terms with your infirmities is a matter of choice; despite ongoing difficulties with illness you can still take charge of your life. Since you cannot alter your inheritance, or past toxic exposures, the only aspect of becoming healed that you have control over is to accept your role as cocreator. In this way you can, from this moment of recognition forward, use your ingenuity, curiosity, courage, and wits to assist yourself to get well.

Living life fully from a place of conscious choice, all becomes precious, despite discomfort and restrictions. You can learn to affect your experience of illness by making choices over how you feel about what is happening. That is the key to empowerment. How you decide to feel about your life sets the stage for everything that follows. Making the choice to see yourself as responsible for your experience offers a tremendous source of information and power that unfolds into the process of healing. The more you see yourself as responsible for creating your experiences, the more you can choose to "discreate" the experiences that do not serve you now.

Making this shift means you can no longer be split off from yourself, living behind the scenes, giving yourself away, changing your personality to blend into the background. From this perspective you can no longer blame yourself for being sick. The fact that you are responsible for creating your life means forgiving yourself both for numbing your compassion and for selling out your true self. It is no easy task to become altruistic, placing your own needs first. This means breaking down dysfunctional ideas and habits acquired early in life.

Recovery is an incremental process that forces you to change your relationship with life. This change doesn't happen all at once; it may take years, and the process can seem endless. You will continue to have ups and downs. Every time you think you've mastered an obstacle, another will appear. After enjoying a long upswing of improved health you may crash. Every time you think you know it all, there is always more to learn. Even when you feel better, there is still much work necessary to sustain recovery. Along the way, obstacles can become welcome challenges offering opportunities for growth.

You never know where healing will come from: a moment of shared laughter; saying "no" when you need to; taking the right supplements; or performing an act of kindness. Each intervention offers a piece of the puzzle. Even in the face of persistent illness, you still possess many options.

The efforts you make on your behalf will set the cause in motion, creating results that are cumulative. Every experience offers an opportunity to learn something more. Even your "failures" can be a useful source of information. Over time you will have the opportunity to learn through a process of trial and error the places where you can take charge and the places where you must loosen the reins. You will need to take risks, venturing into uncharted territories. The process of healing will require that you make a shift in perspective that must accommodate new ways of being and doing.

Eventually, this accumulation of small changes will snowball into an avalanche that can make an enormous difference. Each small change helps to build momentum toward strengthening your body. There may be great times of growth and change and times when you need to rest and retreat. You already know there is no instant cure and that recovery is not a linear progression or a permanent, static state. True healing is not limited to physical health; it includes self-empowerment, increased awareness, and a larger understanding and acceptance of all that exists.

EI and CFS, by their very nature, are isolating illnesses. You have had to cope alone, being too tired to make contact or having to be careful to avoid toxins, which has limited your interactions. Without mirrors reflected by others who share your circumstances, it is difficult to gauge your own progress.

A key aspect of your recovery may include hearing about the experiences of others who have been ill. Observing their struggles may catapult you out of self-involvement, increase your understanding of these illnesses, and enable you to measure your own growth. There are an abundance of stories of courage, growth, and healing that can validate your own efforts to heal. Reaching out can help you develop a rudder by which to steer the course of your healing. Stories of people with EI and CFS appear on these pages to give you hope that recovery is possible.

Don't adhere to their guidelines for your journey. People who have achieved the greatest degree of wellness or those who live in harmony with these illnesses are those who have taken off on their own path, not waiting for someone to come along who will fix them. There are some who are going at their own healing using very unusual, subtle measures. Chanting, visualization, energetic healing practices, and completely revamping dietary practices are some methods. Gaining this information can help move you to new levels in your own awareness.

You may not agree with all that is offered in this book, but this information will increase your options. Try to adapt what is here to suit your needs and adjust to changing circumstances. Use your own judgment and discernment to empower you, allowing a healthy sense of curiosity to steer you while trusting your intuition.

Coming to terms with both the spiritual and emotional aspects of illness is an essential part of the process. True healing is not about the absence of symptoms but rather about the integration of the estranged parts with the whole. Your illness offers an opportunity, a point of departure from the old self and, paradoxically, an opportunity to reconnect with those estranged parts.

What can make a difference in your recovery is to form a team of your healer-self and your survivor-self. Forming this partnership can make it easier to survive the ups and downs of these illnesses. The healer-self is the aspect of you that accepts full responsibility for your life. The healer-self is able to be totally honest, without pretense or judgment; knowing and accepting exactly who you are in this moment and in the next. The healer doesn't worry about making mistakes and holds a space of unconditional compassion that reaches beyond judgment.

While the healer-self is vulnerable, expansive, and accepting, the survivor-self is your feistier aspect that will fight to protect you. The survivor brings you through times of anguish and distress. It is the unruly, tousle-haired child, a part of you that is noisy, argumentative, and willing to stand up for you. It is the survivor-self that believes you are worthy. Particularly handy in difficult times, it is controlling and resistant in ways that keep you from giving up.

Cultivating the healer-self can enable you to take tiny steps toward greater acceptance of what each moment has to offer. This acceptance becomes easier as you learn to surrender to the way things are instead of how you want them to be. The idea of surrender and acceptance may imply abandoning the fight to become well. Yet, acceptance is not about giving away power; it is saying yes to being fully present in life and accepting what is. In fact, the more you resist and deny reality, the more you lose physical energy. This happens most noticeably when you leave the present, to imagine wellness, wishing that things could be different than they are. Acceptance enables you to recover lost energy. Acceptance offers you power which means you are no longer helpless.

The survivor-self, motivated to search for solutions, has great curiosity. This desire to know compels you to seek out books, teachers, and methods of self-help. This doer-self pushes you forward, putting you in charge, while protecting you from being engulfed by trying experiences.

These two aspects form a team that creates a harmonious, balanced whole. The healer guides and shows the survivor where to look for answers, while the survivor provides the energy and inspiration to move forward. It is the healer that uncovers and forces you to face your resistance and the survivor that pushes you to the edge of what is possible.

Balancing on the razor's edge, staying disciplined, focused, and doing, while at the same time staying open and allowing can be tricky. You may find yourself bouncing between the two states. Your work is about finding a balance between acceptance and living full tilt. You may wish to consciously employ both of these forces to help you to move from being a victim toward living fully while in the process of overcoming EI and CFS. Making a team of these two qualities, allowing them to work for you, can make it easier to access and achieve recovery.

*Part
One*

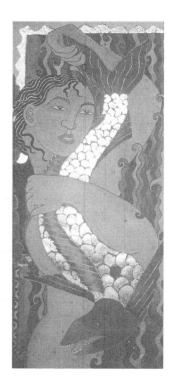

*Understanding
These Illnesses*

Chapter One

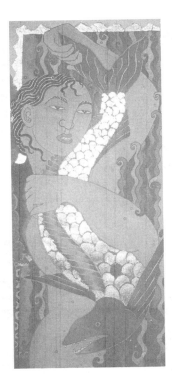

The Immune System

*t*he immune system has an enormous task, namely, to provide protection from the damaging effects of pathogenic bacteria, viruses, molds, fungi, and parasites that can lead to illness. The key to good health depends on how well the immune system does its job. When the immune system is strong the body is healthy; when it is weak the body may be sick. Recovery and staying well means taking care of the immune system by doing everything possible to support its ability to function. With EI and CFS the immune system is not able to perform its protective functions.[1-3] Strengthening the immune system is what directs the care in these illnesses.[4]

Because your recovery centers on helping the immune system do the best job it possibly can, it is important to understand how it works. The immune system is like those old-fashioned Christmas tree lights, the kind where when one light burns out the whole string goes dark. It's not a hard job to fix when just one bulb is burned out, but when two are out, the frustration level can drive even a 12-year-old to tears. In the case of EI and CFS there are at least two bulbs out, and you never know what's going to flare up next. Sometimes it's easier to get a whole new pack of bulbs and start over.

Even when you replace all of the lights, each immune system is unique, reacting differently when it is called into action. This is why there is no one treatment that is uniformly effective with all people. Owing to the individual variations of the immune response, there is no one way to treat all of the problems of EI and CFS. On top of that, individual sensitivity can vary over time; an intervention that once brought relief may no longer alleviate symptoms.

What Is the Immune System?

Natural immunity is provided from your mother at birth through breast feeding. Other sources of immunity arise in the face of illness when antibodies and T cells increase in number, performing their assigned tasks. Further immunity develops as a result of vaccinations you receive during the course of your life.

The immune system is made up of a vast network of interrelated organs and biochemicals, each part carrying a preprogrammed imprint of how it should perform and what a healthy body state is. It is composed of (1) the bone marrow, (2) lymphatic vessels and organs, including the spleen, thymus, tonsils, and lymph nodes, (3) the white blood cells (lymphocytes, monocytes, macrophages, neutrophils, basophils, eosinophils, and other cells), (4) specialized cells found in various tissues (macrophages, mast cells, and others), and (5) specific serum factors.

All of these cells communicate with each other with overlapping functions between various white blood cells, which helps the system to compensate when certain parts are not working properly. The immune cells receive information from the diverse organ systems including the brain.[5-7] This means every aspect of one's being is influenced by and has an influence on immune capability.

The Role of the Immune System

What is of greatest concern is the immune system's ability to perform the job of destroying foreign substances before they cause harm. This system must be ever vigilant to protect you whenever there is contact with potentially harmful substances. Agents that could cause harm are found everywhere in everything; requiring that the immune system discretely work to ward off illness all of the time. Even without your conscious participation, the immune system is constantly working behind the scenes to enable you to recover.

There are two main aspects to immunity: cell-mediated immunity and humoral immunity. Let's first consider the major components of cell-mediated immunity. Cell-mediated immunity is the portion of the immune system that is mediated by the T cells and is important in the defense against malignant cells, viral infection, fungal infection, and some bacteria. The principal protectors against invading organisms are the white blood cells. Each white blood cell, also known as a *leukocyte*, is born in the bone marrow. Some of them migrate to the thymus to become T cells. Others become macrophages, monocytes, granulocytes, eosinophils, basophils, megakaryocytes, B cells, or natural killer cells. These cells are present in the lymphoid tissue of the spleen, the lymph nodes, the gastrointestinal tract, and the bone marrow, or circulate in the peripheral blood.

Lymphocytes are leukocytes found in lymphatic tissue and the whole blood circulatory pool, while *phagocytes* are leukocytes that function as scavenger cells. There are several varieties of scavenger cells. *Macrophages* engulf and destroy invaders, eating debris and diseased tissue and signaling the presence of invaders to other immune cells. *Monocytes* digest antigen particles after an infection and trigger many immune responses. *Granulocytes*, like T-killer cells, are ever vigilant to detect and destroy virus-infected cells.

Eosinophils contain highly toxic proteins and oxygen radicals which fight pathogens. In addition, they release biochemicals called leukotreines and prostaglandins which initiate inflammation in surrounding tissue. *Basophils*, found in the anterior lobe of the pituitary, produce corticotropin, the substance that stimulates the adrenal cortex. *Megakaryocytes* are large cells of bone marrow that help in the formation of platelets.

Types of thymus-derived (T) cells include: T-helper cells, T-killer cells, and T-memory cells. These cells coordinate many immune functions and are the major component of cell-mediated immunity. *T-helper cells* sound the alarm to activate various aspects of the immune system and boost the activation of B cells, which produce antibodies. *T-killer cells* also called phagocytes are each programmed within the body to recognize and destroy a specific virus or bacterium. They do this by recognizing foreign antigens present on the surface of the body's own infected cells and then proceed to destroy the infected cells. *T-memory cells* are long-lived T-helper and T-killer cells that carry the memory of previous contact with antigens, allowing more rapid activation of the immune response.

Natural killer cells (NK) are unique in that they act independently of other immune cells and are able to detect cancerous and virus-infected cells and destroy them. They are able to act even when T-helper cells have stopped sounding the alarm to action and may be an important source of cytokines, which will be discussed shortly. In CFS, the level of NK cells is usually low.[4,8] *B-cells* are responsible for producing antibodies that attach themselves to pathogens and inactivate them.

Antigens and Antibodies

Humoral immunity, the second aspect of immunity, involves the activities of antigens and antibodies. Humoral immunity is the portion of the immune system that is mediated by antibodies produced by B cells. The B cell is the cellular source of antibodies that are released into the bloodstream as well as tears, saliva, genital secretions, and mucus and into the digestive system. Recognizing the presence of foreign viral or bacterial cells, or environmental pollutants, the B cell is stimulated to produce specific antibodies. These antibodies attach to the surface of invading proteins or antigens to neutralize them until a phagocyte arrives and devours the immune complex.

Antibodies are protein molecules in the blood and body tissue capable of recognizing foreign matter in and around the body. When B cells recognize alien substances, they multiply to become large numbers of antibody factories. Each of the classes of antibodies, known as *immunoglobulins,* has a different role. The most common ones are IgG, IgA, IgM, IgD, and IgE. For further information regarding immunoglobulins, consult *The Merck Manual* (Rahway: Merck Sharp & Dohme Research Laboratories).

An antigen is any substance that is foreign to the body or that the body reacts to as if it were foreign which triggers an immune response. Antigens can be invading viruses, fungi, parasites, bacteria, or any other substance, including food and self-produced hormones that the body rejects. One of the remarkable aspects of the immune system is its ability to recognize past invaders, allowing it to respond rapidly to block a second attack.

While some antibodies disable toxins produced by bacteria, others prevent viruses from entering healthy cells. Some activate the *complement system,* which is made up of a series of proteins that cause cells to release chemicals. These chemicals produce the inflammatory response that kills the cells and signals to scavenger cells to destroy and carry away the debris. The chemicals produced in the process of mobilizing the immune response can contribute to the inflammatory reaction responsible for allergic symptoms.

Normally, the body orchestrates the destruction of bacterial, viral, and chemical invaders by igniting protection in the form of macrophages, NK cells, B cells, T cells, and cytokines. Dr. Paul Cheney, researcher and physician whose practice emphasizes CFS, reports that with CFS there is a pattern of chronically elevated T-cell activation, variable B-cell dysfunction, and severe NK cell deficits.[2] There are also elevated cytokine levels and immunoglobulin deficiencies.

Cytokines

Cytokines are hormones produced by the immune cells which help regulate the immune response. They are extremely potent mediators which are active at very low concentrations. A diverse array of these mediators have been identified and different immune cells produce different cytokines. When there is an infection or an allergic reaction, the cytokines are released by cells at the local site of inflammation.

Certain cytokines, such as interleukin 1 (IL-1), tumor necrosis factor (TNF), and interleukin 6 (IL-6), can be found systemically in the circulation during infection, and may be released in high enough quantities so as to cause unpleasant side effects. The chronic overproduction of certain cytokines may result in the variety of symptoms seen in CFS, including profound fatigue, characteristic of the illness.[9-11] High levels of certain cytokines have been found in CFS,[12] and they may be responsible for many of the unpleasant symptoms of EI. Also present may be certain immunosuppressive cytokines such as interleukin 10.

Their activity can make you feel more sick than you actually are, causing aches, flu symptoms, and fatigue, often mistaken for the presence of a virus. In addition, cytokines interact with central nervous system receptors, creating difficulty with memory. The activity of cytokines makes it difficult to differentiate the discomfort caused by the illness itself from the physiological immune response to the illness.[4]

Immune Abnormalities

The immune system is capable of acting in abnormal ways; it can be overactive or underactive in performing its protective duties. The immune system can even react to "normal" substances by either over- or underproducing immune substances necessary to protect the body.

Autoimmunity

Autoimmunity is the overactive response against the body's own tissues, likened to an allergy against the self. Examples of illnesses where this occurs are EI, Hashimoto's thyroiditis, rheumatoid arthritis, multiple sclerosis, lupus, and Graves' disease. In the case of autoimmunity, the immune response goes into high gear and is unable to halt its protective reactivity even when the threat is past. Antibodies then attack healthy parts of the body in the same way they would an invading bacterium or virus.

The body fails to return to a normal state and simply goes on producing antibodies that cause allergic symptoms. Unlike the healthy immune system, which relaxes after handling an immune reaction, in autoimmunity healthy cells are attacked and destroyed. In the healthy individual, when the intruder is destroyed the body sends out a signal to curtail its mobilization efforts. It is not understood why those with CFS and EI never receive this crucial message.

Overactive Immune Response

For unknown reasons the body can overreact to ingested substances and to those in the environment in an allergic manner. With CFS and more commonly with EI, this process escalates to the extent that the body overreacts when in contact with hazardous and even nonhazardous matter. Reactivities to organic foods and seemingly benign materials such as spring water are examples of inappropriate harm caused by overly vigilant immune activation.

Underactive Immune Response

When the system is underactivated, the body reacts only minimally or does not react at all to substances that should trigger the protective action of the immune response. In this case the immune system may be suppressed or the pathogen may be able to alter its form, evading the defense systems, as in the case of AIDS. This underactive response can be to a bacterial or viral infection or to environmental toxins.

Ironically, the indicator that Theresa, a 41-year-old who has had severe EI for over 13 years, is improving is that she is more allergically reactive. Increased allergic sensitivities can signal improved health, and her physician regards it as a sign that her immune system is activated. At her worst she could not summon any protective immune response; her body was simply too disabled to protect her.

T-Cell Defects

T-cell abnormalities are commonly seen in CFS.[4] With immune malfunction there is often a defect in the production of T cells or a defect in their ability to perform their designated function so that antibodies can be over- or underproduced. At times, with CFS, T cells are noted to become active, later returning to normal during periods of improved health.[4] In the face of EI, chemical exposures can damage T cells, interfering with their functioning.

Toxins and Immune Dysfunction

Your immune system mobilizes to protect you from toxins, foreign objects that come in contact with the body and cause a disturbing resonant effect. The environment is full of toxic matter which the body is constantly struggling to detoxify and at times these toxins may not be met with an adequate immune response.

Many household products as well as commonly used materials that you think of as "safe" can endanger your health. Examples of common household toxins include products containing phenol or formaldehyde.[13] The problem of chemical susceptibility and its relationship to the immune system has been clarified by the work of the late Theron Randolph, MD, president of the Human Ecology Research Foundation. His work notes that increasing exposure to the growing number of chemical toxins in the environment places everyone's health at risk.[14]

Environmental pollutants can hamper the body's ability to detoxify substances through the normal immune pathways. The liver, the major organ of detoxification, works to break down toxins into metabolites and harmless waste chemicals. When liver function is hampered by excess toxins, it is unable to remove them through normal routes such as excretion and perspiration, causing an increase in total body burden of poisons.

When the immune system is impaired, the body has difficulty removing toxic matter. Over time, toxins are absorbed and ultimately bound into the cell structure, resulting in a disturbance of normal function. This buildup of cellular toxins may overwhelm the body, making it difficult to overcome their damaging effects, and can lead to physical degeneration. It is possible to dislodge toxins from the cells, but organs may not be functioning at peak efficiency so that the toxins can be difficult to excrete from the body. Even when toxins are dislodged, they may resettle in a new location or back in the same site, causing new symptoms depending on where they end up.

In turn, exposure to toxins further prompts intolerance to foods. Unable to digest needed foods, nutritional depletion ensues, further contributing to immune malfunction. When nutrients are depleted, all systems stop functioning efficiently. A vicious circle of toxic buildup increases as the immune system is less capable of mustering its forces to cope with the damage.

Diet and Immune Capability

The major determinant of the ability to keep the immune system healthy is your nutritional status. Some factors that inhibit immune function are: inadequate nutritional intake, excessive dieting, malabsorption, physical and emotional stress, toxic exposures, medications, street drugs, surgery, illness, or chronic disease. Factors that assist immune function include: heightening elimination pathways, strengthening organ function, assisting overall detoxification, and ingestion of essential nutrients, antioxidants, and carotene.

The simplest way to support immune function is to maximize nutrition while minimizing factors that inhibit immune function. Dr. Theron Randolph, the father of environmental medicine, asserts, "If we're not eating things that make us sick, we tend to stay well."[15] Sugar in various forms—glucose, sucrose, fruit juices, fructose, and honey—can significantly impair immune activities. The body has to work extra hard to break down processed sugars, depleting you of vital energy stores by using up more energy than it has to offer in the form of nutritive support.

In times of stress, such as during illness, it is important to limit sugar intake. Unprocessed foods provide the highest quality and quantity of nutrients. A diet rich in fresh, enzyme-rich, dark green leafy vegetables, raw seeds, nuts, and whole grains can supply bodily needs and replenish immune reserves. Healthy nutritional habits will be discussed further in Chapter Nine.

Personality and Immunity

Toxic emotions can also compromise immune function. Emotional states are believed to play a vital part in immune capability.[16,17] The work of psychoneuroimmunology (PNI) supports the idea that life-style and emotional states impact health. This means that everything is linked; that illness may emerge from unspoken, unmet emotional needs that become translated into physiological imbalance.

This is an interesting concept because so many EI and CFS sufferers share certain similar emotional states. For example, they tend to see themselves as victims of external, out-of-control forces, which may help create unconscious mental disturbances that become reflected in the body. Support groups abound with stories of depression, feelings of isolation and loss, anger and grief. Group members also report acute or prolonged emotional stress prior to becoming ill. Individuals under stress, or those who are depressed, anxious, or lonely show reduced NK activity and those who cope well with stress show increased NK activity.[18]

Dr. George Solomon, psychiatrist and UCLA professor, has searched for links between psychological profiles and the health of the immune system in a study of gay men with AIDS, including long-term survivors of the illness. Patients with the most helper T cells showed less depression, fatigue, anxiety, and stress related to their illness. The most intriguing finding was the correlation of strong immune function with the ability to answer "yes" to the question: "Could you say no to a request for a favor?" In this regard, there appears to be an "immune-competent personality" who is aware of one's needs and who is willing to assert him- or herself. It is no small task to learn to say "no," but doing this can help you reclaim your life. Solomon believes that people are capable of making these personality changes in order to increase immune capability.[19]

One aspect of immune competence includes having a sense that you can control your environment. People with EI and CFS commonly have feelings that out-of-control forces are adversely impacting their health. Recognition that there is much you can do to consciously develop immune competence will have a positive influence on your health.

A starting point toward developing immune competence includes finding meaning and pleasure in life. Yet, the key to improved immune function rests with learning to appropriately express rather than repress emotions and needs. Once you discover the ability to influence external stressors, you can choose to be disturbed by toxic exposures or stressors or not. Recognition of the fact that you are in charge may completely change your life.

Excessive Sensitivity

Many people with EI and CFS have difficulty filtering external influences and managing their sensitive nature. Gloria, a 50-year-old who has recovered from CFS, describes herself as having been overly concerned about the needs of others all of her life. As a caretaker, constantly putting her needs last, she was a clear example of the mind–body influence on health. Her sensitivity made it difficult to protect herself from the suffering of others as well as from physical contamination caused by the environment. She attributes her recovery to the fact that she has learned to set limits and assert her needs.

Constantly internalizing the emotions of others makes it difficult to sort out which conflicts and emotions are your own and places you at the mercy of toxic forces. As a result, you may often find yourself assuming responsibility for the lives of others and cultivating enmeshed, codependent relationships. On top of that, you may be overly ingratiating or thoughtful to the point of self-neglect. The inability to filter out the emotional debris of others goes hand in hand with difficulties filtering out physical toxins as well and these behaviors compromise immune capability.

Assertiveness

Learning to manage and control the way you respond to out-of-control influences can play a big part in your recovery. In order to make the mind–body link, you must wake up to your emotional needs as well as your physical ones. Making small inroads toward self-assertion can give you the confidence that you are able to impact some of the conditions in your life. When you take charge, you can avoid decompensation and depression by learning to express yourself in ways that can increase your sense of hope.

In order to advance in this direction, you may need to ask for support. By giving yourself permission to ask for help, you are taking responsibility for getting your needs met. Asking for help can be a humbling, courageous, empowering experience. This is what makes EI and CFS support groups so helpful.

Appropriate expression of feelings is an important aspect of the biochemical, physiological process. When you deny your feelings, the immune system bears the brunt. Problems don't go away by refusing to recognize them: repeated suppression of needs and feelings can eventually result in physical illness. Expressing uncomfortable, difficult emotions takes courage and practice, but will ultimately cause you to feel better. When left unspoken, they can be driven into the body, making you feel worse.

How do you undo a lifetime of habit? You need a safe way to manifest your feelings. Start by paying attention to how you feel. When you are ready, practice saying what needs to be said with people who will understand. Over time, using your conscious intent, it will become easier to express your needs. Remember that the health of your immune system depends on it.

Summary

Every aspect of your life and health is interrelated with healthy immune function. While you attend to daily existence, your immune system is intelligently communicating, remembering, and protecting you. Even when one part breaks down, it is resourceful in solving problems, activating other parts that can step in when needed. EI and CFS represent an unbalanced immune response. Strategies such as healthy dietary habits and increased awareness of the body–mind connection can help bring the immune response back into balance. Since the role of the immune system is vital to recovery from EI and CFS, the interplay of these factors will be repeatedly emphasized.

Endnotes

[1]Kimberly Kenney, ed., quotes from Antony Komaroff, "The Role of HHV-6 in CFS," *The CFIDS Chronicle* Spring 1991: 31–36.

[2]Paul Cheney, "CFIDS Research Progress Reports," *The CFIDS Chronicle* Fall 1991: 5–8.

[3]Sherry Rogers, *The EI Syndrome* (Syracuse: Prestige, 1991).

[4]Nancy Kilmas, "Diagnosing CFIDS: An Immunologist's Approach," *The CFIDS Chronicle* Sept. 1992: 41–42.

[5]Y. Kusaka, H. Londou, and K. Morimoto, "Healthy Lifestyles are Associated with Higher Natural Killer Cell Activity," *Prev Med* 21 (1992): 602–615.

[6]K. Nekachi and K. Imai, "Environmental and Physiological Influences on Human Natural Killer Cell Activity in Relation to Good Health Practices," *Jpn J Cancer Res* 83 (1992): 789–805.

[7]Nicholas Hall, "Health-Related Pleasures," seminar, Palo Alto, 4 Oct. 1995.

[8]Michael T. Murray, *Chronic Fatigue Syndrome* (Rocklin: Prima, 1994) 133.

[9]Michael Rosenbaum and Murray Susser, *Solving the Puzzle of Chronic Fatigue Syndrome* (Tacoma: Life Sciences, 1991) 100.

[10]William Collinge, *Recovering from Chronic Fatigue Sydrome* (New York: Perigee, 1993) 29, 59, 70–71.

[11]Robert Keller, "Immune Dysfunction in CFIDS: Why You Feel the Way You Do," *The CFIDS Chronicle* Fall 1994: 34–35.

[12]Collinge, 29.

[13]Lynn Lawson, *Staying Well in a Toxic World* (Chicago: The Noble Press, 1993) 188–201, 299–322.

[14]Lawson, 9–10.

[15]"Growing Old with Environmental Illness," *The Human Ecologist* interview with Theron Randolph, Fall 1991: 13–15.

[16]J.K. Kiecolt-Glaser and R. Glaser, "Psychoneuroimmunology: Can Psychological Interventions Modulate Immunity?" *Consult Clin Psych* 60 (1992): 569–575.

[17]S. Schleifer *et al.*, "Suppression of Lymphocyte Stimulation Following Bereavement," *JAMA* 250 (1983): 374–377.

[18]M. Sharpe, "Management of PVFS," *Br Med Bull* 47 (1991): 989–1005.

[19]Henry Dreher, "Are You Immune Competent?" *Natural Health* Feb. 1992: 52–61.

Chapter Two

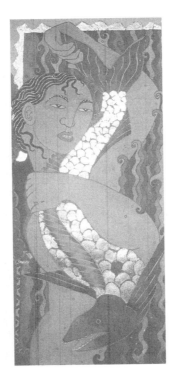

Environmental Illness

*t*he Committee on Environmental Hypersensitivity Disorders in Canada released its 1985 comprehensive definition of EI:

> *Environmental hypersensitivity is a chronic multi-system disorder, usually involving symptoms of the central nervous system and at least one other system. Affected persons are frequently intolerant to some foods and they react adversely to some chemicals and to environmental agents, singly or in combination, at levels generally tolerated by the majority and have varying degrees of morbidity, from mild discomfort to total disability.* [1]

The two primary ways people can develop EI are: through food allergies or through chemical overload, or both. These allergies are not just limited to the occasional hay fever and runny nose, but are the result of increased environmental pollution and the presence of chemicals in foods. These chemicals contribute to chronic illnesses of all kinds.

It is no secret that foods are treated with chemicals to heighten flavor, to add color, and to prolong their shelf life. It is also no secret that the air and water on this planet are increasingly polluted with harmful substances such as heavy metals and pesticides. For those who wish to become well from EI, it is important to understand these sources of chemical contaminants in the food supply and in the environment.

Toxic Chemicals

Over 30 years ago, Rachael Carson, author of *Silent Spring* (Boston: Houghton Mifflin, 1962) wrote:

> *Like the constant dripping of water that in turn wears away the hardest stone, this birth-to-death contact with dangerous chemicals may in the end prove disastrous. Each of these recurrent exposures, no matter how slight, contributes to the progressive buildup of chemicals in our bodies and so to cumulative poisoning. . . . Lulled by the soft sell and the hidden persuader, the average citizen is seldom aware of the deadly materials with which he is surrounding himself; indeed, he may not realize he is using them at all.*[2]

EI is not just about allergic reactivity; it involves all systems of the body and is the result of a compromised immune function. EI can be insidious, its cumulative impact breaking down the body after years of exposures, or it can begin precipitously, the result of an acute exposure, such as to aerial spraying of pesticides. Your immune system does its best to protect you, but ongoing contact with chemicals such as insecticides and disinfectants can damage cellular membranes, causing increased permeability of foreign substances.

Chemicals damage the immune system and the liver, and suppress cellular mediation that controls the way the body protects itself from foreign materials. These chemical compounds are particularly difficult to metabolize and excrete, accumulating in the body and leading to an elevated total burden.[3]

It is easy to underestimate the impact that chemicals have on health, as recognition of human reactivity to chemicals has come only recently. At present, research has not found the tools necessary to diagnose physiological damage caused by these chemicals, so the average person continues to believe that there is no harm. According to the U.S. Department of Health, Education and Welfare, many of the 15,000 chemicals used commercially in the environment have never been tested for toxicity. There can be a latency period of 10–20 years in unmasking environmentally caused illnesses. Decisions as to acceptable levels of environmental agents should be set now to reduce damage that is inevitable in the future.[4]

Consumers have placed trust in industry and the government to regulate and act prudently to ensure their safety by selling products that are ostensibly safe. This trust is being betrayed as occupational, environmental, and accidental exposures are on the rise. According to the National Academy of Sciences, 37 million Americans suffer from EI.[5] They estimate that as many as 15% of Americans can no longer live comfortably in our postindustrial world.[6]

Dr. John Wakefield, whose private practice is in Sunnyvale, California, deplores the lack of research in this field and predicts that "it will become a more and more significant problem."[7] Those individuals who cannot tolerate tap water, food, air, medicines, clothes, consumer products, and buildings have EI, also known as multiple chemical sensitivities (MCS).

Until recently, this field had not been well researched; in the past it was largely regarded by physicians and the public as neurotic, controlling, hysterical behavior. However, two researchers, Nicholas Ashford and Claudia Miller, were commissioned by the New Jersey Department of Health to distinguish the difference between chemical sensitivity and allergic response and the exposure to high doses of environmental chemicals. Their 1990 report notes that medical sensitivity is a very real problem and evidence "does suggest that chemical sensitivity is increasing and could become a large problem with significant economic consequences related to the disablement of productive members of society."[8] As more individuals have become ill, such as Gulf War veterans and people with autoimmune reactions to breast and other body implants, exhibiting a constellation of EI-like and CFS-like symptoms, society has started to take notice.

"The production of environmental illness is not strictly related to exposure to levels of harmful substances that are higher than FDA safety limits," notes Richard Gerber, MD, in his book *Vibrational Medicine*.

> *Conventional safety limits of exposure do not take into account the subtle vibrational effects of toxic substances. Because of their inability to comprehend vibrational levels of toxicity, the orthodox scientific community is more lenient in defining safe levels of exposure to many harmful substances. The inadequacy of conventional scientific testing to measure subtle negative disturbances to human physiology also limits the FDA's ability to define exactly which substances are really harmful to human beings.[9]*

It is impossible to avoid contact with damaging agents. Chemicals are found in the air we breathe, foods and food additives, water, medical drugs, synthetic fibers, gas heat, household cleaners and furnishings, pesticides, and fungicides. Reactivity to chemicals can go undetected, existing alongside multiple other sensitivities such as allergies to food, dust, and pollen.

Outgassing

The insidious damaging effects of chemicals can occur via outgassing from inanimate objects—such as books, plastics, clothes, and treated wood in furniture in the form of vaporized fumes emitted from solid substances. Many of these chemicals such as plastics are thought to be stable compounds that remain unaltered within the material, yet the molecular contents are constantly changing, causing a slow release of unstable chemicals. These chemical fumes are emitted over a period of years, adding to your toxic load.[10]

Seemingly innocuous pieces of furniture such as a couch can pollute; chemically treated clothing can emit formaldehyde and chemicals from the dyes which are then absorbed into the skin; and household cleansers and floor waxes can cause harm long after they have evaporated. Fumes from kerosene, fabric softeners, clothing dyes, and the like can leak into the home, filling it with harmful vapors. Entering a newly painted or carpeted room may cause you to feel light-headed or confused.

On initial contact it's easy to smell the fumes and identify the source; yet when the smell wears off, you are still being bombarded by outgassing fumes. Construction materials such as particleboard are treated with formaldehyde, and volatile compounds such as those used in insulation emit gasses long after they are installed in the home. Soft plastics, rubber, synthetic fabrics, paints, and furniture sealants are further examples of substances that outgas.

Heat and light enhance the outgassing process. For example, when you get into a hot car the fumes from the upholstery are more evident. Laura, who has severe EI and Crohn's disease, an autoimmune disease characterized by chronic inflammation of the digestive tract, places her mail in the sun and washes new garments as many as 50 times before wearing them to speed up the outgassing process.

Chemical Overload

As the number and variety of chemicals used by modern society continue to increase, the ranks of those who are no longer able to tolerate chemical exposures will grow. Those who currently have EI and CFS may be just the tip of the iceberg. Those who are well may also be undergoing unsuspected immune system damage. Still others may have symptoms of illness, but fail to attribute them to damage caused by chemical exposures.

Those who already feel poorly may have subclinical illnesses, not directly measurable by current medical standards, so they believe nothing is wrong. These people live with low energy or exhibit moody, irritable behavior that is never attributed to a specific cause. They may crave foods, feel high from the smell of gasoline and later have a headache, or experience peculiar vague symptoms that come and go, unsuspectingly the victim of damaging exposures.

Understanding Environmental Illness

The human body is capable of becoming allergic to anything, e.g., its own hormones, organic foods, as well as internal organs. As already noted, EI is not about everyday, conventional allergies, hay fever, rhinitis, and food allergies. It is about an immune system that has gone into overdrive, reacting to everything around you as if they were the enemy.

In order to come to terms with this alarming illness, it may help to have contact with others who are suffering from these problems. Meeting those who are also struggling can have a very positive effect toward your recovery. This may mean "coming out," openly acknowledging that you are "one of them."

When you do this, you may recognize parts of your own life, or think you don't have it so bad as you hear about Laura, a 54-year-old with severe EI, CFS, and

Crohn's disease. Near the front door of her house is a sign that reads, "Warning: Chemically Sensitive Persons Live Here." Four pairs of shoes are arranged by the doorstep and a small outdoor table holds a phone book, pens, and a stack of mail that is outgassing. Several articles of clothing hang on a nearby hat tree, airing out from contact with other fumes.

Before she became ill she had been an actress, a career that must have served her well, as much of her current life is spent on this porch in the public eye. It is here that she safely visits with friends whose bodies and clothes reek of fumes that make her sick. Even when it rains she's out there pounding away on her typewriter under an umbrella. When the woman upstairs does her laundry using commercial detergents and when the air is filled with wood smoke, she must retreat inside. Lately she has befriended a stray cat, for which she must don gloves and a mask in order to pet.

At one time there were only six foods she could safely eat. They had to be organic and could not be consumed in combination with each other—she could eat only one food item per meal. One year she became so ill that her weight fell to 78 pounds. During that time she literally lived in her bathroom; it was the only safe place where she was not bothered by toxic fumes. Did she mind this oddball existence? Probably, but she used that time as an opportunity to write and publish a book of poetry.

In order to accomplish the simplest task, Laura must be constantly vigilant to avoid toxic exposures. At times she wonders if her obsessive tendencies help fan the fires of her illness. To counteract this concern, she continuously works to find a balance; enjoying life to the fullest without denying her illness. Refusing to give her infirmities any more room in her life than they already have, she courageously insists on being treated as if she were normal. Her unfailing optimism keeps her whole and sane.

It is the work of Dr. Theron Randolph, the father of environmental medicine, that gave a name to her chemical sensitivities. Randolph proposed that synthetic chemicals in the environment could cause the same allergic symptoms as foods. To that end, he studied 1000 cases of individuals who demonstrated psychotic behavior that directly correlated with toxic exposures.[11]

In his coauthored book, *An Alternative Approach To Allergies: The New Field of Clinical Ecology Unravels the Environmental Causes of Mental and Physical Ills* (New York: Harper & Row, 1989), Randolph established three critical hypotheses. The first holds that health is impacted by total body load; the cumulative effect of food allergies, environmental toxins, and emotional stressors. Second, he asserts that chronic low-level exposures can cause damage to the immune system, prompting inappropriate adaptation. The third hypothesis holds that many toxic chemicals are fat-soluble and stored in body fat, capable of remaining in the body for years, and as a result, chemical exposures can have a cumulative effect.[12] Randolph further identifies the characteristics of (1) total load, (2) masking or adaptation, (3) hidden addictions, (4) unmasking, (5) withdrawal, (6) frequency, and (7) the concept of the "universal reactor," which are little-known, essential aspects of reactivity.

Let's explore these concepts. Understanding the concept of *total load* is essential to healing the immune system. Total load is the cumulative burden placed on the body from multiple factors. Examples of factors that increase total load include environmental inhalants, food allergies, chemical hypersensitivities, reactivity to molds, phenol and petrochemical products, and the presence of viral, bacterial, parasitic, or yeast infections.

Nutritional status plays a vital role in total load, as an unhealthy diet can burden the healing capabilities of the body. Hormone hypersensitivity is often overlooked as an aspect of total load, yet reactivity to one's own hormones can disable the immune system. Toxic exposures, whether they occur gradually or through an acute incident, play an important role in increasing the total body burden of toxins. Stress is another important factor; people with EI and CFS report the onset of illness as having coincided with stressful times, such as the death of a family member or the loss of a job.

Masking or *adaptation* occurs when the body is so used to the presence of a contaminant that it isn't seen to be the cause of the health difficulties. Adaptation is not necessarily a good thing. Dr. William Rea, environmental physician, says, "If you are one of those who can adapt real fast you won't perceive damage until it's too late."[13]

One example of adaptation is that many in our culture are intolerant of lactose, found in dairy products. Yet, they don't identify milk as the source of allergic reactivity until it is removed from daily intake for a time. Most people naturally lose the ability to digest lactose because they no longer synthesize the digestive enzyme lactase. Studies have also shown that milk contains unsafe levels of environmental contaminants as well as antibiotics.[14] In addition to lactose intolerance, people can be allergic to milk or dairy products. If you resume drinking milk, allergic reactivity and discomfort may ensue.

It wasn't until Judy, a 48-year-old woman now recovered from CFS who also has ongoing struggles with EI, stopped drinking milk that she realized how dearly she had paid a price; years of daily dosing kept her body bogged down with constant reactivity. She hadn't realized that milk was a primary source of her chronic chest congestion and joint pain. Adaptation masks symptoms, allowing chronic, low-grade, insidious deterioration. If the stressor is reintroduced often enough, the body reacts by normalizing its acute response to subsequent exposures.[16] The truth is, she was a milk addict, and when she stopped drinking it she experienced withdrawal symptoms, craving the very thing that was causing her harm.

The reason she didn't know this was because milk was integrated into a pattern of constant reactivity. Drinking a glass in the morning had a stimulating effect; when she felt tired later in the day she'd simply drink another glass. It never occurred to her that her milk habit was a problem until she stopped the cycle. This is just one example; any other food can be addictive in the same way.

Hidden addictions are composed of two phases: an immediate improvement of chronic symptoms such as fatigue is noted when an addictive substance is eaten, and the hangover phase which occurs when you fail to ingest the food within a certain time frame. Addictions become evident when you avoid ingesting a food for several hours or days and develop unpleasant withdrawal symptoms, including cravings for that food, irritability, anxiety, muscle weakness, shakiness, fatigue, headache, and general aches.

Coffee is a common addictive substance. Life moves along just fine when you have a cup every day, but try going without for a day or two and you will notice the jitters, a headache, and irritability. Drink a cup again and you'll feel fine. Reexposure to the reactive substance avoids withdrawal symptoms.[15]

Efforts to avoid withdrawals can prompt cravings for sugar, cravings for other addictive substances, or the craving for contact with other toxins. For reasons not completely understood, addictive reactivity can occur to chemicals and objects in the environment as well as foods. Judy, who has EI, craves sugar after exposure to auto exhaust or mold.

The body can lose its adaptive abilities as a result of ongoing exposure to toxins and stress, causing the immune system to go haywire. In *unmasking* there can be a triggering agent such as a newly painted house, or a pesticide exposure, which adds one more insult to the immune system that tips the scales. Once the scales tip in favor of reactivity, minute exposures to seemingly benign objects can trigger other reactions. Sherry, 37-year-old mother of two, became ill with severe EI when exposed to termite fumigants while living in an old house. That exposure unmasked reactivity to many other substances and she has not been well since.

It is important to distinguish between the reaction of *withdrawal* that can occur after a harmful substance leaves your body and an actual allergic reaction. Allergic reactivity is a physiological reaction to the presence of a substance; withdrawal is a physiological reaction to its absence. Though they may feel the same, withdrawal-like symptoms occur when the offending substance is removed from contact or consumption, and an allergic reaction involves the action of antibodies mobilizing in the presence of a foreign invader.

The *frequency* of exposure to substances that trigger allergic reactivity can heighten sensitivity. Gloria, an elementary school teacher, became ill after the carpeting to her classroom was replaced. It took months of daily exposures to wear her immune system down; eventually she had to quit her job. The way to resolve reactivity is to avoid or minimize contact with chemical and food triggers, preventing an allergic response. After you avoid substances that trigger reactivity for a time, brief reexposures can make you feel worse.

Universal reactors experience the phenomenon of allergic reactivity that spreads, igniting into multiple sensitivities. Universal reactors literally react to everything and anything, all chemicals and substances constructed with or treated with chemicals, seemingly benign objects in the environment, and sometimes all foods. Commercial toothpaste, tap water, dust, books, synthetic thread, plastic buttons on clothing, and the tiny plastic parts from the TV that outgas fumes can make these people sick.

In the process of reducing the body's toxic burden, people can become so sensitive that they react to any foreign substance as if it were a harmful invader.

Carried to an extreme, ingestion of even organic foods can cause the body to react in an allergic fashion. Selima is a petite 42-year-old in recovery from EI; at her sickest she nearly died, as everything she ate made her worse, including organic foods, which caused severe intestinal reactions. Her body was under the impression that everything, even life-sustaining foods, were foreign invaders. "I got well by moving to the ocean where the air is clean, by being scrupulously careful about all foods I ate, and by carefully avoiding contact with all chemicals."

Theresa, mother of a 2-year-old, has severe EI and is a universal reactor. She got polio when she was 4, and at 13 she was beset with conventional allergies. These difficulties spread to reactivity to even the most innocuous substances; everything she comes in contact with makes her sick. To collect the mail she must don a mask and run to the mailbox, avoiding car fumes. She has lived in virtual isolation for over 12 years, seldom leaving home. When she does go out, she is inevitably assailed by many toxins. Last year was the first Christmas celebrated with her family in 10 years, afterwards she was sick for weeks. Still, she says smiling, "It was worth every minute."

Food and Allergy

The most common cause of food allergies is faulty digestion. The average healthy body has intestinal tissue that only permits molecules of a particular size to pass through. Yet, food allergies typically begin with a change in the mucous membrane of the digestive tract, often caused by chronic unbalanced dietary practices. Bowel inflammation can also be caused by yeast, excess alcohol intake, the use of street or prescription drugs, food allergies, bacteria or intestinal parasites which are all factors that upset the normal acid–base balance. Prolonged inflammation, caused by ongoing allergic reactivity, alters the permeability of the bowel wall, allowing larger protein molecules, bacteria, viruses, toxins, and, in extreme cases, *Candida albicians*, a yeast found in the intestinal tract, to penetrate and circulate in the blood.[16] Once they penetrate the bowel, they can pass into the bloodstream and set up infections anywhere in the body. Whether candida, proteins, or toxins are the cause, these changes in the bowel membrane result in what's known as a "leaky gut."

When the body detects these proteins and other particles where they shouldn't be, it treats them as foreign objects, causing the production of antibodies and allergic reactivity against once harmless foods. Antigen–antibody activation creates widespread havoc, which commonly leads to extensive food and environmental allergies. This explains why organically pure foods that enter the digestive tract can also be met with allergic reactivity.

When antibodies are produced, they can do many things such as cause an inflammatory reaction, including arthritic symptoms in a joint space. Furthermore, bacterial toxins that leak through the bowel wall can harm the liver, reducing its ability to cope with other chemicals. When the liver is overwhelmed, toxins from the bowel will recirculate in the bloodstream. When allergic sensitivity to foods is at the heart of the problem, recovery lies with restoring the mucous membrane's health and the intestinal flora.

Intestinal Balance

The approach to healing the intestinal tract includes restoring the normal flora and acid–base balance of the bowel. Harmful bacteria and toxic materials resulting from the accumulation of waste are held in check when healthy intestinal bacteria are restored. With healthy bacteria in the intestine, the body is able to maintain a balance against putrefactive activities that are ongoing in the intestines. When there is an imbalance, excessive quantities of unhealthy flora cause large quantities of ammonia to be released, irritating the intestinal walls. The bacteria then produce excessive amounts of histamine, which causes allergic reactivity and the further buildup of toxins.

The intake of favorable bacteria such as *Lactobacillus acidophilus* and bifido-bacteria found in active culture yogurt or in supplemental form helps implant healthy bacteria, reducing the presence of unfriendly bacteria and restoring a favorable balance. *Lactobacillus acidophilus* is a strain of friendly bacteria commonly found in the small intestine and stomach, and bifido-bacteria is a strain of friendly bacteria common to the large intestine. Some believe that ingestion is not enough and that better results are achieved by implanting normal flora directly into the lower bowel. The WIT Kit is a program that has been used by some to support the reintroduction of healthy flora to the digestive tract.[17]

Sometimes the treatment may require the use of antifungal or antimicrobial medication to kill organisms that have proliferated and infected the bowel. Ingestion of antioxidants, pure aloe vera juice, flax teas, and the amino acid L-glutamine can help reduce bowel inflammation and heal the bowel wall. As the bowel becomes less inflamed, it becomes healthier; as a result, foods that previously caused allergic symptoms no longer penetrate the bowel and enter the bloodstream. At times the best thing to do is to permit the gut to rest by fasting.

Eliminating alcohol and carefully monitoring the use of prescription medications can also be effective in controlling the problem. Avoiding alcohol is important because this reduces the burden on the liver to detoxify and because it is seen to be a part of the cycle of addictions. A diet that eliminates allergy-producing foods such as wheat protein and dairy products will allow the intestine to become less irritated and inflamed in order to heal.

It can be an unhappy surprise to learn that the foods you crave the most are the foods you are the most allergic to. One way that you can spot an allergy is when you consume a food and get a temporary high. In order to maintain this high, you must sustain a regular "fix" of the very substance that is harming you. Even when you know certain foods make your health worse, you may have an overwhelming desire to eat them; and as previously noted by the late Dr. Theron Randolph, EI specialist, addiction and allergic responsiveness typically go hand in hand.

Food Addictions

Not having a regular fix of sugar or substance your body craves can leave you feeling irritable and depressed. This is an addiction. Food addictions can take the form of cravings for a certain type of food that is usually harmful to you. The presence of candida overgrowth can make addictive sensations worse when your yeast-infested body begs for sugar to sustain it. So long as you supply your body with allergy-producing foods, your body is never free from reactivity and it continues to crave things that are detrimental.

Food allergies are similar to alcohol addiction; an alcoholic requires liquor in order to feel good and in the case of food allergies you may require certain harmful foods in order to feel good. Once you stop eating substances that cause reactivity, you may experience extreme irritability, low energy, and discomfort akin to withdrawal symptoms. Consequently, consuming more of these addictive substances temporarily sparks you with energy and euphoria. Despite a brief high, the damage to your body continues as long as you ingest substances that cause reactivity.

As a rule, most allergies are to foods you eat the most often. Since they are eaten often you may not recognize them to be sources of reactivity. Foods common to the diet that typically cause allergic reactivity include: corn, wheat, eggs, milk and other dairy products, sugar, soy, chocolate, peanuts, and tomatoes. As with chemical sensitivities, it's possible for your body to adapt so that you can tolerate foods that are harmful—not attributing your lethargy or arthritic pain to foods you have eaten.

The cycle of reactivity is broken when you remove the offending food from your diet. Effective identification of food allergies requires that you understand the symptoms related to reactivity. These symptoms are many and varied, including: headache, ringing ears, chest congestion, postnasal drip, sinusitis, nausea, mental confusion, joint pain, and many more.

Once you identify a food as causative, you must eliminate that food completely from your diet for at least 5 days to see if your symptoms clear up. When you eat it again, note what happens. If you are not reactive, nothing will happen; if you are allergic, you may note dizziness, nausea, feelings of restlessness, muscle weakness, shakiness, fatigue, headache, or general malaise. If you feel euphoric or energized, that food may also be suspect.

It takes willpower and determination to cleanse your body, starting with changing your eating habits. Initial withdrawals can be intensely uncomfortable, even scary, but you are giving your body the opportunity to repair itself. Reminding yourself of the benefits of breaking the cycle of allergic reactivity may make it easier to avoid damaging foods.

The Cocoa Pulse Test

Joanna Brick, certified nutritional consultant, has used the Cocoa Pulse Test, named for its developer, on herself to determine which foods are causing allergic reactions. She notes, "Not everyone has the discipline to test for food allergies and it's success assumes that you are adhering to a rotation diet. This self-challenge is the most accurate of the allergy tests. The RAST, MAST, and ELISA tests all have false-positive and false-negative results."

Here's how it works. Several mornings in a row, take your baseline pulse for a full minute before getting out of bed. This is done by placing the fingertips of one hand on the thumb side of the wrist of the opposite hand and counting the beats. Then before you eat a meal, sit and calm yourself for a minute before taking your pulse for another full minute, writing down the rate. Next eat one food item, one you suspect you are allergic to and take your pulse 5 minutes later, and then 20 minutes later, recording both numbers. If your pulse increases by at least 8 beats a minute above your initial measurement, it is possible you are allergic to that food.

Pinpointing Sources of Food and Chemical Reactivity

When dealing with chronic exposures it is not easy to pinpoint their source. Cumulative effects can be subtle and your body may have adapted over a prolonged period of time. It can also be difficult to isolate the causative agent, as reactivity may not occur until days after contact.

Reactivity can take many forms. Some react to chemical exposures in an addictive manner; you may enjoy the smell of fumes from your gas tank, feeling a burst of energy. Since a toxic exposure can cause a temporary sense of well-being, you may resist correlating it with chemical sensitivity. By looking beyond the superficial sources of reactivity and isolating the causes of more subtle reactivity, you will improve your health. And, even when reactivity is under control, reexposure to these substances can prompt the return of symptoms.

At first it may be hard to believe that newspaper fumes can cause your head to spin. Sherry, who became ill after an acute exposure to fumigants, says, "It took some getting used to the fact that I was allergic to many foods, but that was within my frame of reference. Finding out that I was allergic to things I'd been in contact with all my life...that was too bizarre. Like finding out everything I'd ever believed was a lie." Seemingly benign substances can make you sick.

What an eye-opener to realize that virtually anything can make you sick. By sorting out what is harming you, you may find that the toxin is something you've been in contact with all your life. And you may react differently to the same agent at different times. The more subtle effects of an allergic reaction such as feelings of fatigue may not be easily attributable to allergic reactivity. It's not a simple project to identify sources of allergic reactivity, as the following examples show.

1. If you wake up in the morning tired after an adequate night's sleep, your bedding or pajamas may be a source of reactivity. Most bedding contains formaldehyde "fireproofing." Use bed linens that have been washed repeatedly or fabrics that have not been chemically treated.
2. Your home may be making you sick. Laura's wood frame home, just two blocks from the Pacific Ocean, is damp and during the rainy season the

walls grow dark with mold. Your home may be full of toxins that constantly bombard you. This continuous onslaught can make it difficult for you to recover. If symptoms change with the seasons, or improve when you go on vacation, it is worth closer examination of household factors that influence your health.

3. Note how you react when in contact with different materials. A long list of possible excitants is presented in Appendix I, which is deliberately inclusive because it may alert you to a substance that you hadn't considered to be a source of difficulty.

4. Examine your cravings and aversions, as well as foods and substances that make you feel high, or those that make you feel poorly. Everything is suspect. Before she became ill, Gloria always had to have a cup of coffee and a donut in the morning. Without this seemingly benign ritual she felt agitated and sick to her stomach. As with foods, experiencing a flare-up when exposed to an environmental substance after avoiding it for at least 5 days may indicate allergic reactivity. If you crave certain foods or enjoy exposure to, say, wood smoke, feeling either high or noticeably worse, you are probably allergically reactive to them.

5. Educate yourself as to what taxes your body; noting reductions in energy, heightening of symptoms, or general malaise after contact. Any synthetic can be a source of trouble. Prescription medications may even cause toxic reactions. You may wish to consult the *Physician's Desk Reference* (PDR), often found in the library, to check for potential side effects of medications; from there, consult your physician if you have concerns.

Judy, a 48-year-old who had CFS and still struggles with EI, went to her doctor for relief from intense pressure headaches. The doctor prescribed a painkiller containing aspirin and other synthetic substances. For a while she felt better, but then the headaches grew worse; little did she know she had been increasing her chemical load. It is generally accepted that prescription medications can have serious acute or subtle side effects; consequently, those with EI need to be particularly alert for problems.

Ingestion of recreational drugs can weaken defenses, polluting the internal system which struggles to clean and detoxify itself. Unwillingness to accept the full extent of your reactivity may prevent you from intervening to protect yourself. Everything should be suspect: assuming that a product is safe can interfere with your health.

Healing Crisis

At various stages of recovery, people report feeling worse in the process of becoming well. These disturbing symptoms are part of the cure and should not be suppressed. A "healing crisis," is the exacerbation of symptoms while the body is ridding itself of accumulated toxic substances. It is also termed a "die-off" or a

Herxheimer reaction when the pathogenic flora of the digestive tract is being destroyed through therapeutic interventions. "In some cases old symptoms may temporarily reappear," reports Dr. Julie Carter-Hinson, doctor of Chinese medicine.

A healing crisis occurs when the body is crowded with waste and poisons that have been mobilized out of the cells, carried by the bloodstream into the organs of elimination. Symptoms are caused by the release of toxins from the cells as they move into the circulation. In order to achieve relief, toxins must then be moved out of the tissue and be excreted.

Symptoms can occur while taking medications to kill yeast; when you stop eating allergy-producing foods; when you cut off contact with chemicals that caused sensitivities; and when you fast to help clear the body of its toxic load. When treated for candida overgrowth the yeast is dying off, which can cause intense cravings for substances such as sugar, bread, and alcohol.

Laboratory tests show that the Herxheimer effect is caused by the release of agents from the dying bacteria as they are attacked by antibiotics, which, in turn, stimulates the body's immune defenses. Instead of feeling better, you may feel considerably worse, which can be a fearful experience unless you understand what is occurring. Old symptoms can reappear and current symptoms tend to worsen.

The movement of poisons out of fatty tissue cells into the bloodstream can cause frightening symptoms including intense cravings for allergy-producing foods and clouded mentation, such as confusion, difficulty focusing, tremors, and extreme irritability. Common to this experience is a certain kind of intense, crushing headache. There may also be fatigue, aches and pains, and digestive system disturbances as well as other complaints. A healing crisis can also include the resurfacing of old negative emotional material that has been obstructing your welfare. When this information comes to light, it needs to be flushed out in order to be released.

If you give in to these sensations and consume allergy-producing foods or restimulate your body through toxic exposures, you will only delay your recovery. This can be scary or demoralizing unless you understand that the intensification of discomfort is an indication that a positive shift is taking place. A headache can mean your body is mobilizing to heal itself as toxins are being excreted.

In a healing crisis your most immediate thought may be to call the whole process off; stopping your fast, or the fungicidal medication, or by resuming consumption of damaging foods. After all, who wants to feel worse than they already do? "Cheating" may bring temporary relief, but it just prolongs your suffering. It's easier to hang in there if you are aware that you are experiencing physiological withdrawal from chemicals, candida, or foods.

In homeopathy a healing crisis is a cause for celebration, signifying that pathogens are being mobilized from the inside out. As you achieve greater levels of recovery, as toxins are mobilized out of the body, you may repeatedly experience these crises. When you understand them to be a cleansing process leading to improved health, they may become manageable. Intensification of discomfort can help confirm an elusive diagnosis as to the presence of candidiasis, food allergies, or toxins. A healing crisis can sometimes be dangerous, signifying toxic damage to your system. Some physicians recommend taking measures to support the liver. Taking more antioxidant supplements and herbs, increasing water intake, and helping toxins to flow out of your intestines may help reduce toxic symptoms.

Herbal remedies such as willow bark can relieve symptoms without interfering with the healing process. When Sherry, who has EI, underwent candida treatment, she became so uncomfortable that her homeopath cut down the remedy dose to slow the healing process down.

Brain-Fogging and Emotional Matters

The term *brain-fogging* may be familiar to you through firsthand experience. Brain-fogging, similar to the neurocognitive difficulties with CFS, is marked by moodiness, confused thinking, and an inability to concentrate. Some experience this as a lack of coordination, a disturbance in balance and perception, or excessive drowsiness. An important aspect of brain-fogging is an acute loss of memory. If you find yourself walking to the refrigerator several times and cannot recall why you are standing there with the door open, you may have brain-fogging. With acute or long-term toxic exposures, brain-fogging can fluctuate in character and intensity and can be an indication of cerebral reactivity to a food consumed or a substance in the environment.

Testing can reveal sensitivities to foods or substances in the environment as the culprits, and treatment focuses on identifying causative factors and then avoiding them. When the brain is clouded, it is common to reach for a food that will give you a brief period of clarity or an energetic lift. Giving in to this inclination will only enhance the problem.

EI and Stress

Removing agents that provoke reactions is perhaps the easiest part of the job. Even after minimizing the damaging effects of the environment and eating properly, there may still be hidden sources of allergic sensitivity. These hangers-on will force you to look further to unseen sources of reactivity, which may include excessive emotional stressors or undetected chemicals.

In the face of ongoing stress, life becomes one big blast of adrenaline and the activation of other stress hormones such as cortisol which can deplete the body.[18] Unrelenting emotional or physical stress such as abuse, overwork, constant allergic reactivity, or an onslaught of viral invaders erodes the body and interferes with its adaptive capacity to the extent that biochemical systems break down.

Josh, a gay nurse working in an oncology unit, became ill with EI and CFS when his house collapsed around him in an earthquake. Four years later he developed facial cancer. Illness has forced him to extricate himself from a life filled with multiple, ongoing stressors. Today he meditates regularly, is not afraid to break dates, or to let his family know who he is, and he takes time out to go for long relaxing walks in the woods.

Stress leads to significant suppression of the immune system and the level of immune suppression has been found to be proportional to the level of stress.[19] People with EI and CFS frequently report that stress precipitates a relapse. Though stress heightens symptoms, it is not the cause of them.[20] Your body is more capable of coping with toxic exposures when you're more relaxed and stress-free. Unclenching from the tension in your life is a matter of conscious choice. You may wish to employ stress reduction techniques appropriate for people with EI and CFS which include visualization, meditation, breathwork, and energetic healing.

Clinical Ecology

Clinical ecology (CE), with its roots in conventional medicine, studies the environmental causes of illness in the belief that people are being adversely affected by inanimate, toxic objects. CE differs from allergy and toxicology medical practice with its emphasis on Dr. Theron Randolph's postulates regarding total load, time factors which include frequency of exposures, and adaptation as key factors that influence health.

As the environment becomes more damaged, CE seeks to minimize the impact of harmful factors by educating patients to reduce stressors and maximize function of the pathways through which the body becomes overloaded with poisons. To alleviate symptoms the clinical ecologist works to detect all factors that trigger illness and to remove the offending substances from the immediate environment.

Diagnosis

There is no single lab test used to determine the presence of EI; primarily diagnosis is achieved through extensive patient reporting, as well as testing. Two main types of confirmatory testing involve intradermal and inhalation challenge. Provocative neutralization testing is commonly used to detect food allergies, chemicals, inhalants, microbial substances, and individual bacteria. If an individual is allergic to wheat, for example, she may respond to the testing process by coughing or wheezing. Once a reaction is provoked, the clinical ecologist can find the appropriate neutralizing dose of the same substance.

The Dallas Environmental Health Center, described in Appendix II, gives patients the opportunity to enter an environmentally safe setting in order to achieve a comprehensive health work-up and indicated treatment. Laboratory tests include immune studies, blood tests, and vitamin and mineral evaluations, as well as diagnostic scans. Perhaps the most important part of the program includes preservative-free antigen skin testing. Laura has been there for extensive testing and experienced relief of some allergic symptoms, reporting her stay to be an excellent educational opportunity.

Another recently developed test useful in both assessing and treating EI is the Functional Liver Detoxification Test, which measures how the liver metabolizes aspirin, acetaminophen, and caffeine. Most patients with EI have evidence of abnormal function of their liver detoxification pathways. This testing, offered by Great Smokies Diagnostic Laboratory of Asheville, North Carolina, also shows how an individual's liver detoxification can be supported with various nutrients.

The EI Cure

In the face of the growing deterioration of the environment, it may surprise you that people with EI can be helped. Adjusting to the notion that food and chemical susceptibility may be the cause of your illness is the first step. Moving from there to identify the sources of your problem comes next. Yet, the real solution is found in avoidance; staying away or minimizing exposure to harmful substances that are making you sick.

Adhering to dietary habits that avoid addictive foods and provide contaminant-free nutrition will make an enormous difference. The elimination–rotation diet is a sensible way for the body to rest and repair from allergic reactivity, and will be discussed in Chapter Nine. Symptom neutralization involves the injection or ingestion of the offending substance in a homeopathic-like dilution. You can also do a great deal to assist by strengthening your overall health and supporting the detoxification process. It may be a long uphill battle, but many with EI are able to enjoy healthy, active lives.

Summary

EI is a complex, multifaceted illness that will force you to wake up to the fact that the environment is ill. The complexity, coupled with the fact that the illness is externally caused, doesn't mean you have to lose hope. It means empowering yourself, by purifying and strengthening your own body. Identification of dietary and chemical hazards will enable you to act on your own behalf in a protective manner and will go a long way toward recovering health.

Endnotes

[1]Richard Leviton, "Environmental Illness: A Special Report," *Yoga Journal* Nov.–Dec. 1990: 44.

[2]Rachael Carson, *Silent Spring* (Boston: Houghton Mifflin, 1962).

[3]Theron Randolph and R. Michael Wisner, "Detoxification: Personal Survival in a Chemical World," *Healthmed* 1988: 173–74.

[4]U.S. Department of Health, Education and Welfare, "Preventing Environmentally Related Diseases" (Washington, DC: National Institute of Environmental Health Services, 1976).

[5]Sara Shannon, *Good Health in a Toxic World* (New York: Warner Books, 1994) 44.

[6]Leviton, 44.

[7]Denise Franklin, "Allergic to the 20th Century," *Santa Cruz Sentinel* 7 Sept. 1986: B-4.

[8]Leviton, 50.

[9]Richard Gerber, *Vibrational Medicine* (Santa Fe: Bear, 1988) 451.

[10]Sherry Rogers, *The EI Syndrome* (Syracuse: Prestige, 1986).

[11]Leviton, 49.

[12]Theron Randolph and Ralph Moss, *An Alternative Approach to Allergies: The New Field of Clinical Ecology Unravels the Environmental Causes of Mental and Physical Ills* (New York: Harper & Row, 1989).

[13]Lynn Lawson, *Staying Well in a Toxic World* (Chicago: The Nobel Press, 1993) 36.

[14]J. McDougall and M. McDougall, *The McDougall Plan* (Clinton: New Win, 1983) 51–52.

[15]Dennis Remmington and Barbara Higa, *Back to Health: A Comprehensive Medical and Nutritional Yeast Control Program* (Salt Lake City: Vitality House, 1994) 82.

[16]Jeffery Bland, "Candida Albicans: An Unsuspected Problem" (Tacoma: Nutritional Biochemistry).

[17]Write to WIT Kit, Healing Arts Associates, 121A West E Street, Encinitas, CA 92024 or call (619) 753-4174 for information about their program.

[18]Michael Murray, *Chronic Fatigue Syndrome* (Rocklin: Prima, 1994) 144.

[19]Hans Selye, *Stress in Health and Disease* (London: Butterworths, 1976).

[20]David Bell, *The Doctor's Guide to Chronic Fatigue Syndrome* (Reading: Addison–Wesley, 1995) 59, 151.

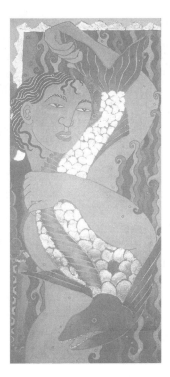

Chapter Three

Chronic Fatigue Syndrome

*C*FS is the most common of about 50 names used to identify an illness that has only recently been recognized as a specific syndrome. It has been variously called *chronic Epstein–Barr virus syndrome* (CEBV), *chronic mononucleosis,* the *"yuppie flu,"* and *chronic fatigue immune dysfunction syndrome* (CFIDS). In Britain, Australia, New Zealand, and other parts of the world it is called *myalgic encephalomyelitis* (ME). There is growing evidence that fibromyalgia is the same illness as CFS.[1]

CFS has been surrounded in controversy, even since physicians began to accept it as a real entity in the mid-1980s. For instance, many people suffer from "chronic fatigue," but this is not CFS. There has been much questioning as to what constitutes the illness of CFS. This uncertainty has led to clarification by the Centers for Disease Control (CDC) regarding specific diagnostic guidelines, which will be examined later in this chapter.

Adhering to the CDC guidelines, the incidence of CFS in the United States is about 11.5%. British and Australian standards for diagnosis are less strict, with 15% of people meeting the British criteria, while Australian criteria yield an incidence of 38%.[2] In 1990 Dr. Hugh Fudenburg, an immunologist noted, "There are at least one million Americans currently carrying a diagnosis of CFIDS, and possibly another five million who are ill and yet to be diagnosed."[3] Estimates are that 60 to 70% of adults who are ill with CFS are women.[4] It is speculated that women are more likely to seek help than men.

The controversy regarding CFS also carries over to symptoms because they are numerous and varied. Disabling fatigue and exhaustion are the most notable and consistent symptoms. "There are many degrees of fatigue. Nearly everyone knows what its like to experience mild fatigue where you can function. At these times you can't envision how it would feel to be more tired. When you're tired it's hard to imagine anything worse, but CFS is at the far end of worse," attests Selima, a 42-year-old former Episcopal minister who has had CFS and struggles with EI.

Other symptoms include: sleep disturbances; headaches; muscle pain; cardiac irregularities; fever; night sweats; joint pain; visual disturbances; emotional changes including euphoria, agitation, and lability; confusion and memory loss; abdominal pain; muscle spasms; or lymph node pain.[5,6] Symptoms may vary, worsening in response to stress, climate changes, and overall health and can persist for years. They can be completely disabling or just be a minor nuisance.

Understanding Chronic Fatigue Syndrome

Audrey, a graduate student now in recovery from CFS, was able to pinpoint the exact date of onset of her illness to be one morning when she just couldn't get out of bed. Prior to becoming sick her friends had called her "Wonder Woman," for she was always taking care of everything and everybody. She believes it was her approach to life that led to CFS. "I got cancer at age 24. Did that make a difference in how I lived my life? No. Getting CFS made a difference though. Like upping the ante, it knocked me down, forcing me to take stock of my life."

Prior to the onset of CFS she wasn't able to set limits and was completely overextended. Once she got CFS the life in which she had been so capable and in charge was suddenly gone. Simple matters such as going to the bathroom required great effort. Audrey says, "I brushed my teeth about every four days because I didn't have any more energy than that. My memory was totally gone. One day it took me three hours to call the disability office. When I finally got hold of them, they asked, 'What's your Social Security number?' I could no more remember it than fly. I had to call back another day." When she became ill she had to reexamine her life-style choices, paying attention to the needs of her heart and mind first. Today she is healthy, working as a Health Educator at the Cancer Support Institute in Menlo Park, California, and as a graduate student in psychology, but she must constantly prioritize her life.

The controversy extends to the heated debate as to the cause of CFS: is it genetic or environmental?, emotionally based?, or is it caused by one disease or by many? The medical community—including immunologists, researchers, physicians who specialize in this illness, as well as The CFIDS Association, the largest CFS-related organization—has been attempting to elucidate its etiology. For the most part they are focusing on viruses as the causative agent. Despite the diversity of opinions as to cause, there is general agreement that the illness involves a compromised immune system. Some theories are examined below.

Viral Theory

"There is an increasing consensus the CFS is a virally induced, cytokine-mediated psychoneuroimmunologic disorder that occurs in genetically predisposed individuals,"[7] offers Dr. Jay Goldstein, director of The Chronic Fatigue Institute in Beverly Hills, California.

The DNA molecule is the basis of heredity. When cells divide, DNA duplicates and thus passes on its genetic code to the daughter cells. There are also RNA viruses that interrupt a cell's "messages" to reproduce genetically. A virus is a packet of genetic material that is capable of taking over the enzyme system of the cell in order to reproduce itself. The survival of these "parasites" is dependent on living inside your cells.

Immune dysfunction occurs when a virus is freed from a dormant state. For example, with chronic stress, the human body becomes debilitated and this enables viruses to proliferate. Evidence of viral presence is found in nearly all persons with CFS. Capable of hiding out in body tissue and reproducing indefinitely, it is possible to have a virus and not show any signs of disease. The virus can remain dormant for many years, reemerging, particularly in times of debility and stress, or can activate illness such as a bacterial or viral infection.

Once inside the body, a virus tends to inhabit the brain and nervous system tissue. In the central nervous system, the virus is not attacked by the immune system, which makes it a safe place to hide undisturbed for long periods. Viral illness is particularly resistant to standard medical interventions because the virus becomes part of the genetic material of the host cell. Treatment that would eradicate the virus can subject the host cells to injury or death.

The viral theory holds that CFS is an immune system illness triggered by one or more viral agents. CFS usually emerges after the abrupt onset of an acute viral infection, and there is no single infectious agent that is known to cause CFS.[8] Part of this theory regards CFS to be a disorder of the activation of T-cell function which causes the cells to react abnormally to viral antigens.[9–11] In turn, this results in the production of abnormal cytokines which alter cellular function.[12]

There are several variations of this scenario, all related to compromised immunity which can lead to reactivation of dormant viruses including: Epstein–Barr virus (EBV), herpes simplex virus, cytomegalovirus, and viruses such as polio, Coxsackie, echo, entero, and retroviruses.[13] Polio, and vaccinations against polio have been cited as possible culprits. Secondary infections also seem to play a role. The clinical picture of CFS shows high levels of viral antibodies that indicate an abnormal immune system response, typically a sign of a bacterial or viral infection.[14]

Initially, it was thought that prolonged persistence of EBV was the cause, based on the observation of high titers of anti-EBV antibodies. Follow-up investigations showed that people with CFS have elevated antibody titers to many viruses.[15] EBV is a member of the herpes family of viruses, capable of establishing lifelong latent infections after the initial onset of illness. Great Britain has also been investigating the Coxsackie B virus as the possible cause.[16]

It may be that no single infectious agent is responsible for the illness, but rather the synergistic effect of several viruses causes immune dysfunction.[17] A healthy immune system can keep latent infections in check, but when the immune system is compromised the virus can be activated. The current belief is that one or more latent viruses become active and cause the symptoms of CFS because the immune system is unable to keep the viruses in check.[18]

Retroviral Theory

As a subset of the viral theory, researchers are looking at a class of viruses known as retroviruses. After penetrating a cell, the genetic material of the retrovirus—RNA—is transformed into DNA. With this transformation, the DNA becomes a part of the human cell. The Wistar Institute in Philadelphia found evidence of retroviral presence in 80% of CFS patients in a small study and no such evidence in a group of healthy people.[19] However, retroviruses are typically transmitted by bodily fluids, which does not fit the CFS profile.

In 1991 there was excitement that the CFS culprit had been found by Dr. John Martin, who cultured the spumavirus, a subfamily of retroviruses, from the cerebrospinal fluid of people with CFS.[20,21] Other known retroviruses include the human immunodeficiency virus, which causes AIDS. Originally, the spumavirus was thought to be rare in humans, being predominantly found in sick animals that exhibit many symptoms similar to CFS. This report has now been disputed, as it is believed that a cytomegalovirus was isolated instead of the virus in question.[22]

Immune Theory

Respiratory allergies often precede the onset of CFS,[23] which suggests an immune system that already has trouble turning off. Enhanced reactivity to allergens tends to accompany increased reactivity to other infectious agents. Allergies such as hay fever, sensitivity to foods and to house dust are common to CFS sufferers; they occur because the immune system overreacts to substances commonly seen to be harmless.[23]

There is speculation by researchers that some allergic people may overreact to infectious pathogens which are then the cause of CFS.[23,24] At the same time, the individual overreacts to environmental pollutants, viruses, and hormonal changes, resulting in symptoms common to EI. Ongoing reactivity causes progressive weakening of the immune system, which permits a multitude of bacterial, viral, yeast, and parasitic infections to take hold. The fundamental concept behind this theory overlaps with the viral theory; namely, that a compromised immune system leads to reactivation of latent viruses.

Cytokine Theory

As already noted, a hyperimmune disturbance in the immune system can lead to the production of an excessive amount of chemicals known as cytokines, which are believed by some to be the cause of CFS symptoms.[25] This theory holds that CFS is caused by an unknown agent stimulating the production of cytokines, which then cause CFS symptoms. This provocative theory is not focused on identifying the triggering agent, but on examining how the symptoms of CFS are caused. Despite a limited understanding of the function of cytokines, their presence helps explain the symptoms of the illness.

Hormone Theory

Research has also revealed that in the brain–adrenal hormone feedback system, hormonal deficiencies of the endocrine system and the brain occur in people with CFS.[26] On the average, levels of cortisol, a hormone produced by the adrenal gland, are lower in the blood and urine of CFS patients.[26] The body secretes cortisol in response to stress, and a deficiency of cortisol can cause lethargy and fatigue.

In addition, people with CFS have been noted to be deficient in corticotropin-releasing hormone (CRH).[26] The hypothalamus in the brain secretes CRH, which activates the pituitary gland to secrete adrenocorticotropic hormone, which in turn stimulates the adrenal gland to produce cortisol. CRH helps to increase energy levels through a direct effect on the brain, and a deficiency may contribute to the lack of energy seen in CFS. Further studies may help determine what contributes most strongly to CFS fatigue: CRH deficiency or a cortisol deficiency, or both deficiencies acting in tandem.

Mental Theory

The most controversial, least popular theory relates to the role of the mind in creating illness. The mental theory suggests that the illness may be in part subliminally activated and that nearly all unexplained chronic fatigue can be linked to emotional disturbance. One CDC study noted that half of the individuals interviewed reported a significant bout with depression during the course of their illness.[27] Dr. Ian Hickie, psychiatrist at Prince Henry Hospital in New South Wales, Australia, has performed studies that repudiate this report, and he notes, "If you contract any medical illness you will become depressed."[28]

Whether depressed mental status leads to the development of the illness or whether persons with CFS become depressed because of the longevity and nature of the illness has yet to be established. Both supportive advocates of CFS as well as those who are ill believe the concept of emotional disturbance as the cause of CFS to be nonsense. However, the pathophysiology of major depression can lead to immunological defects and thus increase susceptibility to the illness.

Unified Theory

The unified theory holds that a spectrum of viral, environmental, and genetic factors assault the body, triggering immune breakdown. Nonviral causes that are suspect include chemical or environmental contaminants which can damage the immune system. Initial toxic exposures may go unnoticed, but can activate a dormant virus that results in CFS for some and EI for others. It may also be that genetic factors predispose the body to act differently to unknown causative agents.[29]

This theory gives consideration to the fact that many with CFS and EI are predisposed to candida overgrowth. Persistent, prolonged treatment with antibiotics is one way that immune function is downgraded, leading to systemic imbalance. The presence of excessive amounts of candida can weaken the immune system, creating an entry route for viral and bacterial infections. Many people with EI and CFS also have intestinal parasites which suppress immune function, and the presence of parasites often goes undetected. Anything that acts to suppress the immune system should be regarded as a possible contributing agent to this illness.

Neurally Mediated Hypotension Theory

Neurally mediated hypotension (NMH) is another possible cause of CFS. At the Johns Hopkins University School of Medicine in Baltimore, a pilot study demonstrated that CFS patients experienced reductions in heart rate and blood pressure that typically should have been increases. This condition typically occurs when the autonomic nervous system, which controls heart rate and blood pressure, misinterprets the body's needs during periods of upright posture, sending a message to the heart to slow down and lower blood pressure, which is the opposite of what is needed. This could account for the symptoms of fatigue, fainting, nausea, and lightheadedness found in CFS. What is intriguing about this study is that 9 out of the 23 patients recovered when treated with medications to regulate blood pressure.[30]

It is a process of trial and error to find the correct drug and dosage for the individual, and careful monitoring by the physician is necessary because of the risk of serious side effects. One of the most commonly used drugs for NMH is Florinef, a corticosteriod that helps the kidneys to retain sodium. As with other steroids, Florinef can affect mood and cause depression or irritability. If these symptoms occur, check with your physician. A key part of therapy includes an increase in fluid and salt intake. Those who increase their fluids seem to respond better to therapy than those who do not change their intake habits.[31] Despite optimistic responses to this approach, this is an intervention that treats symptoms, rather than resolving the cause.

Heredity, environment, life-style, overall medical health, physical and emotional exhaustion, abnormal red blood cells, encephalitis, and acute toxic exposure may all be causative. Any one or all of the causal theories may be correct. Despite major efforts on the part of a small, dedicated medical community, there is no known cause or cure for CFS. It is still not understood why some people get it and others don't. It also remains a complete mystery why some get well quickly, while others take years to recover, and still others have remissions and recurrences.

Whatever the causative agent, it is certain that the immune system is compromised. As a result, there is intense biological activity that depletes the body's energy at a molecular and cellular level. So for our purposes, CFS involves immune dysfunction.

It is also unclear if CFS is contagious. Clusters of cases in families, workplaces, schools, and communities have occurred. What makes this confusing is that most people in close contact with people who have CFS do not become ill. Some researchers believe that CFS may be contagious in the acute phase of illness, while others speculate that continuous, long-term exposure may prompt illness.

What is stressed is that those with CFS not donate blood, blood products, or organs. Some doctors believe that those who are ill should not share food, utensils, drinking glasses and should practice "safe" sex. Since individuals with CFS often have overactivated immune function and may not manufacture antibodies after receiving immunizations, they are at risk for adverse reactions to vaccines.

Demographics

A CFS surveillance study performed by the CDC in four U.S. cities, spanning from September of 1989 to September of 1991, yielded the following data:

1. 82% of patients were female
2. The average age at onset was 30
3. Average duration of the illness at the time of entering the study was 7.1 years
4. Median household income was $41,200
5. Median energy level on a scale of 1 to 100 before illness was 95; at the worst point during illness it was 12
6. 50% reported a viral-like onset to the illness; other triggers included auto accidents and death in the family[32]

Symptoms

The most prevalent symptom of CFS is intense, crippling exhaustion and weakness. Prolonged episodes of this sort of fatigue make it difficult to maintain a normal life-style. With CFS you feel as though you are constantly experiencing the aftereffects of the flu. Elaine, a gifted psychic who struggles with EI and CFS, reports that on many days, she has only a couple of hours a day where she has the energy to be up and about. "My life used to be so busy. Now I spend all my time resting."

Many report difficulties with digestion, and others have endocrine involvement. Worse still, symptoms can change over time, or combine to involve multiple systems. There is often an assortment of disturbing neurological and cognitive symptoms. "For the most part I didn't mind the fatigue. What upset me the most was trying to get my brain to work. I couldn't count on myself for anything; names, faces, dates, all eluded recall," asserts Audrey who is now well from CFS. Magnetic resonance imaging of the brain shows evidence of lesions in some subjects.[33] Topographical brain mapping is often abnormal in CFS, revealing abnormalities of the temporal lobes, particularly the left lobe.[34]

For some, the act of moving or talking can be intolerable, as there can be muscle and joint pain as well as spasms. Lymph node pain and joint pain are present in 70% of CFS patients.[35] Driving a car, walking, or tolerating human contact can become things of the past and the illness can become a wedge that destroys relationships. There are unusual pressure-like headaches. Because of an intolerance to alcohol, one becomes inebriated quickly, and symptoms can worsen. Many are sensitive to medications; even the smallest dose can cause toxicity.

The problems with sleep are varied and contradictory. Logic suggests that if you are tired, you should be able to sleep. Despite exhaustion, many have insomnia and cannot sleep for more than a few hours at a time. Some cannot stay awake, but when they do sleep they awaken unrefreshed and often more tired than before. Sensitivity to light, fever, chills, night sweats, shortness of breath, and palpitations add to the list of discomforts. All of these symptoms can wax and wane on a daily basis. On top of this, you may appear to be perfectly healthy.

Diagnosis

The physician must rule out other causes before deciding on CFS. The illness can be difficult to diagnose, in part because its symptoms are similar to those of many other illnesses, such as multiple sclerosis, Lyme disease, interstitial cystitis, and polio. CFS can resemble clinical depression, as it shares many of the same symptoms. Being chronically tired doesn't mean you have CFS and not everyone has the most severe form of the illness. Then there are the walking wounded who may never receive a diagnosis of CFS, despite the obvious presence of illness.

Once Josh, the registered nurse with CFS, received a definitive diagnosis, he felt enormous relief, as this made him eligible for disability and helped him assert that it's not all in his head. CFS is difficult to diagnose because medical testing that would confirm the condition remains nondefinitive. However, studies of T-cell function, depressed NK-cell function, with an increase in NK cell numbers, as well as other abnormal lab findings can help confirm the illness. The main tool for diagnosis is the CDC's working case definition of CFS, which is as follows:

1. Fatigue: Severe, unexplained fatigue persistent, or relapsing for 6 months; which is not caused by exertion or relieved by rest; which has a new or identifiable onset; which results in a substantial reduction in previous levels of occupational, educational, social, or personal activity.

2. Symptoms: The presence of four or more of the following symptoms must have persisted or recurred during six or more consecutive months of illness, and must not have predated the fatigue:

    a. Memory or concentration problems
    b. Sore throat
    c. Tender lymph nodes
    d. Muscle pain
    e. Joint pain with normal-looking joints
    f. Headaches of a new type or severity
    g. Unrefreshed sleep
    h. Postexertional malaise

3. Exclusions: People may be excluded if they have an active medical diagnosis or physical findings suggestive of a medical diagnosis or previous nonresolved medical diagnosis; a major psychiatric disorder, including depression or psychosis; severe obesity; alcohol or substance abuse occurring within 2 years before the onset of fatigue, or at any time afterwards.

4. Inclusions: Conditions defined solely by symptoms without confirmatory diagnostic tests (i.e., fibromyalgia, untreated depression, neurasthenia, multiple chemical sensitivities, and anxiety), treated conditions with fatigue extending beyond expected resolution (i.e., hypothyroidism, asthma, both with normal lab studies), conditions following completion of definitive therapy with continued fatigue (i.e., treated Lyme disease or syphilis), any physical examination or laboratory finding that does not suggest an exclusionary condition.

The CFS Cure

As of this writing there is no cure for CFS; but this does not mean you can't achieve relief. Although the process is long and gradual, it is encouraging to note that large numbers of sufferers have fully recovered or have returned to a nearly normal level of function. So far, treatments emphasize alleviating symptoms. This includes paying attention to the messages issued by your body: limiting your activities, as well as resting as you need to, developing healthy dietary habits, undertaking a program to strengthen your immune system, reducing the influence of stress, exercising as tolerated, taking steps to reduce depression, seeking pharmacological relief, and many more interventions. Employing a multifaceted approach includes learning to live in harmony with your rebellious body with hope and courage.

Fibromyalgia

Research studies show that about 2% of the population is afflicted with fibromyalgia (FM), a syndrome characterized by widespread pain and aching muscles.[36] The

American College of Rheumatology defines FM as a history of widespread pain, lasting for over 3 months, on both sides of the body, and pain on manual palpation in 11 of 18 tender point sites.[37] Known to occur as a secondary aspect of other diseases such as lupus erythematosus or rheumatoid arthritis, FM may also occur as a primary illness.

As a primary illness, FM shares many symptoms with CFS, and likewise is a disease without a known cause or cure. Owing to these similarities, there is little question among researchers that CFS and primary FM are the same illness. Drs. Dedra Buchwald and Goldenberg noted that 63 to 70% of CFS patients met criteria for FM.[38] However, in another study, researcher Dr. Wysenbeek found that only 21% of FM patients met the criteria for CFS.[39] Though nearly all CFS patients suffer from muscle pain, there is often not enough muscle pain to reach the criterion for FM diagnosis.

Common precipitating factors for FM are similar to those for CFS, including infectious triggers, physical and emotional trauma, and medications that suppress the immune system, such as corticosteroids. As with CFS, some experts believe FM is the result of chronic stress brought on by an underlying emotional disorder. Like CFS, those who have FM suffer from depressed mood as a result of the restrictions and discomfort caused by the illness.

Similar to CFS, the symptomatic focus for FM includes sleep disorders, tender swollen lymph nodes, joint pain, anxiety, and depression. With FM, muscle pain is described as a flulike achiness that worsens with exercise. Josh, the oncology nurse, has had prolonged muscle and joint pain, without the brain-fogging and neurological deficits common to CFS. Symptoms related to cognitive impairment are not as frequent or severe in FM as they are in CFS. Though Josh has a CFS diagnosis, the constellation of his symptoms fits the FM profile more closely, as he describes sharp pains in specific muscle groups coupled with muscle weakness. In FM there can be muscle atrophy, yet paradoxically muscle strength testing is often within normal range.

As with CFS, FM sufferers report unrefreshed sleep. Unrefreshed sleep is defined as sleeping so lightly that the individual doesn't know if he has been sleeping or not. Exhaustion without the ability to sleep is a variant of unrefreshed sleep. Unrefreshed sleep can affect immune function and, in turn, heighten pain, fatigue, and other symptoms. One interesting study was able to induce the muscle pain of FM by depriving the subjects of sleep.[40]

FM Therapy

As with CFS, interventions are largely palliative, directed at reducing symptomatic discomfort. Physical therapy, coupled with exercise to tolerance can offer relief. Josh, who has CFS, experiences relief from joint and muscle pain by performing gentle stretching exercises. Antioxidant supplements such as carotene, chlorophyll, vitamin C, and B vitamins may assist with pain reduction. Prescription medications include antidepressants, anti-inflammatory drugs, and muscle relaxants. Treating the sleep disorder may help resolve problems with fatigue. Doxepin, an antidepressant medication, has been particularly useful in relieving pain and correcting the sleep disturbance. While many improve, the majority of people with FM have chronic symptoms.

Several other illnesses share similar clinical findings and/or symptoms with EI and CFS, including lupus, Lyme disease, porphyria, rheumatoid arthritis, multiple sclerosis, Hashimoto's thyroiditis, and postpolio syndrome. There is also mounting evidence that supports the induction of CFS and EI-related symptoms in the case of implants, such as pacemakers, silicone as well as saline breast implants, and artificial valves and joints. While medical science has yet to determine exactly how these illnesses are linked, interventions that offer relief for EI and CFS may help alleviate some of these other health problems.

Brain Involvement

CFS is not just about physical incapacity; many sufferers have difficulties with memory and mental acuity as well. With brain involvement there is a disturbing sort of sensory rawness and vulnerability. Suddenly you may be unable to remember how to operate the TV channel changer, or what to do when you see a stop sign, or how to decipher a string of words. In conversation you may find yourself not making sense. It's possible to get hopelessly lost driving home from work. At times, you may have trouble remembering familiar names and faces. The persistence of brain-fogging is frightening and baffling. Perhaps the most disturbing symptom is the inability to cope with stress, which is the most common reason people have difficulty working.

Brain symptoms come and go without rhyme or reason. Mental fogging, described by people who are ill, can abruptly resolve into clarity. Fogginess can make it impossible to complete simple tasks. CFS patients demonstrate varied memory problems, spatial disorganization, as well as attention and concentration deficits.[41] Dr. Jay Goldstein, CFS specialist, says that dementia seen with CFS is typically caused by the presence of the wrong types, or excessive amounts, of cytokines in the brain. Coupled with that, these patients show significantly abnormal brain mapping studies. He also notes that short term memory loss can be marked, yet long term memory remains unimpaired.[42,43]

It is possible to compensate for many of the drawbacks of these illnesses. You can hire people to perform tasks you cannot do. You can compensate for a lack of energy by reorganizing your life. Yet, it is not possible to compensate for fuzzy thinking, getting your brain to work when it cannot. Brain impairment is the most difficult and complex symptom to cope with.

Cognitive Dissonance

Since you don't look as sick as you feel, it is difficult to get others to comprehend your memory lapses, fatigue, and discomfort. At one point, frustrated by the lack of acceptance, Jamie, a therapist with EI and CFS, shaved her head so she would look as terrible as she felt. When there is external damage, a deformity, or an obvious crutch, empathy flows with greater ease. When this evidence is lacking, there can be judgment. Looking normal means you are expected to perform as though you are healthy.

It can be exhausting to put out idle energy in conversation. Jamie, mentioned above, avoids casual conversations altogether, noting that the simple act of listening is exhausting. "I have to work extra hard to digest incoming information and to cover-up when my brain feels like mush. At times I find myself with the refrigerator door open, unable to recall why I am there. At other times I am flooded with rage and irritability that has no bearing on external circumstances." You may feel you have little control over mercurial emotions; an upsurge of rage can give way to tears, or you may be inappropriately giddy. You are not alone, these emotion-flooded states affect people with EI and CFS as well.

Acting on these impulsive swings can have a destructive impact on interpersonal relationships. Jamie has a strategic plan that includes retreating from contact during these times in order to reduce the potential for negative interaction. By informing others that you are prone to these deficits and mood changes, you may avert conflict, or prevent others from judging you or from taking your irritability personally.

Cognitive Restructuring Tips

Cognitive restructuring offers techniques that make information retrieval easier, and can make it easier to memorize and retain information. In addition, restructuring can enable you to compensate for losses by increasing your ability to process and use information. A few simple tricks for people with CFS have been adapted from Dr. Tarras Onischenko, a North Carolina specialist in evaluations and treatment of the neurologically impaired.[41]

1. Reducing background stimuli makes it easier to focus on the task at hand and to retain information. When overstimulated, the brain may close down to protect itself, so turn off the radio while driving or studying. Some people work best during early morning hours, while others work best at night when there is less stimulation and fewer distractions that the brain must block.

2. Attack a task well before the deadline so you can work at your own pace. You may want to break down the job into realistic flexible increments.

3. Accomplish as much as possible when you are in a clear, relaxed mental state and stop working when you become tired. You may work unproductively if you continue to push on. Table a project when too many mistakes occur, take frequent breaks, and pace yourself by limiting periods of intense brain activity.

4. Emphasizing what you have accomplished will enable you to feel productive even if you haven't completed the entire job. Try to do tasks that require your immediate attention, interspersed with enjoyable tasks. Don't beat yourself up for the things you haven't done.

5. If you have trouble focusing when reading, cut a rectangular shape out of the center of a piece of cardboard, a little larger than the length of a written line and about the height of the written text. Using this to frame reading material will make it easier to focus.

6. Repetition and categorization can help with the retention or retrieval of information. Creating an image in your mind's eye of the environment or emotional state you were in when the information was received will increase recall. Information is often learned or retrieved by association or the pairing of a similar image.

7. External cues can help keep you on track. A calendar, appointment book, photographs, writing yourself notes, making lists, and the use of an object to serve as a cue can facilitate memory. "Post-it" notes can also be a valuable crutch.

8. Making lists will make it easier to focus and prioritize, enabling you to accomplish much more in the course of a day. However, don't allow an incomplete list to serve as a reproach when you're out of energy; just hold the task over until a more convenient time.

9. Prepare a list of passive activities that you can engage in when you move into low gear. Like rainy day activities, these might include reading, listening to tapes, crocheting, or TV.

10. Save tasks that don't require clarity for later in the day when the brain is more tired. Exercise can be one pastime saved for times when you don't need to engage the brain.

The Search for Credibility

The controversy as to whether CFS is a legitimate illness stems from the notion that fatigue is not a true pathological state. The illness has been derisively called the "yuppie flu" following an epidemic of the illness in the Lake Tahoe area and "Royal Free disease" after a similar outbreak in London over 35 years ago. It has been dismissed by physicians and the press as a trivial psychological problem elevated to the level of illness. Since fatigue is a normal aspect of existence, it raises the question as to what separates CFS symptoms of fatigue from ordinary fatigue found in those who don't see themselves as ill.

Yet, there is increased evidence of viral presence and abnormal T-cell and NK-cell activities, indicating a tangible physiological basis. It helps that the past director of the CDC, Dr. Walter Gunn, has validated CFS as a legitimate illness, largely because of the neurological changes that are not seen in the average person who is tired or depressed. He notes, "Our surveillance study does not support the notion that CFS is a psychiatric illness and in fact, suggests that it has an organic basis."[44] Studies that compare serum, immunologic, and psychological profiles of those who are clinically depressed don't match the profiles of those with CFS. With clinical depression there is a pervasive sense of helplessness and hopelessness. People with CFS, like Josh who spends his days writing poems and stories, demonstrate a strong sense of will and desire.

From a biochemical perspective, immune system suppression and depression can go together, with depression as a common feature of chronic illness. Chronic illness is a good breeding ground for depression and most people with CFS become depressed at some time during the illness. Along with the isolation imposed by the illness and its ups and downs, it is easy to despair of becoming well. It is not clear if the depression experienced with CFS is caused by the physiology of the illness or if it is a by-product that develops as a result of experiencing the downside of any chronic health problem.

Summary

Although the etiology of CFS is not known, it is a relief to know that competent specialists are working hard to uncover the cause(s) of CFS. It can also be a relief to know that medical science is taking this illness seriously and that you are not alone in your struggles. Interventions are geared toward doing all you can to support your immune system, as well as finding relief from the discomfort of this illness.

Endnotes

[1]Donald Goldberg, "Fibromyalgia and CFS," *The CFIDS Chronicle* Winter 1995: 38.

[2]D. Bates *et al.*, "Prevalence of Fatigue and Chronic Fatigue Syndrome in a Primary Care Practice," *Arch Intern Med* 153, 24 (1993): 2759–2765.

[3]Kimberly Kenney, ed., quote from Hugh Fudenburg, Los Angeles research conference 16 Feb. 1990, reprint *The CFIDS Association* Sept. 1991.

[4]David Bell, *The Disease of a Thousand Names* (Lyndonville: Pollard, 1991) 8.

[5]David Bell, *The Doctor's Guide to Chronic Fatigue Syndrome* (Reading: Addison–Wesley, 1995) 9.

[6]William Collinge, *Recovering from Chronic Fatigue Syndrome* (New York: Perigee, 1993) 36–41.

[7]Jay Goldstein, "Chronic Fatigue Syndrome," *The Female Patient* Vol. 16 (Jan. 1991): 39–50.

[8]Kimberly Kenney, ed., quotes from Anthony Komaroff, 17 Nov. 1990, "The Role of HHV-6 in CFS," *The CFIDS Chronicle* Spring 1991: 31.

[9]J. Goldstein, "Limbic Encephalopathy in a Dysregulated Neuroimmune Network," and M. Loveless, "Immunologic Activation Syndrome and its Association with Chronic Fatigue Syndrome," CFS Conference Chronic Fatigue Syndrome: Current Theory and Treatment, Bel Air, 18 May, 1991.

[10]Collinge, 29.

[11]Nancy Klimas, "Diagnosing CFIDS: An Immunologist's Approach," *The CFIDS Chronicle* Sept. 1992: 41–42.

[12]Michael Rosenbaum and Murray Susser, *Solving the Puzzle of Chronic Fatigue Syndrome* (Tacoma: Life Sciences, 1991) 100.

[13]Kimberly Kenney, ed., "A CFIDS Model: Compromised Immunity," *The CFIDS Chronicle* Spring 1991: 33.

[14]Bell, *The Doctor's Guide* 94.

[15]L. Calabrese *et al.*, "Chronic Fatigue Syndrome," *The CFIDS Chronicle Physician's Forum* Sept. 1992: 6–10.

[16]Bell, *The Doctor's Guide* 202.

[17]Kenney, ed., Komaroff, 31.

[18]Collinge, 27.

[19]Collinge, 28.

[20]John Martin, "Spumavirus Associated Myalgic Encephalomyelopathy: Research Breakthrough in the Study of CFIDS," *The CFIDS Chronicle* Fall 1991: 2–4.

[21]Geoffrey Cowley and Mary Hager, "A Clue to Chronic Fatigue," *Newsweek* 30 Sept. 1991: 66.

[22]Kimberly Kenney, ed., "Martin's Findings Questioned," *The CFIDS Chronicle* Winter 1995: 59.

[23]Irwin Landau, ed., "What Causes CFS? A Lineup of Suspects," *Consumer Reports* Oct. 1990: 674.

[24]S. Strauss *et al.*, "Allergy and the Chronic Fatigue Syndrome," *J Allergy Clin Immunol* 81 (1988): 791.

[25]Bell, *The Doctor's Guide* 210.

[26]M. Demitrack *et al.*, "Evidence for Impaired Activation of the Hypothalamic–Pituitary–Adrenal Axis in Patients With Chronic Fatigue Syndrome," *J Clin Endocrinol Metab* 73 (1991): 1224.

[27]Kimberly Kenney, ed., quotes from Ian Hickie 18 Nov. 1990, "The Assessment of Depression in Patients with CFS," *The CFIDS Chronicle* Spring 1991: 92.

[28]Kenney, ed., Hickie, 91–95.

[29]Bell, *The Doctor's Guide* 203–213.

[30]Ridgley Ochs, "Researchers find Chronicle Fatigue Link," *San Francisco Chronicle* 27 Sept. 1995.

[31]Vicki Carpman, ed., notes from The Neurally Mediated Hypotension Working Group, Johns Hopkins Hospital, "Patient Information Brochure on Neurally Mediated Hypotension and its Treatment," *The CFIDS Chronicle* Fall 1995: 15–16.

[32]"CFS Surveillance Study . . . and Beyond," *Fibromyalgia Network* Jan. 1993: 4.

[33]Jay Goldstein, "The Diagnosis of Chronic Fatigue Syndrome as a Limbic Encephalopathy," *The CFIDS Chronicle Physician's Forum* Sept. 1992: 20–34.

[34]Goldstein, 30.

[35]Bell, *The Doctor's Guide* 35.

[36]F. Wolfe *et al.*, "Prevalence and Characteristics of Fibromyalgia in the General Population," *Arthritis Rheumatism* 38, 1, (Jan. 1995): 19–28.

[37]Calabrese, 8–9.

[38]D. Buchwald, "The Chronic Active Epstein–Barr Virus Infection Syndrome and Primary Fibromyalgia," *Arthritis Rheumatism* 30 (1987): 1132–1136.

[39]Calabrese, 9.

[40]David Bell, *The Doctor's Guide to Chronic Fatigue Syndrome* (Reading: Addison–Wesley, 1995) 209; research by H. Moldofsky and F. Lue, "Sleep and Symptoms in Fibrositis Syndrome after a Febrile Illness," *J Rheumatol* 15 (1988): 1701–1704.

[41]T. Onischenko, "Cognitive Rehabilitation: Strategies, Tasks, Theories, and Games," adapted from lecture 14 June 1990, *The CFIDS Chronicle Physician's Forum* Aug. 1991: 7–18.

[42]J. Goldstein, "The Evolving Hypothesis: The Brain and CFIDS," *The CFIDS Chronicle* 1988: 10–14.

[43]M. Handelman and J. Goldstein, "Brain Mapping," *The CFIDS Chronicle* 1988: 15.

[44]Kimberly Kinney, ed., *CFIDS Chronicle* quote Walter Gunn, Feb. 1992.

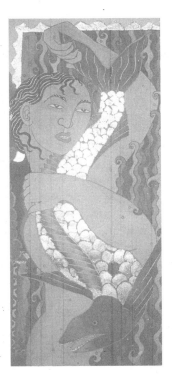

Chapter Four

The Commonalities of EI and CFS

*t*his chapter examines the similarities between EI and CFS and what you can do to aid your recovery. The subject matter is not grounded in scientific fact, but rather comes from observations that people with EI and CFS have similar symptoms, similar laboratory changes, and in some ways, similar personality traits. This will help to establish a basis for intervention and to keep sufferers from feeling overwhelmed. Although the etiologies of EI and CFS are unknown, both are believed to be different aspects of the same physiological malfunction, namely, immune dysfunction. The latter term refers to an immune system that is either over- or underactivated in its efforts to help the body cope with invading pathogens such as bacteria, viruses, parasites, or environmental chemicals. Such states are common to those suffering from EI and CFS. When the immune system is overcharged, the body does not halt the production of cytokines, antibodies, and other factors in its protective efforts. This excessive activation produces many disturbing symptoms and ultimately may result in an "allergy" to the self, or an autoimmune process.

When the immune system is underactivated, it is not performing its job of protecting the body. For example, T cells may not be produced in adequate numbers, or there may be reduced NK cell function, or protective antigen–antibody reactions may fail to occur. AIDS patients, CFS sufferers, as well as others with EI are vulnerable to pathogens because they are not able to mount an effective immune response. Multiple insults, such as environmental toxins and ongoing viral infections, can render the immune system immobile or can trigger inappropriate, ineffective overreactions, suffocating the healthy immune response.

Dr. Lapp, an internist who has been treating CFS patients, notes that allergic reactivity such as asthma and hay fever are common in people with CFS probably because the immune system is overactivated.[1] Allergies can become more apparent when the body is burdened with CFS because of the overall impairment of immune capability. In turn, allergies common to EI may prompt increased susceptibility to CFS.

Dr. Heuser, who primarily works with people with chemical injuries, noted at an annual CFS conference, "We conclude that toxic chemical exposure can cause CFIDS."[2] Environmental pollutants can overload the immune system to the point of collapse, contributing to the onset of either illness. Other physicians, such as Dr. David Bell, speculate that CFS is probably the cause of chemical sensitivities that are believed to develop after the onset of illness.[3] A 1994 study comparing patients with CFS, EI, and fibromyalgia was performed by Drs. Dedra Buchwald and Deborah Garrity and revealed that these illnesses might be similar, if not identical, conditions.[4]

What is also confusing about both EI and CFS is that they share characteristics with several other medical conditions such as multiple sclerosis (MS), lupus, and polio. Owing to diagnostic limitations, it may be difficult to determine what is actually occurring in the face of so many other related health problems present in the same individual such as bacterial infections, candidiasis, and parasites.

For example, consider that some unknown agent has impacted the body, causing immune dysregulation. From there, it may be that genetics and environmental factors then dictate the pathway by which illness develops. This means these illnesses could be triggered by one or multiple causative agents, leading to immune problems which result in either EI or CFS, or both illnesses. Though EI and CFS may be overlapping syndromes that have common features, their mechanism of activation is different. EI may emerge because of disability of the detoxification capabilities of the body, whereas CFS may be caused by the inactivation and, or disturbance of various body systems.

The Roller Coaster Ride

Both CFS and EI symptoms are varied and unpredictable. Elaine, who has EI and CFS, feels poorly much of the time, yet there are days when she feels normal. On days when she risks contact with allergic sources, she comes through unscathed, and at other times she is reactive to everything. She has "up" days in which she has the energy to accomplish many tasks. A downside to such days is that they provoke a raised brow here and there, calling into question the reality of her ongoing malaise. Even worse, she may end up paying for these good days with several days of weakness and exhaustion.

Remission and relapse are an expected way of life. EI and CFS have ups and downs, varying in intensity from one day or month to the next. Both illnesses have been referred to as "terrorists," striking anywhere at any time without warning. Just when relief is in sight you can find yourself backsliding. These ups and downs make it difficult to sustain hope.

You may try to do everything just right, taking perfect care of your body. You may have covered all of the bases by attending to your spiritual and emotional growth. After a time, you may have felt pretty good, cocky enough to decide you were well. This declaration may invariably cause you to become more casual about your health, taking it for granted.

But, like a terrorist attack, newly recovered health can be torn to shreds without warning at any time. Decompensation occurs after scheduling too many dates, or eating too many preservative-filled foods, or forgetting to pace yourself at work, or when you take on too much. In resuming the fast-paced life, you may forget to take care of yourself. Reexposure to pollutants and chemicals can cause deterioration for both EI and CFS sufferers, triggering a resurgence of viral and allergic symptoms.

At times it is possible to identify the cause of decompensation; at other times it is a mystery why illness has returned. It is difficult to link these cycles with any particular environmental or stress-related influences. Changes in emotional and hormonal states, weather, temperature, and humidity affect people with both illnesses. These changes can be confusing to family and friends who never know what to expect, and your limits may vary daily as symptoms fluctuate.

The good news is that EI and CFS are not necessarily progressive illnesses. There is currently no evidence that these illnesses cause permanent tissue or organ damage. Many can look forward to full recovery, yet there is no consensus as to what "recovery" means. Gloria, who considers herself to be well from CFS, continues to remain vigilant in efforts to avoid a relapse. Her symptoms have diminished to the extent that she has a full, happy life. Still, she has not returned to her pre-illness level of activity.

Bargaining

Bargaining is a common pastime among those who are ill. Theresa, who has severe EI, was determined to get through the Christmas holidays without incident. Later she paid the price and was ill for weeks. You may find yourself asking the Universe to supply you with energy to carry you through an important occasion, even though this often means accepting the price you will have to pay, suffering for days to come. The fact that you can will yourself through a particular stressor points out the tremendous influence that the mind has over the body.

In times of crisis you may be able to summon the energy to do things you may not be able to do with your baseline energies. Some report that multiple chemical sensitivities and fatigue disappear while recovering from surgery or during pregnancy, only to return later in full force. Mobilizing to support her brother through his ordeal with cancer enabled Jamie, a therapist with EI and CFS, to summon her own physical resources. She had energy to fix meals, care for his children, and drive him to appointments. When he was out of danger, she suffered a relapse.

Diagnostic Skepticism

Because there are so many seemingly unrelated symptoms that come and go, clear clinical and causative diagnoses may not be possible. With both EI and CFS, physical discomforts may change daily, making it difficult to link symptoms with each other in order to establish a cause-and-effect relationship. The complexity of one of these illnesses alone, involving so many physiological systems—immune, neurological, endocrine, and digestive systems to name a few—can be baffling. Add to that a second illness, just as complex and variable, and you can have great confusion.

The effectiveness of treatments can vary between individuals. What is even more perplexing is that an intervention that brought relief a few months ago may afford no comfort at all today. Furthermore, although two people can have the same amount of exposure to an offending agent, when the more sensitive person is reexposed the reaction can be rapid and intense, while the other person may not experience any change in the magnitude of reactivity. Small wonder that these events are confusing and unaccountable to the logical mind of the physician.

Medical science typically believes in the relation: no supporting empirical evidence = absence of that particular problem. When physician after physician could not uncover relevant clinical data, Jamie, the therapist who later was diagnosed to have EI and CFS, was told to seek psychiatric care. It was frightening to have her emotional stability questioned; that had always been one thing Jaime could count on. In part, because elusive symptoms make it difficult to reach a clinical diagnosis, both EI and CFS have been stigmatized as "fad illnesses" or hysteria. Because it is so difficult to achieve credibility, you may blame yourself for the presence and persistence of either illness.

If these illnesses are the workings of a disordered mind, you have to wonder how so many people could have manufactured these complex illnesses in isolation. Thankfully, increased publicity in the form of news articles and public education, particularly regarding CFS, has enabled these illnesses to gain greater acceptance.

EI and CFS as Mental Illness

CFS is seen by some as a treatable mental health problem because of the high incidence of depression reported among those with the disorder. It should come as no surprise that proponents of this view are very unpopular with those who are suffering with EI or CFS. Allergic reactivity seen in EI, as well as the neurological changes common to CFS can make it difficult for sufferers to control their emotional states. They may act erratically, exhibiting mood swings, hyperirritability, and difficulties with appropriate self-expression.

Is, it important whether depression is a secondary or a primary characteristic of both EI and CFS? The important point is that these illnesses make it difficult to control and direct the normal functioning of the brain in order to prevent depression and emotional lability. It is certainly cruel to suggest that the sufferer is responsible for creating the problem. Blame doesn't elicit a cure and the reality of disturbing symptoms should be enough to prompt compassion.

Political Implications

It is obvious that if both EI and CFS were to achieve recognition as legitimate illnesses, there would be serious political and economic implications. In 1994, studies found the incidence of CFS to be between 98 and 267 cases per 100,000, and that of plain chronic fatigue between 2316 and 6321 per 100,000.[5] In a 1987 estimate, The National Academy of Sciences asserted that 15% of the U.S. population could no longer live comfortably in our industrialized world, and those numbers are steadily growing.[6] Add those who suffer undetected illness who may eventually become overtly ill, and we are faced with enormous economic implications.

With the numbers who suffer from EI and CFS growing, it is difficult to speculate how many millions of once productive individuals might be lost from the ranks of the working world. Forced to drop out, they may have to be cared for, sometimes for many years, at great expense to the taxpaying public.

It is understandably not in the best interest of insurance companies and government to accept and validate the existence of these illnesses. Insurance companies would be faced with huge potential costs. Once EI and CFS are accepted as legitimate illnesses, there can be no turning back. Once identified as real, insurance companies would have to reimburse claims, and disability payments would have to be made.

Dr. Byron Hyde, a physician in Ottawa, Canada, reports that he has treated 1000 CFS patients with an average income of about $30,000 a year, which translates to a loss of $30 million in productivity to that community alone. He further estimates a loss of $100 billion in salaries in the United States and Canada.[7] This has far-reaching economic implications.

Thanks to efforts by The National CFIDS Association and politically active groups such as the CFIDS Action Campaign for the US (CACTUS), $10 million was funded for 1994 research. Government-funded research specifically earmarked for EI is not known to exist. This lag in interest may be related to EI being a new entity, reflecting the fact that never before in history have we been so overwhelmed by the presence of chemicals in the environment.

These are not sexy illnesses: no one is dying, there is no external deformity to elicit compassion, the illness lingers long past the time for sympathy, and symptoms can cause irritability or eccentric behaviors. The need for vigilance, coupled with the need to stand up for your rights—asking a smoker to go outside, or telling someone her perfume is making you sick—these things do not endear you to the general public.

Illness of Life-Style

What if these are life-style illnesses triggered by chronic stress? Perhaps EI and CFS are manifestations of the decline in the support of the human ecosystem, coupled with a life-style that fails to nurture and support. In the morning you throw yourself out of bed, getting your motor started with a cup of coffee. From there you may eat on the run, consuming foods lacking in life-supporting qualities. Rushing through the workday, regular exercise is often sacrificed to an overly scheduled life. When your energy slumps you may drink another cup of coffee or eat a candy bar. Relationships may bear the brunt of irritability and mood swings. In the evening you may unwind with alcohol, and perhaps take a pill to get to sleep.

This scenario has become the human condition, and chronic stress is inherent in everyday life. Yet, an important part of recovery for those with EI and CFS has been to buy out of that loop. Josh had to quit his job and go on disability because of the debility of CFS. For Gloria, who has recovered from CFS, getting well has meant reevaluating her priorities, putting her own needs first. Reevaluation of life-style choices is essential to improved health.

An Interrupted Life

What causes these illnesses is secondary to the amount of disruption they cause to your life. In the face of sickness, the goals you have cherished, and the carefully ordered routines unravel. Many have depleted their life savings on unsubstantiated fixes. Jamie, who has EI and CFS, was sick for 12 years and spent $5000 a year on nonreimbursable health interventions. In all, she spent $60,000; to say nothing of the fact that she was too sick to work for 2 years.

Rest and obsessive avoidance of potential toxins can become your main preoccupation. You probably avoid shopping malls as much as the detergent aisles at the grocery store. Ever vigilant to avoid fatigue-causing stressors, your social life has likely become as flat as a pancake. You may avoid friends for fear they will want something from you that you cannot give. For many, their social life comes to a screeching halt. Still more are unable to work, or incapable of performing simple tasks. You may have to change your life-style to fit the changing needs of your nervous system, allowing recovery time from external stressors. In both illnesses, no area of life is left untouched.

The Twelve Point Recovery Plan

EI and CFS are complex diseases with many variables. Coupled with this, each person reacts differently to a specific intervention and the constant change of symptoms can make any cure elusive. So what can be done to achieve relief? Healing must involve a comprehensive approach including a variety of multilevel interventions. The overall goal with both illnesses should emphasize detoxifying the body and strengthening the immune system.

What has also become apparent is that achieving greater spiritual and emotional health is an essential aspect of healing. "The people who seem to be getting well are those who strengthen their spiritual life," notes one former CFS patient. In order for the body to heal completely, interventions have to be equivalent to the degree of imbalance present. Superficial treatment aimed only at symptom relief will not be adequate to sustain health, and it can take years of repair to undo damage that has accumulated over a lifetime. Conditions often return if you have failed to move to deeper, nonphysical levels of self-examination and change.

Learning to live in ways that reduce stress, thereby heightening immune support, can enable you to gain control over some symptoms, particularly allergic reactions and fatigue. Coming to accept that hidden allergic reactivity could be part of the cause of fatigue may prompt your interest to investigate further to discover more subtle sources of reactivity.

A good deal of your focus should be on maximizing the detoxification process. Detoxification is achieved through increased elimination of body waste, avoiding contact with harmful substances, changing your dietary habits, the use of nutritional supplements, physical exercise, counseling, stress management, and immunotherapy. Adhering to this program, your immune system is allowed to strengthen and regain competence. As the body is strengthened on all levels, it is more resistant and resilient to pathogens.

The following *twelve point recovery plan* is a synthesis of multidimensional interventions to consider in developing your own plans for your return to health.

1. It is vital to *treat allergies*, even hidden allergies, because they constantly drain and overburden the immune system. By avoiding toxins, environmental irritants, and allergy-producing foods, the body is able to rest and repair. This task also applies to those with CFS who may not perceive allergies to be their primary problem.
2. The next task is to *clean up* the environments you spend the most time in, starting with your bedroom. Keep your living space clean and dry to prevent the growth of mold and bacteria. Sniff for mildew; check sheets, towels, clothes, mattresses, and closets. The self-help section, "Creating a Safe Zone" (see Chapter Eight) provides specific directions on how to do this.
3. *Palliative treatments* emphasize reduction of discomfort. This part of the plan may include the use of prescription medications, energy work such as Reiki, and strengthening emotional supports. Medical treatment includes: pain medications, fungicidal preparations, antivirals, anti-inflammatories, and antidepressants. Narcoleptic pain medications, while they help in the short term, are not helpful for long-term relief. Ampligen achieves significant relief for some with CFS who have brain involvement. Kudipressin, a liver extract, can give relief from viral symptoms. In addition, intramuscular and intravenous injections of vitamin B_{12} and gamma globulin have been used with some success.

4. Aggressive *rest therapy* and *stress reduction* are important interventions, particularly with CFS. This means stopping when your body tells you to and getting plenty of sleep. You may be particularly sensitive to stress and must learn to recognize your limits and act protectively. Ongoing efforts to reduce stress may be the missing piece toward accelerating your recovery, as stress can compromise immune function. Simplifying your life-style can help reduce emotional strain and external stress that robs you of energy. Letting go of an overabundance of "shoulds" can also enable life to be more stress-free.

5. Resolving an existing *sleep disorder* is one of the simplest means of heightening responsiveness to other treatments. A full satisfying sleep can reduce the intensity of pain, brain-fogging, and other symptoms. Hot baths and hot tub soaks help to relax muscles, reduce night sweats, and can make it easier to sleep.

6. The next step is to engage in a program that includes actively *taking care of yourself*. Pay attention to the choices you make that influence your health, what you eat, what you think, as well as the people you spend time with. Efforts to actively seek pleasurable experiences on a regular basis should be an integral part of your recovery program.

7. Engaging in *daily exercise* helps you to detoxify and strengthen your natural defenses. Gentle exercise can lift your spirits and help you to relax. This may mean challenging your comfort zone in some small way so that life is more than just surviving; you want every cell to thrive. Start with an easy form of exercise that you can gradually increase. Stretching may be all that you can do. True, exercise can make symptoms worse and has been noted by some to prolong the illness. Some contend it's impossible to exercise at all, because slight exertion makes them feel worse. The key is moderation, so if you can, get out and do what feels right.

8. Vitamin and nutritional *supplements* play a vital role in helping to mitigate exposure to damaging chemicals and to rebuild the body. Most people with CFS and EI have vitamin and mineral deficiencies. Certain vitamin and mineral supplements help boost the immune system, increase energy, and balance the body. In pursuing this option you may come up against physicians who contend that supplements are of no value, and then it's up to you to decide what's best.

9. Wise selections of *whole foods* will help strengthen the body. This includes raw or steamed organic fruits and vegetables, and a balanced selection of grains and proteins. Minimize intake of foods that contain pesticides, additives, and those that have been processed. Additives, sugar, processed, and preserved foods weaken the immune system, increasing susceptibility to viruses and infection. Dietary controls emphasize eating balanced meals and eliminating foods that require more energy to digest than they offer in nutritional value. Avoiding foods that cause allergic reactions, paying attention to foods that deplete you, and which ones

energize can make a big difference in how you feel.

10. When stronger, you may be able to tolerate brief exposures that gradually allow your immune system to mobilize on your behalf. This only works if you *limit toxic exposures*. In time, occasional intake of small quantities of foods or contact with substances that cause reactivity may become tolerable; whereas large amounts or ongoing contact can bog your body down.

11. *Support* in the form of individual or group counseling can help you to reframe the experience of illness. Support groups can be of tremendous value in helping you to adjust, and most of these groups don't cost money. In a later chapter the role of support groups will be examined in detail.

12. *Spiritual empowerment* is an important part of the picture and can include any of a variety of forms, traditional or nontraditional. Meditation is frequently used to access inner awareness. Visualization can enable you to create the life you wish. Chanting can help you to relax and vibrationally recharge on a cellular level. Breath-work combines the healing powers of oxygenation with the experience of being fully present in the moment. Traditional religions with their organized format also offer support for the searching pilgrim.

Throughout the rest of these pages, interventions will continually emphasize various points of this 12-point plan. Remember, the overall focus of treatment is to boost the immune system so that the body is strong enough to cope with ongoing stressors. As the body becomes stronger it is more capable of fighting off the onslaught of harmful forces.

Summary

Not only do EI and CFS have common physical symptoms, but they also are responsible for complete disruption of the lives of those who are affected. Both illnesses have a lack of credibility at the present time. If they were to be taken seriously, the economic fallout would pose an enormous burden to society. For both EI and CFS, the 12-point pathway to recovery as outlined herein holds important keys for your return to health.

Endnotes

[1]Charles Lapp, "Feedback Forum," *The CFIDS Chronicle* Spring 1992: 127.

[2]Janet Dauble, ed., Chronic Fatigue Syndrome Institute's Conference, *Share Care and Prayer* May–Oct. 1993: 17.

[3]David Bell, *The Doctor's Guide to Chronic Fatigue Syndrome* (Reading: Addison–Wesley, 1995) 62.

[4]Janet Dauble, ed., *Share Care and Prayer* Oct.–Dec. 1994: 24–25. Article notes, Dedra

Buchwald and Deborah Garrity, "Comparison of Patients with Chronic Fatigue Syndrome, Fibromyalgia, and Multiple Chemical Sensitivities," *Arch Intern Med* 154, 18(26 Sept 1994): 2049–2053.

[5]Kimberly Kenney, ed., conference notes, Dedra Buchwald, "Epidemiology," *The CFIDS Chronicle* Winter 1995: 47.

[6]Richard Leviton, "Environmental Illness: A Special Report," *Yoga Journal* Nov.–Dec. 1990: 44.

[7]Kimberly Kenney, ed., conference notes, "CFIDS Historical Perspective and World View," *The CFIDS Chronicle* Spring 1991: 64.

Chapter
Five

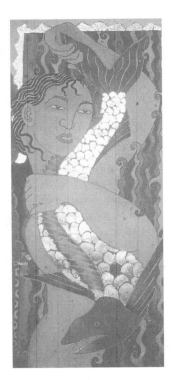

Cofactors

*J*ust as EI and CFS seem to be influenced by viruses and environmental hazards, so parasites, yeast, and bacterial infections can have a tremendous impact on health. Shown on the next page is a schematic of the interplay between these seemingly unrelated maladies and their impact on the health of those with EI and CFS. Many who are ill have the picture clouded by the presence of parasites, yeast overgrowth, and bacterial infection. Once you grasp the inter-relatedness of these other maladies, you may see that, like peeling the layers of an onion, you must address each of these issues in order to recover.

Candida

Candida albicans is a yeast found on the surface of all living things. Normally, yeast live in healthy balance within the digestive tract, functioning to recycle organic material in the body. For the average person with CFS or EI, candida-related health symptoms develop because of four main causes: (1) the presence of candida toxins, which weaken the immune system, (2) a leaky gut, which permits the absorption of

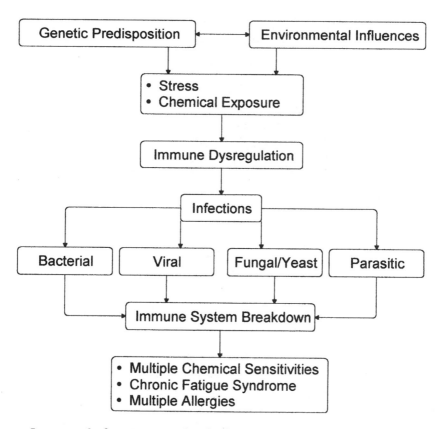

Immune dysfunction in individuals with chemical sensitivities and chronic fatigue syndrome.

food antigens and other toxins, (3) candida allergies, and (4) a compromised immune system, which can also prompt the proliferation of yeast.

When the immune system is compromised, yeast proliferation can cause your health to deteriorate. With abnormally high levels of yeast present in the body, over time the immune system is taxed as proteins pass through the bowel wall into the bloodstream and subsequently into various organs of the body. Candida overgrowth then interferes with the health of these organs, causing further systems to break down.

The reason why yeast tends to proliferate in immune difficulties is not understood. It isn't clear if candida overgrowth is the primary cause or merely the effect of a dysregulated immune system, or if its presence suggests ongoing viral activity. When the body loses its immune protection or the acid–base balance of the bowel is altered, yeast can proliferate, producing toxins which can heighten allergic reactivity. In allergic reactivity, histamines suppress the T-cell immune response to candida which, in turn, interferes with the metabolism of fatty acids. The activities of the T-suppressor cells eventually become impaired, causing excessive proliferation of antibodies which react to the presence of candida.

Candida Triggers

Factors that weaken the immune system include high dietary intake of carbohydrates and sugars, repeated use of antibiotics, the use of birth control pills and hormonal medications such as corticosteroids, and parasitic infestations. Pollution of air, water, and food, alcohol ingestion, and chronic food and chemical allergies put a strain on the immune system that can cause yeast overgrowth. Women are more susceptible to candidiasis secondary to hormonal changes. Pregnancy can alter hormonal balance upsetting the presence of healthy flora in the intestine.

Antibiotics alter the acid–base balance of the bowel and destroy friendly bacteria that are normally found there, also causing an overgrowth of yeast. Consumption of meats that have been treated with antibiotics can also kill off healthy bacteria and cause problems. Emotional stress that suppresses the immune system can leave the body open to the invasion of yeast. William Crook's book, *Chronic Fatigue Syndrome and the Yeast Connection* (Jackson, TN: Professional Books, 1992) can help you understand this problem and its relationship to CFS. CFS and EI commonly exhibit symptoms similar to candida, including food intolerance, chronic diarrhea or constipation, and mental and emotional manifestations.

The Sugar Connection

Candida thrives on sugar. The combined presence of yeast and sugar in the intestine causes fermentation, leading to excessive bloating and gas commonly experienced after eating. When yeast are not fed, they undergo "die-off." Like hungry piranhas, they wait to tear into the food you send down the digestive tract. When you stop eating these foods, the yeast seem to turn and attack you, causing uncomfortable symptoms. "Die-off" can cause great discomfort that may make you feel like eating more sugar. In the face of efforts to control yeast overgrowth, you can experience craving for foods that are off-limits.

Avoidance of processed foods and all substances that contain sugar is necessary for full healing to take place. Chemical exposures can also increase sugar cravings. Work in the garden invariably gives Elaine a nose full of moldy leaves, leading to allergic irritability and the desire for sugar. Avoidance of all toxic exposures can help calm your unhealthy longings.

Candida/Yeast Treatment

Effective treatment of candidiasis includes these steps:

1. Following and, if necessary, maintaining a yeast control diet
2. Taking medication to kill yeast
3. Healing the intestinal tract
4. Taking supplements that support and rebuild the immune system

The Candida Diet

Common sense dictates that you avoid foods that cause the proliferation of yeast. Yeast feed on dietary carbohydrates and sugar in the body. You must make a commitment to stop eating foods that contain sugar, ferments, dried fruits, caffeine, fresh fruits, and anything that is processed. Cheeses, dairy products, alcohol, breadstuffs, and essentially all processed foods, canned or packaged, or those that contain sugar or yeast, are off limits. Herbal teas are not allowed because of the presence of mold on the dried leaves. When meat containing antibiotics is forbidden, is anything left?

What's left is a basic diet composed of vegetables and other complex carbohydrates such as grains of rice, millet, buckwheat, corn, and legumes. Lean meats and fish can also be included. Treatment for candidiasis includes a diet that also removes allergy-stimulating foods; avoiding these foods offers a boost toward healing.

The first few days or weeks on a yeast-restricted diet can be very uncomfortable. "Die-off" symptoms increase as dead candida are released into the bloodstream. Craving the very foods that harm you, it's not unusual to feel spaced out and irritable to the extent that you may have a murderous longing for the taste of sugar. If you break down and eat a candy bar, there may be temporary euphoria, but the last thing you need is more sweets. It only prolongs the process; when the high wears off the cycle of craving returns. You will sabotage the "die-off" process if you sneak the slightest amount of forbidden food. Despite the discomfort of "die-off," remind yourself that the experience is temporary.

Medications and Other Interventions

The health of your liver is said by herbalist Michael Tierra to offer one of the keys to overcoming yeast overgrowth. "The main issue with candida has to do with faulty digestion. Without proper liver and pancreatic enzymes, digestion is incomplete and this creates accumulation of gas and bloating and food allergies which in turn affect the immune system." Studies show that poor liver function encourages candidiasis so that supportive cleansing of the liver is a vital part of treatment. Continuing to crave sweets, even after adhering to rigorous dietary restrictions, may indicate a chromium deficiency. This mineral, found in brewer's yeast, whole wheat, oysters, potatoes, chicken, and apples, can also be taken in supplemental form.

Fungicidal medications such as nystatin, ketoconazole (trade name Nizonal), or fluconazole (tradename Diflucan) help destroy candida. The drawback to these interventions is that they may weaken the immune system, interfering with the ability to fight pathogens. Nonprescription antifungals include: caprylic acid, citrus seed extract, vegetable tannates such as Tanalbit, and Mycocidin, an undecyclenic acid from castor bean oil. Garlic, with its strong fungicidal capabilities, can be ingested raw or in odorless capsules to destroy candida. Taheebo or Pau d'Arco tea from the bark of a South American tree functions as a natural fungicidal agent.

Dioxychlor™, one of a class of inorganic oxidants, has been useful against viruses, fungi, and bacteria. Biotin prevents candida from converting to the invasive rhizome or mycelial form, which can penetrate the bowel wall. It should be noted that a fungus can become resistant to a medication that it was formerly responsive to; and yeast can mutate, changing their structure to avoid destruction.

Supplements that support and rebuild the immune system assist the body in healing from fungal overgrowth. Beta carotene is one such bodybuilder. Topical applications of tea-tree oil can help reduce localized fungal problems. Evening primrose oil stimulates the thymus to produce T cells. This oil also helps balance the production of prostaglandin and the processing of fatty acids which facilitate the removal of toxins. Sherry, an EI sufferer, has found homeopathic dilutions of *Candida albicans* to be effective. Chiropractic adjustments and acupuncture treatments also stimulate the immune system.

Since the normal flora of the bowel is damaged, it must be replaced with healthy microflora. Mega-acidophilus in capsule, liquid, or powder form helps restore the normal balance of the bowel. *The Body Ecology Diet* by Donna Gates (Atlanta: B.E.D. Publications, 1993) is a helpful resource regarding the restoration of the inner ecology of the digestive tract in order to enhance immunity. Aloe vera juice reduces inflammation, assisting the intestinal lining to mend. Elaine uses DAG, a solution that contains Irish moss, to heal and reduce bowel inflammation. Vaginal yeast infections are commonly seen in women with candidiasis, typically occurring between ovulation and menses. Some women replenish normal flora and prevent overgrowth by inserting a capsule of *Lactobacillus acidophilus* into the vagina. Once yeast overgrowth is under control, allergic sensitivities can diminish.

Parasites

Jamie, a therapist, took various fungicidal medications for 8 years in an attempt to rid her body of candida overgrowth. After some time, each drug ceased to effectively kill the yeast. Several thousand dollars and years later, she was finally able to report a cure, namely, the concurrent treatment of intestinal parasites the presence of which had kept the yeast in place. The normal acid–base balance of her bowel had been continually upset by the presence of the parasites, which made it impossible to completely heal her body.

Thinking that candida was the sole cause of her illness kept her stuck in a vicious circle, taking fungicidal medications ad nauseam. It can be difficult to cure candidiasis in the presence of other disorders such as parasites. If your primary health problem seems to be candidiasis, yet repeated treatment does not make you well, you must look further. Perhaps you have intestinal parasites.

Not all parasites are pathogenic. Much of the world's population live healthy lives, not suspecting that they are hosts to parasites. However, the presence of parasites in the intestine is believed by some to be the primary cause of CFS. Though this has yet to be substantiated, many with CFS and EI do have intestinal parasites. Parasite infestation is commonly seen in the presence of immune dysfunction, and in particular, allergic disorders.

Sources and Symptoms

In order to protect yourself from parasitic infections, you need to know the sources of such infestations:

1. Contaminated water and food sources, including raw meats and fish
2. Household pets
3. Antibiotic use which destroys normal flora, setting the stage for infestation
4. Sexual contact
5. Poor hygiene, including fecal contact

Parasites exist not just in unsanitary living conditions, but can attack anyone in a weakened state. Symptoms of parasitic infestation span a wide range including fever, cough, food intolerance, bloating, and diarrhea. Anemia, abdominal pain, apathy, and malnutrition are a few more examples. Protozoa such as amoebas can cause arthritic-like pain. Generalized weakness is prevalent in most forms of parasitic infestations. The multiple symptoms can be baffling, often misdiagnosed as bacterial infestations.

Successful cures are dependent on having accurate parasite test results and laboratories that specialize in parasitology tend to have the most accurate results. Such laboratories include: The Institute for Parasitic Diseases in Phoenix, Arizona; Great Smokies Laboratories in Asheville, North Carolina; and Dowell Laboratories in Mesa, Arizona. Your physician can contact them for further information.

It is common to get false-negative results when tested for parasites. Testing by stool sample is often inconclusive; the sample may not show evidence of parasites even while the ova or eggs are hiding out in the intestinal wall. Parasites reside in mucus, so the most accurate tests employ mucoid matter in the stool.

Parasite Treatment

Traditional treatment using Flagyl is the most common intervention, yet ingesting Flagyl can be a disagreeable experience, particularly for those with sensitivities. Aside from feeling terrible as a result of increased candida symptoms, there can be depression. An alternative is Yodoxin, a quinine derivative that is easier to tolerate. Herbs including gentian violet formulas such as Biocidin, black walnut, garlic, grapefruit seed extract, and artemisia are antiparasitic in some cases.

It can be difficult to rid the body of parasites. Treatment must span a long enough interval so that the ova can be killed off, not just the parasites themselves. The first step in ridding the body of parasites naturally is to cleanse the gastrointestinal tract. Since many parasites are embedded in the intestinal wall, treatment can only reach them when the waste matter surrounding the parasites is softened. Substances such as flax seeds, bentonite clay, citrus pectin, beet and comfrey root, and psyllium husks sweep out bowel debris.

The next step concerns dietary modifications which include daily intake of essential fatty acids via safflower, sesame, and flax seed oils. These oils lubricate the gastrointestinal tract and help strengthen cell membranes. Vitamin A and foods rich in vitamin A, such as carrots, squash, yams, and greens, increase tissue resistance to the permeation of parasitic forms. Parasites thrive on processed sugar so you should eliminate all sources from your diet.

Fresh pineapple and papaya contain high amounts of protein-digesting enzymes such as bromelian and papain and have long been used by Hispanics to cure worm infestations. Papaya, lemon, and pumpkin seeds can be taken to eliminate tapeworms or roundworms. Garlic is also a deworming agent; two raw cloves a day can be effective against several types of worms.

Herbs such as black walnut, butternut, ficus, mugwort, and wormwood are effective against parasites or worms. The combination of green-black walnut hulls, wormwood, and ground cloves is recommended by Dr. Hulda Clark in her books, *The Cure For All Cancers* and *The Cure For AIDS* (San Diego: ProMotion Publishing, 1993). This specific combination is available as a tincture.[1] Stanley Weinberger, certified metabolic technician and expert on the treatment of parasites notes that any intervention should be carried out for a minimum of 2 months. This will ensure complete elimination of ova which were not hatched during the first month.

Acid–Alkaline Balance

Selima, a 42-year-old who is now in recovery from EI and CFS, also had a history of severe digestive problems, including parasites and candida. She reports that controlling her pH has been one of the most effective means of achieving relief. pH is the concentration of hydrogen ions in solution; a pH under 7 indicates an acidic state and a pH above 7 indicates an alkaline state.

Controlling the pH of the body means maintaining a balance between acid and alkaline body states. Normal pH varies with the individual and surrounding circumstances: acidity is associated with illness and alkalinity with health. When the acid–alkaline balance is correct, serum pH is about 7.4. However, any prolonged extreme of pH, whether acid or alkaline, strains the body's adaptive capabilities. The pH of EI patients tends to be alkaline, more toward the 7.4 to 7.6 range.[2] As the pH changes, metabolic functions are turned on or off. For example, enzymes, which are the catalysts for all biochemical activity, are active only within specific pH ranges. With the stress of pH extremes, metabolic processes tend to be less efficient.

The presence of parasites and candida alters the acid–base balance of the bowel. Restoring proper pH can prevent recurrence of parasites and candida. Blood, saliva, urine, or colon pH can be monitored to avoid strongly acid or strongly alkaline states and urinary pH is easiest to measure. By determining the range in which your symptoms are least prevalent and coupling this information with urinary pH, you may be able to determine what factors contribute to imbalance.[3]

Healing the bowel wall is an important step. Anticandida supplements such as acidophilus, and grapefruit seed extract, an antiparasitic, should be instituted toward the completion of your regimen to prevent fungal overgrowth. What finally resolved Jamie's parasites was a 7-day milk fast, coupled with herbs offered by Light Harmonics, whose address is given in Appendix II. It wasn't until she was successfully treated in this manner for parasites that she was also cured of chronic candida problems. The resolution of these two problems caused her health and energy to take a giant leap forward, relieving an immense burden on her immune system.

When you are well it is important to avoid reinfestation. Common sources of parasitic infestation are other people and water, and restaurant food handlers have been known to carry them. If you have had parasitic infections in the past, it is advised to avoid salads and raw foods when you dine out. When eating at home, thoroughly clean fruits and vegetables and wash your hands with soap and water after going to the bathroom or handling pets.

You will know you are better when you have regular, healthy bowel movements, without gas or bloating. Once you are successfully treated for parasites, there may be a dramatic reduction in allergic symptoms. In some cases, when the parasites are eradicated, difficulties with candidiasis also resolve. General improvement in health may occur when parasites are eradicated because the overall immune system becomes stronger.

Bacterial Infections

What is the relationship of hidden bacterial infections to EI and CFS? Common bacterial infections such as strep throat, sinusitis, bronchitis, cystitis, tonsillitis, and acne are thought to be contributors to CFS.[4] Many people with CFS and EI report extended treatment with antibiotics for acne, chlamydia, strep, and staph infections. As an infant, Jamie, the therapist with EI and CFS, had been treated with large doses of penicillin. "I believe the stage was set for my chronic health problems when I first got that staphylococcal infection, and perhaps that initial infection was never fully resolved, or it paved the way for later opportunistic infections."

Many who are ill report having been treated repeatedly with antibiotics for various problems, and they may show improvement for a time, yet the symptoms often recur. This may indicate use of the wrong antibiotic or the wrong dose. Or it may have been the correct antibiotic, but it killed too many normal bacteria, setting up an environment conducive to candida overgrowth and parasitic invaders. Or a secondary bacterial infection may have arisen. Clostridia, staphylococcus, and gardnarella, also known as bacterial vaginitis, are examples of opportunistic infections that are often stubbornly resistant to intervention.

It is suggested that hidden bacterial infections may hold CFS and EI in place. When the immune system is compromised, the host is an easy target for the introduction of a bacterial infection. Chronic bacterial infections may go undiagnosed with current clinical testing. For example, there may be nonspecific bacteria such as chlamydia which are difficult to diagnose because they are so hard to culture. When the bacteria cannot be isolated, these conditions are often treated by trial and error with different antibiotics until the correct match is found.

There are several bacterial infections that may contribute to CFS. Among the most common is acne, a chronic bacterial infection of the oil-secreting glands of the skin. Antibiotic treatment for acne is often prolonged and can result in candida and parasite infestations. Interstitial cystitis is another infection involving the cells lining the urinary bladder. Judy, who has EI, but is well from CFS, notes that she had repeated bouts of cystitis, leading to repeated treatments with antibiotics prior to becoming ill with EI and CFS. Prostatitis can take the form of a chronic infection and irritation of the prostate gland and chronic sinusitis is a stubborn infection of the facial sinuses. Another example is Lyme disease caused by the bacterium *Borrelia* which is introduced in a tick bite. Penicillin, doxycycline, or erythromycin are useful in treating Lyme disease, but most effective when used early in the illness. These are just some of the many infections that begin the vicious cycle of treatment, recurrence, and possible attenuation of other illnesses, such as EI, CFS, and candida.

Jody, a 35-year-old acupuncturist who had CFS for 2 years before getting well, struggled for years with tonsillitis and recurrent strep infections. Only after undergoing a tonsillectomy did her symptoms of fatigue disappear. Because fatigue is frequently caused by infection and infections can have surprising adverse effects on the entire body, it is important to consider their possible presence contributing to your health status. Laboratory studies may help identify any likely suspects. And it is important not to dismiss bacteria as the problem just because lab studies fail to detect them.

Minocycline Trial Results

The pioneering work of Dr. Thomas McPherson Brown, former chairman of the Department of Medicine at George Washington University School of Medicine in Washington, DC, treated rheumatoid arthritis (RA) as an infectious disease for over 52 years with great success. He believed that RA was caused by small bacteria known as mycoplasma which settle in connective tissue. The mycoplasma model considers arthritis to be an allergic response not to the organism itself but to the mycoplasma toxin as the organism dies or multiplies, it releases toxins, which cause inflammatory reactions that result in the disease. His protocols and techniques are described in his coauthored book, *The Arthritis Breakthrough* (New York: M. Evans & Co., 1988).[5]

In January, 1995, the *Annals of Internal Medicine* published the details of a study regarding the use of antibiotics in the treatment of RA. That study reported:

> *Benefit became evident after 12 weeks of therapy, and the proportion of patients treated with minocycline showing improvement continued to increase through week 48 of the study. Along with clinical improvement in joint swelling and tenderness, objective laboratory features of active inflammation such as hematocrit, erythrocyte sedimentation rate, platelet count, and IgM rheumatoid factor level showed favorable changes. No serious toxicity occurred.*[6]

A subsequent study in The Netherlands supports the contention by Dr. Harold Paulus, UCLA rheumatologist, "that a well-protected infection may be at least partially responsible for rheumatoid arthritis manifestations and the treatment may suppress this infection."[7] What does the treatment of RA have to do with EI or CFS? This work has heightened investigation of infectious causes in CFS and EI, as well as lupus and other syndromes.

Minocycline and Other Interventions

Dr. Vincent Mark, specialist in EI, notes, "Patients who fail to respond well to intravenous therapy alone have been helped when tetracycline has been added to their regimen. 80 to 90% of those with long-term arthritic-like symptoms report they're feeling better." Along with the ability to attack certain microorganisms, tetracyclines have anti-inflammatory capabilities, can block certain enzymes, and can suppress the immune system. Minocycline is a member of the tetracycline family. Tetracycline is used to kill the organism and to modulate the formation of the toxin. The major tetracyclines used in the treatment of RA, lupus, and scleroderma are: minocycline, doxycycline, or tetracycline. The antibiotic can be taken in low doses for months, years, or permanently without building up resistance to the drug and without serious side effects.

There may be a concern about the potential for tetracycline to cause yeast infections. It is reported that Dr. Brown's work never found yeast overgrowth to be a problem. Yet, individuals who take repeated or prolonged courses of tetracyclines or broad-spectrum antibiotics tend to develop secondary yeast-related problems. Some physicians recommend taking prescription or nonprescription antifungal medications or probiotics such as *Lactobacillus acidophillus* along with the antibiotics to prevent fungal overgrowth.

If all other possible culprits have been dismissed, a trial of an antibiotic most specifically fitting the clinical picture may be advised. The risk of taking an antibiotic must be weighed against the alternative of doing nothing. Natural measures emphasize boosting the immune system. Sherry takes echinacea and goldenseal, antibiotic herbs used to fight bacterial infection, in order to help resolve the abscesses she often has in her nose and mouth. She also wears magnets on areas of her skin when she has pain, which help increase blood flow and reduce discomfort.

Summary

When the immune system has been weakened by battling any of these conditions, it can become more susceptible to EI or CFS. It is important not to unknowingly feed microorganisms such as yeast and parasites. In this regard, dietary habits, food selection, and personal hygiene play an important part in protecting an immuno-suppressed individual. Exploring the connection that yeast, bacteria, and parasites have to EI and CFS can greatly aid understanding the types of therapeutic interventions necessary for healing. The presence and persistence of each of these cofactors can greatly influence overall health and subsequent recovery.

Endnotes

[1]This tincture, Clarkia 100, is available through Klabin Marketing at (212)877-3632.

[2]Richard Leviton, "Environmental Illness: A Special Report," *Yoga Journal* Nov.–Dec. 1990: 97.

[3]"The pH Work Book" is available by writing to CDIF, P.O. Drawer JF, College Station, TX 77841-5148.

[4]M. Rosenbaum and M. Susser, *Solving the Puzzle of Chronic Fatigue Syndrome* (Tacoma: Life Sciences, 1992) 62.

[5]For more information about their rheumatoid arthritis organization or to order the book, *The Arthritis Breakthrough,* send a SASE to: The Road Back Foundation, 4985 North Lake Hill Road, Delaware, OH 43015.

[6]Barbara Tilley *et al.,* "Minocycline in Rheumatoid Arthritis," *Ann Intern Med* 122.2 (15 Jan. 1995): 81–89.

[7]Harold Paulus, "Minocycline Treatment of Rheumatoid Arthritis," *Ann Intern Med* 122.2 (15 Jan. 1995): 147–148.

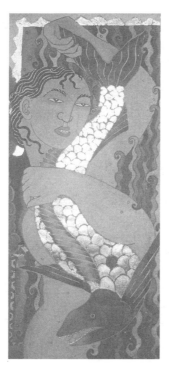

Chapter Six

Understanding the Body

*t*he pieces of the immune puzzle will make more sense once you grasp the impact that these illnesses have on specific body systems. The health and functioning of each organ is vital to your overall health; when one organ is damaged, other systems must go into overdrive to compensate. This chapter will examine some of these systems, how they work and what you can do to return them to health. Once you understand how these systems interact with your illness, it may become possible for you to intervene to strengthen and assist those organs and systems to heal.

The Liver

The liver is the largest gland and the most complex organ in the body, with numerous vital responsibilities which impact EI and CFS. Its many and varied tasks include energy balancing and regulation and immune modulation. Another major function is filtering the blood and removing harmful chemicals and bacteria.

There are several ways that improper liver function can affect these illnesses. The liver converts thyroid hormone, which helps regulate biochemical reactions.

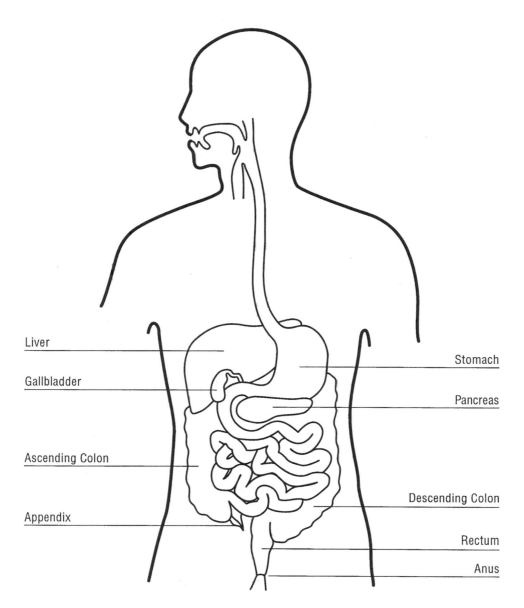

Liver

Gallbladder

Ascending Colon

Appendix

Stomach

Pancreas

Descending Colon

Rectum

Anus

The digestive system.

Inadequate conversion of thyroid hormone results in hypothyroidism, which, in turn, results in chronic fatigue. It's the liver's job to transform fat-soluble chemicals into water-soluble compounds so they can be released by the kidneys and bowel. This process is conducted by a complex system of enzymes manufactured by cells of the liver. The liver also has filtering channels lined with special cells that break down foreign debris, bacteria, and toxic chemicals.

When the liver is burdened with toxic chemicals and pathogens, it is less capable of processing and eliminating these substances. A healthy liver eliminates impurities into the colon, but it cannot do this unless the colon is clean and functioning well. It is important to make sure that the colon is in good shape before stimulating the healing of the liver. If toxins cannot be excreted, the liver may store them, over time causing irreversible harm. With EI, toxins that accumulate in a sluggish liver can heighten the total load. Bio-Magnetics, a form of hands-on healing, hypothesizes that causative viruses for CFS hide out in the liver. In the face of EI and CFS, optimal liver function can greatly improve health.

Liver and Toxic Detoxification

For the purposes of EI and CFS, one of the most important liver functions is the detoxification of poisons. "When I feel my health sliding, I know I have to go to work on detoxifying my liver. Doing this makes all the difference in my health," says Selima who is nearly well from EI and CFS. Through the production of specific enzymes, the liver detoxifies virtually all external and internal matter that poses a health threat. When a chemical exposure occurs, the liver must work to detoxify these substances, breaking them down into less toxic matter.

The liver is responsible for breaking down and processing toxins such as pesticides, herbicides, heavy metals, drugs, alcohol, chemicals found in processed foods, and other chemicals in the environment. In addition to a diet of processed foods, such as cold cuts and canned foods, factors that contribute to liver dysfunction include coffee, alcohol, smoking, auto exhaust, birth control pills, and bacterial and candida infections.

Because of the increasing number of poisons in the environment, such as polluted air, contamination of water supplies, and chemical cleansers, the liver has to work harder and harder to detoxify the poisons. It is the organ most directly strained by pollution and environmental damage. Any substance that inhibits the liver's detoxifying capability may increase the risk of illness.

Mount Sinai School of Medicine in New York has reported abnormal liver tests in painters and those working with chemicals.[1] Others who are at risk include artists working with paint and paint removers, house painters, auto shop workers, fiberglass and plastic fabricators, and highway maintenance workers.

Diet, Digestion, and the Liver

A diet full of devitalized foods that have been overcooked, processed, or that contain preservatives will not supply the liver with adequate levels of activating nutrients vital to carrying out its functions. Inadequate diet compromises the detoxifying capability of the liver, eventually exhausting the supply of detoxifying nutrients not supplemented by diet. In order to have a healthy liver, processed sugar, alcohol, and saturated fats are to be avoided. Since your energy levels are directly correlated with the quality of foods eaten, it makes sense to have as healthy a diet a possible.

The liver works closely with the digestive system. Toxins absorbed through the intestinal tract enter the blood, where the liver must detoxify them. The intestines play a major role in permitting vital nutrients to be absorbed, while rejecting harmful toxins. In order to assist the liver toward optimal functioning, the intestines must work efficiently. Factors that strain the digestive system, thereby taxing the liver, include constipation, overeating, a diet rich in meat, consuming mucus-forming or refined and fried foods, lack of exercise, and long-term laxative use.

Bile salts are produced by the liver, helping to emulsify dietary fats and fat-soluble vitamins such as A, D, E, and K for absorption. The liver secretes bile into the gallbladder where it is stored and eventually excreted into the small intestine, while removing fat-soluble toxins from the body. Excessive amounts of fat and protein in the diet make it difficult for the liver to break them down because their presence calls for greater production of bile and digestive enzymes.

It is speculated that many with EI and CFS have subclinical liver dysfunction, meaning there is functional impairment that is not detected by liver function studies. This subtle inefficiency can have wide-ranging effects on overall health, impairing the ability of the liver to transport nutrients to the cells. Liver dysfunction is known to result in fatigue, acne, tenderness and pain in the liver area, weakness in tendons and muscles, depression, mood lability, allergic reactivity, anger, and premenstrual symptoms.

Healthy Interventions for the Liver

Whatever you can do to alleviate stress placed on the liver will have a beneficial effect on overall health. Exercise, saunas, intestinal cleansing, and juice fasting are useful adjuncts to detoxification. Various supplements and interventions have been found by herbalists and nutritionists to be effective in detoxifying and stimulating liver function. Some suggest drinking organic apple juice on a daily basis to help with liver and gallbladder detoxification, but this has also been known to cause stomach pains. Selima recommends Liv-Alive Tea by Crystal Star as a more gentle form of liver detoxification. Interventions that can strengthen and detoxify the liver include:

1. Milk thistle, or its active ingredient, silymarin, helps fight liver damage by stimulating protein synthesis, stabilizing cell membranes, and accelerating the process of liver tissue regeneration. Silymarin works as an antioxidant by inhibiting the amount of toxins that can penetrate the cell walls of the liver. Among other things, it has powerful antihistamine, antiviral, and

antiallergy properties. Gloria, a CFS activist, notices increased energy and physical stamina when taking this product.

2. Vitamin E is a major fat-soluble antioxidant that can help detoxify the liver. Other useful supplements include cystine, a liver protective nutrient found in egg yolk and mammal meat (N-acetyl cystine is a particularly helpful form); glutathione, a combination of three amino acids, has detoxification properties; and coenzyme Q10, which protects and energizes the liver.

3. Avoiding red meats, concentrated fats, processed sugar, preservatives, and food additives increases liver cell regeneration.

4. Nutrients that support liver function include the trace minerals: zinc, copper, manganese, selenium, and molybdenum. Magnesium is an important alkaline mineral which assists in the excretion of toxins.

5. Foods that are beneficial for the liver are: lemon, dandelion greens, mustard greens, black radish, saffron, watercress, beets, parsley, artichokes, cherries, grapefruits, parsnips, garlic, onion, horseradish, lime, wheat germ, and lecithin.

The Liver and Emotional Balance

An important role of the liver is removing excess hormones from the blood. When the liver is not able to function properly, its ability to remove hormones is hampered. Since hormones have a large impact on mental states, it is thus possible for you to be flooded with out-of-control mood swings if your liver is unable to do its job.

In traditional Chinese medicine (TCM), anger is associated with liver and gallbladder function. If the liver is flooded with hormones and toxins, you may be aroused by rageful, angry feelings that seem to emerge from nowhere. While there is no clear evidence that holding onto or denying anger causes liver dysfunction; there is a biochemical basis for the notion that an overburdened sick liver can prompt emotionally labile states. Part of your healing experience may include learning to notice and accept feelings of anger as they surface, learning to channel them into appropriate expression.

The Thyroid

Low thyroid function is a common cause of chronic fatigue, yet is often overlooked because the serum measurement of thyroid hormone may not accurately reflect low thyroid hormone levels. Mild, or subclinical, hypothyroidism can go undetected. Low thyroid hormone levels can mimic CFS, but differ in that the malaise of CFS includes flulike symptoms. The primary symptoms of hypothyroidism include fatigue and feeling deep-in-your-bones cold, without flulike symptoms. Hashimoto's thyroiditis, an autoimmune disease, does include the flulike symptoms of CFS.

In the case of thyroiditis, the immune system attacks the thyroid gland; as a result, inadequate amounts of thyroid hormones are produced, resulting in fatigue, weight gain, and other CFS symptoms. Hypothyroidism is common in CFS because of the changes in the hypothalamic area of the brain (which affect the hormones of the body) and the upregulation of the immune system (causing the production of antibodies to the thyroid).[2]

The thyroid, located in the lower portion of the throat, produces thyroid hormones which are essential to the regulation of metabolism, or the rate that cells burn oxygen. Because thyroid hormones are important in all bodily functions, their deficiency has widespread effects. Hypothyroidism causes decreased utilization of fat, which means a moderate weight gain in those who are ill. Women with mild hypothyroidism tend to have a history of heavy menses, with irregular cycles. Depression is common, as well as difficulty thinking clearly. There can also be muscle weakness and joint stiffness. Dry rough, scaly skin, as well as coarse, dry brittle hair are common in hypothyroidism. Cravings for sugar and carbohydrates are also noted.

The old-fashioned way to determine thyroid functioning, developed by Dr. Breda Barnes, is to take your basal body temperature. This is done by shaking down a thermometer at night and placing it beside your bed. When you wake up in the morning, before getting up, place the thermometer under your armpit for 10 minutes. Don't get up until the results are read. Record the results for three consecutive mornings. Women who menstruate should perform the test during the second, third, and fourth days of their menses; all others can take the test at any time. Your normal, resting temperature should be between 97.6 and 98.2. People who are hypothyroid tend to have a pattern of lower basal body temperatures.

Healthy Thyroid Interventions

Thyroid replacement allows the gland to rest and repair, easing its constant job of hormone production. Some physicians prescribe thyroid replacement without having abnormal laboratory results. That was done for Theresa, a 41-year-old with severe EI, who reports, "After taking desiccated thyroid for 2 years I have enough energy to keep up with my 4-year-old. My fatigue used to be worse in the mornings, I couldn't get out of bed until ten, and my hands and feet were always cold. By taking a small dose of thyroid replacement I have a higher baseline energy and I am slightly less sensitive to some substances."

Treatment involves the use of synthetic thyroid hormone, or desiccated thyroid extract; however, people who are chemically sensitive tend to do better using the desiccated form. Health food stores also offer a milder form of thyroid extract. A diet rich in vitamins A, E, C and most B vitamins, and particularly iodine can help stimulate the production of thyroid hormone. Kelp is a good source of iodine. The amino acid tyrosine is necessary for the production of thyroid hormone, which is comprised of tyrosine and iodine. Tyrosine supplements can help stimulate thyroid function. Exercise also stimulates the secretion of the thyroid gland. Some foods can inhibit its production; these include cabbage, turnips, soybeans, peanuts, pine nuts, and millet.

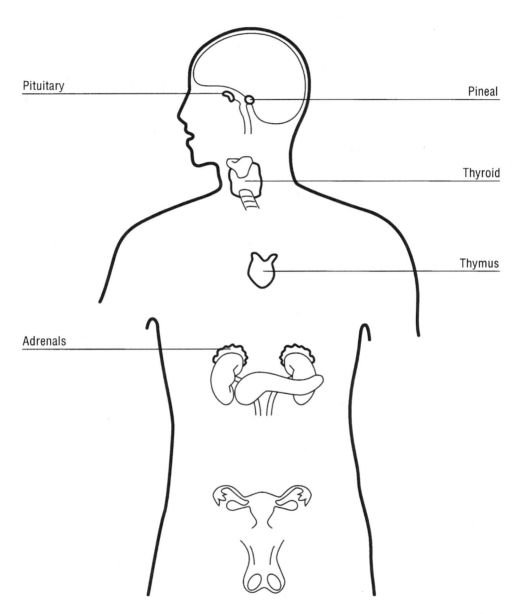

Pituitary

Pineal

Thyroid

Thymus

Adrenals

The endocrine system.

The Thymus

The thymus gland is located in the upper anterior chest. To a great extent the health of the thymus dictates the health of the immune system, as it secretes hormones and produces specialized white blood cells, known as T lymphocytes, that control cell-mediated immunity. Cell-mediated immunity refers to immune activity that is not controlled or mediated by antibody activity. In its role of optimizing immunity, the thymus is crucial in the resistance to infection by yeast, parasites, and viruses.

For many years the thymus was thought to be superfluous in adults. In the aging process it gradually shrinks to a fraction of its original size. Some scientists believe this shrinkage is directly linked to the amount of coenzyme Q10 as well as zinc available in the body. Coenzyme Q10 is an enzyme, produced by the body, that is essential to the production of cellular energy. It is theorized that zinc is needed to activate the thymic hormones and that deficiencies of zinc could be responsible for immune dysfunction as well as cause decreased function of thymic hormones even when it is present. Because the thymus is vital to the function of the immune system, its diminished capability directly affects the ability of the body to produce antibodies needed to fight pathogens.

Healthy Thymus Interventions

Optimal function of the gland involves preventing shrinkage of the thymus through dietary intake of antioxidant nutrients such as carotene, vitamin C, vitamin E, zinc, and selenium; consuming nutrients needed for the action of thymic hormones such as vitamins B_6 and C and zinc; and ingestion of products such as concentrates of calf thymus extract, which stimulate and restore thymus function. Theresa, who has severe EI, takes these supplements in doses above their recommended daily allowances, enhancing immunity by reversing thymus depletion.

The Thymus Thump

The thymus can be stimulated by increasing circulation to its location. Theresa, mentioned above, recommends a simple exercise to stimulate the thymus and increase energy and awaken immune function. Several times a day, use your fingertips to gently tap the area of the thymus, located in the middle of the chest about an inch below the collarbone. Don't rub or knock too hard, just gentle taps. Though the effects may only be subtle, it doesn't cost a thing to try.

Adrenal Glands

The adrenal glands, located above the kidneys, secrete hormones important to regulating and maintaining a balance of bodily processes. The adrenals are actually two glands in one. The adrenal medulla secretes epinephrine and norepinephrine, hormones that stimulate specific body functions to do their work. These hormones stimulate the body to react to "fight or flight" situations, maintaining control over the involuntary bodily functions such as cardiac rate, respiration, and digestion.

The other portion of the adrenals is the adrenal cortex, which secretes a group of hormones known as corticosteroids. Of the three corticosteroids, the one we are most interested in acts to increase serum glucose, reducing inflammation and the allergic response. When this gatekeeper to both the inflammatory and the allergic response is impaired, the body is less capable of directing and controlling these activities. When you are under stress, the adrenal glands act by producing corticosteroids, which can, in turn, deplete the thymus gland. Stress and nutritional deficiencies accelerate adrenal depletion, resulting in the involution of the thymus.

Because of the chronic nature of EI and CFS, great strain can be placed on the adrenals. The continued stress of illness can shrink the adrenal cortex to the point of "adrenal exhaustion." Temperature changes, infection, drugs, stress, exercise, and overtaxing your body can also exhaust the adrenals so that they can no longer perform their function. The following are primary factors that stress the adrenals:

1. Low blood sugar
2. Low blood pressure
3. Low body temperature
4. Low body weight
5. Low endurance
6. Prolonged emotional stress

Adrenal exhaustion that accompanies chronic stress can be difficult to diagnose, usually determined by conjecture rather than by laboratory data. However, the adrenocorticotropic hormone (ACTH) stimulation test can accurately measure the adrenal's ability to produce cortisol. Blood levels of cortisol are measured before and after injection of ACTH, revealing the status of adrenal reserve.

Measurements of dehydroepiandrosterone sulfate (DHEA-S) can also help assess adrenal function. Another useful test measures the level of cortisol in the saliva, which is directly proportional to serum levels, four different times during the day (The Adrenal Stress Index from Diagnos-Techs in Seattle, Washington.)

The adrenals control blood pressure by secreting cortisone and adrenaline. Cortisone causes water and sodium retention, while adrenaline constricts the arteries. Adrenal exhaustion commonly seen in the face of excessive or prolonged physical, emotional, or chemical stress results in flaccid blood vessels. When this happens, you can feel lightheaded because of a drop in blood pressure, resulting in neurally mediated hypotension, currently being treated with blood pressure medications, and increased fluid and salt intake. This intervention, as well as the use of adrenal supplements may give the adrenals an opportunity to recuperate.

Overconsumption of refined carbohydrates has a negative impact on mechanisms that control blood sugar. Caffeine and other stimulants push the adrenals into overdrive and should be avoided to allow the adrenals the opportunity to recuperate. There are also nutrients, herbs, and adrenal extracts that can support healthy adrenal function.

Adrenal Interventions

The adrenals require zinc, magnesium, and vitamins C and B_6 for hormone production. Pantothenic acid, also known as the antistress vitamin and particularly important in strengthening the adrenals, is found in whole grains, cauliflower, broccoli, salmon, sweet potatoes, legumes, and tomatoes. Adrenal cortical extract (ACE), an extract of beef adrenal glands, is used in cases of low adrenal function. There are reports of people who feel instantly revitalized on taking ACE. For Elaine, who has EI and CFS, Apex Energetics's homeopathic adrenal remedy has been particularly helpful (see Appendix II).

Siberian and Panax ginseng are adaptogens that protect against mental and physical fatigue. In Oriental cultures, ginseng is believed to provide resistance to stress, normalizing body function, and in the process enabling the adrenals to release hormones that are needed by the body.

Additional support for the adrenals may come from learning how to manage stress. Helpful interventions include exercise and relaxation techniques such as biofeedback, deep breathing, and meditation. Progressive relaxation is a practice that involves progressively contracting all muscle groups of the body, alternately tensing and relaxing them. Start at your head, contracting the facial muscles and then relaxing them; next contract your arm muscles and then relax them, working your way down to your feet. This procedure can also reduce anxiety and insomnia.

DHEA

The adrenal gland also produces diehydroepiandrosterone (DHEA), one of the most abundant steroid hormones found in the body. Often called the "mother hormone," it converts to other hormones such as estrogen and testosterone. Blood levels of DHEA decline as one ages. Current research suggests that DHEA may help prevent immune system disorders, memory disturbances, chronic fatigue, as well as several other disorders.

Dr. George Fletchas of Hendersonville, North Carolina, has treated CFS patients with DHEA. In his practice, patients with CFS commonly show low DHEA levels.[3] Symptoms suggestive of low DHEA levels include dizziness, dry skin, loss of hair on the legs, underarms, and pubic area, loss of sex drive, impotence, brittle nails, increased weight, cold extremities, and loss of cognitive function. On treating patients with replacement DHEA at 25 to 50 milligrams a day for 3 months, he notes improved laboratory findings. As a source for DHEA, Dr. Fletchas recommends the Belmar Pharmacy because of its safety record.[4]

Free Radicals

It is impossible to avoid stress in your life. Environmental stress comes in many forms: water and air pollution, chemicals, pesticides, heavy metals, radioactive wastes, drugs, and even food. Everyday stress taxes your health, taking an emotional and physical toll. The main way stress causes harm is by manufacturing toxic molecules. These molecules, known as "free radicals," are distinctive because they have an unpaired electron in their outer orbit.

Healthy molecules typically have electrons that spin in pairs, which makes them electrically balanced. Free radicals are unstable and highly reactive as a result of their unpaired electron. This instability causes reactions that impede the function of normal cellular metabolism and produce cellular and tissue damage. Atoms lose electrons because of the effects of radiation and chemical pollution, creating unstable atoms that wreak chemical chaos in nearby tissue. Free radicals are capable of breaking old chemical bonds and forming new ones that wouldn't have existed under healthy conditions.

Free radicals damage fats or lipids in our cell membranes, causing them to become rancid. The membranes thus become rigid and impermeable, preventing the cells from receiving nutrients and preventing them from disposing of waste. Eventually the cells become useless and die.

Free radicals also have beneficial qualities. The immune system uses their destructive effects to destroy viruses and bacteria. It is natural for a limited number of free radicals to be generated through oxidation, the result of normal cellular metabolism. The difficulty occurs when several factors such as pollution, allergic reactivity, and infections combine to cause free radical overproduction. When there are too many free radicals, the body cannot adapt, causing cumulative damage that harms the cells faster than they can be repaired.

The Effect

A major reason free radicals play such a large role in our illnesses is because of pollution. All kinds of pollution—solar radiation, radon gas, alcohol, tobacco, chemicals, medications, pesticides, heavy metals, car exhaust, and emotional stress—increase free radical production in the body. Although free radicals are manufactured as a normal body process, poor dietary habits, including eating junk foods and consuming unsaturated fatty acids found in vegetable oils, increase free radical load.

Common symptoms of free radical activity seen with EI and CFS include inflammation, painful muscles, and delayed healing. Aging and wrinkling of the skin are other examples of excessive free radical presence.

The Fat Connection

Consumption of unhealthy fats such as margarine and certain cooking oils can lead to the formation of harmful free radicals. It is therefore advisable to avoid unsaturated fats and oils, particularly fried foods. These fats combine with fat compounds in our tissues, causing molecules to oxidize and turn rancid which in turn produces more free radicals. Free radicals also disrupt DNA and RNA function, leading to production of protein molecules that are perceived as foreign to the body. The immune system attacks these proteins and tries to neutralize them.

Antioxidants

The good news is that there are substances known as antioxidants that can neutralize, alleviate, and minimize the damaging effects of stress on your body. Antioxidant enzymes are the first line of defense against free radicals, donating electrons that enable the unstable atoms to become stable which prevents further tissue damage. These enzymes are normally manufactured by the body's own cells to minimize damage.

A second group of antioxidants include vitamins E, C, and A and the trace minerals copper, selenium, manganese, molybdenum, and zinc. The trace minerals are not actually antioxidants themselves but work by activating the antioxidant enzymes. Aloe vera and pycnogenol, an extract from pine tree bark or grape seed pips, also serve as antioxidants. Coenzyme Q10 is another one, capable of rapidly neutralizing free radicals.

It is also possible to control excessive free radical activity by eating wholesome, unrefined foods. When your body is overwhelmed with free radicals, you can assist their mobilization and removal by ingesting antioxidant food sources and supplements. The thymus is particularly vulnerable to free radical damage and can be protected by the use of these supplements.

Gloria, who has recovered from CFS, is an advocate for green tea, drinking it throughout the day. The health benefits of unfermented green tea have generated increasing interest. This tea shows potent antioxidant effects, anticancer properties, antiviral and antibacterial activity, cholesterol and body-fat reducing capabilities, and regulatory effects on blood pressure.[5] It can also enhance the body's ability to metabolize dietary sugars, while supporting the growth of beneficial intestinal bacteria and aiding in nutrient absorption. Though low in caffeine, it can give you a more healthy energy boost than coffee.

Elimination Pathways

EI reactivity can be reduced by using various tools that enhance the elimination pathways. A healthy body is constantly cleansing and eliminating waste from the system, and when this cleansing process is inefficient, as with EI, toxins stay in the body, inviting illness and interfering with healthy bodily functions. The primary function of the intestines is to absorb vitamins, water, minerals, and nutrients from digested food, transferring them to the bloodstream. These nutrients are then carried throughout the body, building and nourishing it.

Reabsorption

The bowel can be a major contributing factor to poor health. Prolonged allergic reactivity leading to irritation and inflammation of the intestinal wall can impede absorption and the elimination of waste materials. Over time, because of poor health, poor dietary habits, lack of exercise, irregular eating habits, poor fluid intake, and wrong combination of foods, the intestines accumulate debris. They can then become encrusted with old fecal matter and layers of mucus that impair proper absorption of nutrients. This material sticks to and thickens the wall of the colon, interfering with the normal process of digestion.

Debris that remains in the bowel blocks the ability to absorb nutrients; the body thus becomes depleted and malnourished because it cannot absorb the nutrients needed to sustain itself. If waste products stay in the body too long, they putrefy and toxic matter enters the blood, eventually being absorbed into body tissues, including those of the organs, thereby increasing the toxic load. When this happens, fatigue, amorphous aches and pains, and irritability gradually erode energy. In the presence of EI, these toxins cause continuous allergic reactivity, forcing the body to use about 30% of its energy to battle rotting fecal matter that can form into fungus and mold.

Maximize Those Pathways

The body is able to cleanse itself properly when there is maximum function of the channels of elimination. The colon eliminates solid unused food and waste from the body. The kidneys filter acid and metabolic waste from the blood, excreting this through the urine. The liver also purifies the blood as well as being a source of energy storage and digestion. The skin is the largest organ that mediates elimination; taking place through the pores by perspiration, disposing of moisture, toxins, and oils through sweat and secretion. Your skin must be kept clean in order for it to breathe.

The more readily you eliminate waste by supporting and assisting avenues of elimination, the more your health is enhanced. There is much you can do to assist and encourage the elimination of waste. Ingestion of foods that contain fiber and bulk facilitates removal of intestinal debris. Drinking fresh water will help flush out waste products, moving toxic matter through the bowel, urinary system, as well as the blood. Rest enhances the process of repair; and fasting reduces the incoming burden placed on the body, allowing organs to rest and heal. Perspiration via exercise or saunas can also heighten the removal of toxins.

Intestinal Cleansing

There are various programs to assist your body to eliminate waste. Jody, an acupuncturist who has had EI, periodically uses the "Lighten-Up" program, which is a gentle method of intestinal cleansing that can be safely repeated as often as necessary.[6] Elaine, who has CFS and EI, finds Eden's Secrets "Cleanse and Detoxify Program" easier to use on a busy schedule.[7]

Any cleansing program should be undertaken with care. When the body is loaded with accumulated toxins, the blood has to transport this waste to elimination sites and if there are many toxins, rapid cleansing can overburden the body and cause increased discomfort. Some feel more ill when implementing a detoxification program, experiencing diarrhea, headache, nausea, and increased fatigue. These symptoms signify a "healing crisis," i.e., temporarily, you feel worse despite the fact that the cleansing process is working. It is easy to become concerned if you experience increased discomfort to the extent that you may want to stop the process prematurely.

At the end of the cleansing process you should feel stronger and have increased energy. Your body may be able to digest nutrients more efficiently. Those who submit to the cleansing process often find they feel more alert, more awake, and more alive.

Digestive Enzymes

Many people of all ages with EI and CFS have trouble digesting and absorbing nutrients. In fact, some are not able to digest much of anything at all. Even with a carefully planned, nutritious diet, if you cannot absorb and digest good foods, they are useless. The key to digestion rests, in part, with the presence of digestive enzymes.

How Enzymes Work

A healthy digestive system breaks down proteins, carbohydrates, and fats to provide nourishment and energy for the body. The organs and glands responsible for the digestive process must secrete adequate amounts of enzymes to enable you to fully digest your food. People who are ill with EI and CFS often show impairment of some aspect of the digestive process and cannot efficiently digest the food they consume.

When you take the first bite of food, digestive enzymes in saliva begin breaking down the starches as you chew. After swallowing, food enters the stomach where it sits for an hour, while the stomach mixes the chewed food and digestive juices. When the body is able to produce enough acidity and enzymes, the digestion of carbohydrates, fat, fiber, and protein ensues. Once the stomach finishes, the partially digested food moves into the small intestine where enzymes secreted by the pancreas continue the digestion and breakdown of food. These enzymes are essential to the digestive process.

Digestive enzymes help release nutrients from the food, allowing them to be absorbed into the blood. They are then used by the body to repair and build organs and tissue to produce energy and maintain immune function. Enzymes comprise the basis of all metabolic activity; that is, every biochemical reaction is dependent on the presence of enzymes. Enzymes enable each organ, gland, tissue, and cell of the body to do its job and without them it would be impossible to sustain life.

Without enzymes, the body could not use any of the foods and vitamins you eat in order to produce fuel for your body. Enzymes are essential for breaking down toxins into substances that can be eliminated from the body. Your digestive system counts on enzymes to prevent foods from putrefying in the colon. Enzymes are used for more than just digesting food: they move muscles, enable hormones to do their work, make your heart beat, allow your brain to work, stimulate nerve activity, and even enable you to breathe. They destroy free radicals, miscellaneous toxins, and antigens in the liver and blood. When your body lacks enzymes, these processes cannot be carried out.

Finite Stores

The body obtains enzymes in two ways: by manufacturing them and by eating foods that contain them. The number of enzymes your body produces is finite and you cannot force the production of more when you run out. Nature placed enzymes in food to facilitate digestion so that the finite stores in animals are not depleted by doing the work of digestion.

Approximately half of the body's total enzyme production is used for digestion. Oddly enough, the body places a greater priority on digestion than on overall health. Thus, if your diet is lacking in food-source enzymes, your body appropriates them from other sites in order to attend to the digestive process. As a result, your immune system dispenses with some enzymes, preventing those enzymes from doing the work of protection. The body eventually is weakened to the point that it can no longer protect against outside invaders.

Consumption of enzyme-deficient foods inevitably leads to poor health. You are continually draining your natural stores, causing your body to work harder and leaving fewer enzymes free to support your general metabolic welfare.

Dietary Enzymes

The best way to reduce this problem is to eat a diet containing rich sources of enzymes. Foods that are enzyme rich can essentially digest themselves. The problem is that most foods common to our diet have little enzymatic value. Enzymes are temperature sensitive so that cooking and processing foods destroys their enzymes; and steaming, baking, broiling, or microwaving food also destroys them. The best source of enzymes is raw foods.

If your diet is lacking in whole raw foods, supplements may provide a solution. Digestive enzyme supplements aid in the digestion of foods, and the presence of pancreatic enzymes when taken between meals can help clean out antigens in the blood, thereby alleviating arthritic as well as other symptoms. Enzyme supplements help balance body chemistry and help alleviate the stress placed on your digestive organs as well as your immune system. In addition, they can make it easier for you to eat foods that previously caused allergic sensitivities because most food allergies are linked to the body's inability to digest and absorb what has been eaten.

Supplements protect your body from having to call on its limited supply of enzymes, allowing your natural enzyme stores to last longer and thereby encouraging greater health and longevity. When selecting enzyme supplements, it is important to understand their differences. A beneficial enzyme supplement should contain a balance of all enzyme groups in order to completely assist in the digestion of all foods.

These digestive enzyme groups relate to the food groups common to our diet—proteins, carbohydrates, fats, and sugars—and include: lipase, which breaks down fat; protease, which helps break down protein; cellulase, which assists in the breakdown of cellulose; and amylase, which breaks down starch. Lactase helps break down lactose, a carbohydrate found in milk. Selima, who has had severe digestive problems, finds the use of plant enzyme therapy effective in alleviating some of her difficulties, and uses NESS enzymes for this purpose.[8]

Mucus Reduction

Enzyme supplements can break down mucus that has been stored in the body for many years. It is noteworthy that different groups have reported that the average body stores between 5 and 50 pounds of cellular mucus. Bacteria proliferate mostly on mucus-forming foods that you have consumed.

When you get an infection, the organism will grow and multiply in a region of the body that holds mucus, such as the sinuses and intestines. Bacterial, viral, and fungal infections can gain a foothold with greater ease in mucoid matter. Allergic sensitivities are heightened by a diet full of mucus-forming foods. Mucoid matter is produced from seed foods such as grains and nuts, but mostly from dairy and flour products.

Strict avoidance of mucus-producing food is one of the keys to renewed health. Fasting and colon cleansing can amplify the results. Remember to proceed with caution under your medical practitioner's supervision as you mobilize toxins out of your body. These poisons have built up in your body over many years, and rapid mobilization and removal of toxins can cause discomfort in the process of cleansing.

Summary

Recovery is directly linked with the health of the organ systems discussed in this chapter. With the liver and digestive systems, detoxification is the key. The adrenals, thymus, and thyroid may require rest in order to undergo repair, as well as nutrients to support their recovery. The presence of free radicals can be reduced with supplements, dietary support, and avoidance of environmental hazards. And digestive enzymes can be supplemented by proper nutrition. As you come to understand the specific characteristics and needs of each of these body systems, you should also have a better understanding of how to keep them healthy.

Endnotes

[1]Robert McCaleb, "Protect Yourself with Milk Thistle," *Natural Health* Mar.–Apr. 1992: 54.

[2]Kimberly Kenney, ed., speech by Charles Lapp, Fall 1991 Research Chronicle, *The CFIDS Chronicle* Spring 1992: 132.

[3]"DHEA," The CFIDS Association of America: The CFIDS Information Line, 1994.

[4]Your physician may contact the Belmar Pharmacy at (800) 525-9473 for information about ordering DHEA.

[5]Kate Maddrell, ed., reprint "Vitamin Research Products," *Nutritional News*, "Green Tea Helps Regulate Blood Pressure, Prevent Cancer," *HEALTHwatch* 1 Summer 1995: 14.

[6]Barbara Rose, *Cleanliness is Godliness* (Birmingham: Purity, 1991). For this book containing the "Lighten-Up" program, a two-week intestinal cleanse, write: 10525 Falk Road NE, Bainbridge Island, WA 98110, (206) 780-0924.

[7]Contact Eden's Secrets, "Cleanse and Detoxify Program," a program for colon and blood purification, (800) 952-7873.

[8]The NESS Company can be contacted at 2903 NW Platte Road, Riverside, MO 64150, (816) 764-0110.

Part Two

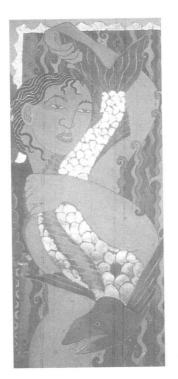

Complementary
Interventions

Chapter Seven

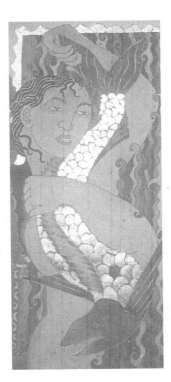

Therapies to Consider

*O*ne of the most important questions you can ask in your search for recovery is, "Who are the people who are getting well, and what are they doing to get there?" Investigating the answer will give you clues as to what you should be doing as well. People who are getting well and those who have come to live in harmony with their ills are taking charge, setting out on their own as active participants in the recovery process. These people have disciplined themselves to avoid the "victim" mentality; regardless of their difficult circumstances they are saying "yes" to life.

A good place to start is with your own medical care. As medical care is becoming more client driven, people who are getting well are proactive, speaking out on their own behalf and demanding a full spectrum of care as well as credibility. The relationship formed with your physician is the responsibility of both participants. You may have been taught to be a good, dutiful patient, afraid to disagree or question your physician, because you think she's your lifeline. In the past, your very survival seemed dependent on her good graces; you may have been afraid to offend by asking too many questions or by disagreeing.

Taking charge means that you form a vital team. You may not be accustomed to investing the time and interest in your body that true healing requires. In the past, you may have been dependent on your physician to do the work for you, but now it's time to take charge. As you already know, with EI and CFS there are no easy answers for the physician to hand you.

One "alternative" Santa Cruz physician, Dr. Randy Baker, always has a waiting room full of people who wait for hours to see him. He gives all patients as much time and attention as they need and they are encouraged to ask him to define medical terms and to explain his conclusions. He's not afraid to level with his patients when he doesn't know what to do. Patients are free to inform him that they are using other methods. He encourages them to undertake comprehensive healthcare, fostering a relationship of mutual respect and responsibility. This is how it should be.

Educating your physician as to how you want to be treated can be energizing as you request information about the full spectrum of complementary modalities. Ask questions about your treatment, take notes, and even help keep your physician abreast of the latest in care. Your welfare is at stake, so don't be shy. Assertiveness should become part of the take-charge attitude that will get you the help you need. Don't be intimidated by the busy airs of your physician; you are as important and as valuable as she is.

It is such a revelation to realize that the power of healing has always resided within yourself. Without ignoring sound medical advice, you may choose to become your own health advisor. Read and learn everything you can about the treatment of these illnesses. Get curious, get excited, become an expert on the subject; after all you are the creator of your own journey. Much can be done to heal, including more than just fixing the physical body. This may mean employing unusual and exciting means, discovering the potential and truths of other modalities.

You may already be self-directed, gobbling up medical literature, tuning in to the latest advances, and trying to come to terms with your symptoms. Yet, the complexities of EI and CFS require a multilevel approach that gives consideration to all aspects of your being. There may be no single, perfect form of treatment, but some options may be more suitable for your unique circumstances and personality. Or, it may take a synthesis of several healing methods in order to cover all of the bases.

Laura, who has severe EI, knows so much that she's become an expert on how to create healthy nontoxic environments. She has founded The Environmental Health Information and Referral Service, assisting fellow sufferers with vital information by phone. Selima, a retired minister, is now a lay healer in recovery from EI and CFS. She notes, "Mainstream medicine saved my life back when I was acutely ill, but there is really nothing it's able to offer me anymore. I have learned many wonderful interventions that medical science would think were pretty far-out. Those are the things that help me now that I've become responsible for my health."

At your inner core you are well, whole, and untouched by illness. As you become acquainted with this central core of wellness, you begin to know who you are and that it's possible to take responsibility for healing. When you become acquainted with this central core, you will trust your own intuition to know which interventions are right for you and which are not.

There is an exciting change in the direction of medicine with a heightened reliance on preventive measures that give consideration to the causes rather than the effects of illness. Growing numbers of alternative or complementary health practices are becoming integrated with traditional medicine and accepted by the mainstream. These models include the whole being and consider subtle energies as a source of disease, yet they work well alongside the traditional medical model. These forms of healing can assist you to understand the more subtle relationships between vibrational energy and illness. By informing you as to what is available, you may elect to explore further on your own.

Only you can be responsible for the choices you make regarding your health. Some procedures may be contraindicated in a particular situation, so make certain an intervention is appropriate for you before you proceed. It's possible to become more confused and worn-out than you already are by participating in fads and complex healing modalities. Seek to make sensible, educated choices when implementing any program and avoid being skunked by the promise of a quick fix.

This brings to mind the story of the guru who concocted Breatharianism and claimed there was no need to eat: all that was needed to survive was the nourishment of air. People immediately followed his practice, starving themselves in order to reach enlightenment. Shortly thereafter, this individual was seen eating at a fast-food restaurant. The point is that even sensible people can forget to think for themselves once they find what they believe to be the answer.

There is a lot of expensive, attractive, "New Age" nonsense out there that can distract you from your true goal. Hold onto your sense of discernment; use good sense and healthy skepticism as a guide in choosing whom and what to trust. Taking charge of your own health will enable your skills of discernment and intuition to grow as you sift through to find out what works and resonates with your truth.

Elaine, the psychic who has CFS and EI, describes herself as being addicted to the chase. "It's become my hobby to frantically go from one intervention to another. When I try something new at first I get the same euphoric high as an allergic reaction. Sometimes I'm so crushed when what I think is the answer doesn't work." This type of thinking inevitably places the answer outside yourself, eventually dissolving into disappointment. As long as you chase after external solutions to your health problems, the source of recovery will not be visible, making it difficult for you to get well.

Like the ripple effect, everything you do, including the things that don't work, will affect your next undertaking. Even when you try a method that produces no tangible results, some kind of subtle shift has undoubtedly taken place. Everything you do forever changes what and who you are. The synergy of each intervention builds on the next, taking you toward increased understanding and wellness.

The greatest benefit of having a handful of interventions to try is that they instill a sense of autonomy and hope. So long as you have choices, you can actively shape your recovery. The worst predicament is to experience unending pain and lethargy when there is nothing you can do about it. A crushing headache can become tolerable if you have a few tricks up your sleeve to try in order to reduce discomfort.

When you do undertake a new path, your physician and other healthcare practitioners should be alerted to the interventions you are using. Some treatments can work against each other. For example, prescription drugs can render homeopathic remedies useless.

Acupuncture

Acupuncture is a branch of Chinese medicine that involves the insertion of needles into specific points in the body. These treatments stimulate the function of the organs and help to balance energy by drawing it either to or away from the organs when there is evidence of deficiency of the blood and ch'i.

Ch'i is an invisible energy known as "life force energy" which permeates the whole person and extends outward to protect the individual. Ancient traditions hold that this innate energy must be present for the body to sustain life. EI and CFS are seen to be the result of stagnation of the flow of this energy and acupuncture heals and balances this stagnation.

The principles of Chinese medicine include a system of channels and points on the body that, if touched correctly, relieve pain and accelerate healing. These channels are called *meridians*, invisible lines that conduct the body's energy. If the channels or points along the channel are out of balance, the energy flows too slowly, too fast, or not at all. The goal in Chinese medicine is to restore balance.

There are 12 major meridians, each linked with a specific organ. There are another set of meridians, known as the *extraordinary channels*, that are not directly related to the major organs. Acupuncture remedies typically combine points near the area of discomfort with points that seem to have no obvious relation to the specific problem. The nearby points are called *local points* and the faraway ones, *trigger points*. Various combinations of points are stimulated through the insertion of needles in a treatment. Along with the use of needles, moxibustion seems to enhance the therapeutic effects. Moxa is a plant resin that is burned at the point of needle insertion, improving the effectiveness of treatment.

"I get the most refreshed sleep of my entire week from an hour's acupuncture treatment," reports Jamie, who is on the road to recovery from EI and CFS. "It's one of the ways I take care of myself and one of the main things that has helped me get well." Research data show that acupuncture causes the release of endorphins from the pituitary gland.[1] One type of endorphin is a morphine-like protein that is thought to mediate pain relief. Following a treatment you may feel that you have just awakened from an exceptionally sound night's sleep, feeling relaxed, revitalized, and more alert. Over time, treatments have a cumulative effect, energizing the body and stimulating its own ability to heal.

Health food stores often sell acupressure guns which can be used in the same way to stimulate acupuncture points on yourself. An inexpensive form of acupuncture is acupressure, where you can manually stimulate the points. If you decide to use acupressure on yourself, don't press too vigorously to the point of discomfort.

As you gently press a tender area, use firm pressure with your thumbs, knuckles, palms, or fingers. Hold the area for 1 to 3 minutes, gradually releasing to come off the points. Doing this will ease muscle tension and muscle fibers will lengthen and relax. When the area is more relaxed, the blood flows more freely to the site of discomfort. Since you are addressing chronic conditions, you may want to continue weekly pressure point stimulation even after obtaining relief. An excellent resource to learn pressure points is the book *Acupressure's Potent Points* by Michael Gach (New York: Bantam, 1990).

Acupuncture and acupressure can be invaluable in allowing the energies of the body to flow freely and stimulate healing. Unlike taking a pill, which offers immediate results, the effects of acupuncture are often subtle and cumulative, and what you notice depends on your level of sensitivity. For some, the treatments are subtle and the effects aren't so noticeable. For others, with the right practitioner, the treatments can reap rapid results. The body is strengthened from deep within the cells as they become healed and this process may take time.

Bio-Magnetics

Bio-Magnetics is a simple, hands-on healing method that uses light touch directed to specific points to stimulate the body's ability to heal itself. The light touch in combination with these points activates the body's healing capabilities, which, over time, resolves illness. Bio-Magnetics is a potent form of healing, often with immediate results. At the same time, a treatment can leave a feeling that more old debris has floated up to the surface waiting to be released.

About ten years ago, Norman Cochran, a coal miner, came on a hemorrhaging pregnant woman who would have bled to death if not for the series of touches that Norman suddenly felt compelled to perform. This marked the beginning of Bio-Magnetics. Over time, more healing interventions came to this humble, simple man.

One woman with crippling scoliosis reports that her spine has straightened over years of repeated treatments. Initial photographs of her spine reveal a very deformed back, with a 33° and 22° "S" curve. More recent photographs show the curvature has shifted to 20° and 18°. Spinal curvatures are not known to straighten out on their own; the only explanation she has is the Bio-Magnetics treatments.

This is not a self-healing technique; it involves one person touching another to activate the natural healing resources of the body. This practice doesn't require any special gift or elevated consciousness on the part of the practitioner and the procedures are easy to learn. All that's necessary for healing to occur is for two people to come together with compassion and love. If you cannot find a trained Bio-Magnetics practitioner, contact the address in Appendix II.

CFS Treatment

Bio-Magnetics employs a specific pattern of touch designed to treat CFS. Norman Cochran believes that Bio-Magnetics chases the virus out of the body, the liver in particular, interrupting the viral replication process. The protocol for treatment includes a daily routine, spanning seven consecutive days. It is important to adhere to this schedule, as the virus is thought to replicate within 24-hour intervals and the treatments prevent this from happening. After the first 7-day routine, treatments should be tapered off to twice a week.

When Selima, who had CFS and still struggles with EI, undertook this treatment, she felt so stirred up that she could not sleep during the first 3 days of the series. Something was shifting and coming to the surface. "It was as if a gigantic iceberg was breaking up, moving and shifting from the inside. Many years of illness were waking up and mobilizing out," she notes. This experience can prompt mood swings, heighten old symptoms, and cause perplexing sensations. This is typical of the healing process: when this happens it is easy to want to stop, but try to stick with it. Over time you will notice a shift in energy, increased stamina, and a reduction in physical ailments.

The days that followed Selima's initial series of treatments filled her with wonder. It was fantastic to have so much clarity and so much more energy! CFS, that immovable iceberg, had moved out of her body and 5 years later has not returned!

Body Work

The need to be nurtured through touch is part of the universal human condition and is a powerful way to nurture yourself. Massage offers one such option. How often do you get to just lie there while someone else does all the work? Better yet, there is nothing to give back and no need to be in control. Greater relaxation and optimal benefit often come from just experiencing the moment and flowing with the silence with no need to talk or entertain.

It is important to feel safe and comfortable while receiving a massage. Select a certified practitioner who offers safety and comfort. Don't be shy informing the practitioner about the type of pressure you prefer; the results of a grin-and-bear-it attitude can be worse than having no massage at all.

There are several types of body work that can benefit those with EI and CFS. Deep tissue massage, such as Rolfing and Hellerwork, focus on chronic tension in muscles far below the surface, seeking to reeducate the body regarding these areas of tension. These sessions can be painful, but people often report increased energy as a result.

Cranial-sacral therapy attends to the skull and spinal column where the practitioner applies light pressure to release energy trapped in the bones, membranes, and fluids. Amini Peller, hypnosomatic therapist, reports, "My clients with chronic illnesses of any type experience cranial-sacral therapy that releases tension which clouds the mind, restricts the body, and immobilizes their spirit. This gentle touch helps restore normal motion of the brain and spinal cord which allows us to live more fully."[2]

Reflexology is a form of massage that applies acupressure to the hands and feet. Points on your hands and feet correspond to specific body parts, and when those areas are stimulated there is a positive impact on the corresponding part of the body. If an area on your foot that links with your liver is tender, it may indicate congestion in that organ. Although a trained reflexologist will thus work only on your feet, your entire body will be given a workout. Health food stores sell credit-card-sized maps of the hands and feet, detailing the location of each organ system if you wish to identify reflexology points for yourself.

More common forms of massage include shiatsu and Swedish massage which involve a relaxing series of maneuvers that have far-reaching health benefits. Some of these benefits include:

1. Reduced swelling and inflammation
2. Relief from chronic pain
3. Increased flexibility and mobility of joints
4. Improved digestion and intestinal activation
5. Improved circulation and lymphatic drainage
6. Heightened skin health
7. Stimulated or soothed nervous system
8. Muscle relaxation

The Skin

During a massage the skin receives needed contact. The skin is the largest organ of the body and is stimulated through touch. However, massage works on both physical and psychological levels. Physically, it works on all parts of the body to increase body heat, heighten circulation, and to enable increased nourishment of the blood by dilating the red blood cells, which causes enhanced oxygenation. Touch increases hemoglobin levels, reduces pain and tension, increases muscle tone, and improves the complexion. Touch also affects the nervous system and the circulation of hormones. Psychologically, massage promotes relaxation and stress reduction. Emotional blocks are freed through tissue work which promotes a relaxed, meditative state, accompanied by heightened alertness.

Lymphatic Drainage

Lymphatic massage is a specialized form of massage that stimulates the activation of the lymph glands, heightening the elimination of poisons. This form of massage also works to cleanse the body, helping to discharge toxins through sweat, urine, and mucus. Cellular toxic wastes in the form of toxic chemicals in our air, food, and water and in the form of preservatives and hormones are flushed out in the face of heightened lymphatic drainage through massage. The lymph system doesn't have the ability to move toxins on its own, but massage and exercise can move lymphatic debris. Lymphatic circulation is stimulated through exercise, and the process of perspiration and increased oxygenation also helps remove toxins from the system.

Lymph nodes destroy bacteria, foreign particles, and cellular debris. In turn, purified lymph is carried back to the heart, where it acts like a vacuum cleaner, absorbing liquid that moves out of the capillaries, cleaning and depositing clean plasma back into the bloodstream. Stimulation of the lymph nodes through massage increases the production of cellular components of the body's immune system, resulting in the release of serotonin, which helps to relieve anxiety and irritability.

Emotional Release

Typically, massage focuses on releasing observable muscular and tissue rigidity. Massage does not include processing emotional material that surfaces as a result of freeing musculoskeletal tension. You may have experienced massage work that caused a flooding of distressful emotions so you know how important it is to have a skilled practitioner on hand to guide the process. Most massage therapists are not trained to help you process feelings that can arise from a massage. Yet, there are forms of body work, such as bioenergetics and Continuum, that incorporate breath work, sound, movement, silence, and psychological processing.

Continuum work has enabled Audrey, now well from CFS, to take a giant leap forward in her life. "On all levels this work has enabled me to make changes, releasing old negative patterns and opening me up to a part of myself I never knew existed. In some ways my illness was a safe haven, its narrowness gave me certainty, order, and ordinariness. Continuum work has busted my life wide open, as a result I am full of energy and hope, and life has many exciting possibilities."

Beth Pettengil, teacher of Continuum workshops, notes, "This multifaceted work is particularly effective for chronic pain and autoimmune illnesses, and releasing restrictive patterning on many levels, as it interrupts nervous system patterning." Insight therapy tends to move the individual to deeper levels of healing when it is coupled with body work release. It appears that a deliberate shift in the psyche can facilitate changes in the nervous system.

Exercise and Strengthening the Body

Half of your physical health is derived from dietary practices and the other half from exercise. The rewards acquired from regular exercise exceed the physical experience of strengthening the body; it improves the quality of life, promoting healing on all levels and making it easier to have energy to do the things you want.

Maintaining a healthy relationship with your physical body includes more than just staying trim and working out regularly. It means putting your body in places that are safe and comfortable and removing it from situations where it isn't safe. It means paying attention to the messages that you get, resting when it says to do so, and nourishing it when needed. Paying attention to your body means not taking for granted the work it's doing to sustain you. Taking care of your physical body is not just narcissistic, obsessive, overindulgence; it's a form of prayer and thanksgiving, allowing you to attend to deeper needs. Movement and care of the body permits subtle energies to flow and has a beneficial impact on the development of your spiritual core.

Exercise and Breath

One way to achieve increased understanding of the physical body is to follow the movement of your breath. Doing this allows you to come into contact with blocks and areas of discord that usually go unnoticed. Often, physical discomfort causes you to try to leave your body, whereas following your breath draws you back in.

When used in conjunction with exercise, attention to the breath connects the body with the part of the mind that is watchful and wide awake. This makes it easier to be present when performing physical exercise as well as more mundane activities. The more you permit yourself to pay attention to what your body is telling you, the easier it is to create and maintain healthy boundaries necessary in order to protect yourself out in the world.

Using proper breathing while exercising—employing deep, rhythmic, controlled breath—is an efficient way to reduce the buildup of toxic residues. Aerobic exercise coupled with good breathing technique enables toxins to leave the body by increasing circulation which aids the detoxification process and supplies oxygen needed to regenerate cells. Regular exercise also enables you to increase staying power at many other tasks and makes sleep more restful. Built-up tension is released, allowing greater relaxation.

Poor health typically causes a sedentary life-style which reduces lung efficiency to an extent that simulates an anaerobic state. Disease processes are often promoted in the absence of oxygen which provides a medium for bacterial and fungal growth. Exercise increases oxygenation of cells, strengthening the immune system and increasing metabolism. Therefore, the stronger the body becomes, the more capable it is of fighting off potential invaders.

The brain is also able to work with greater fluidity and clarity after exercise, which, incidentally, can also improve your outlook. It causes the release of the hormones serotonin and norepinephrine by the brain; for that you feel better emotionally, as these hormones counteract depression. If mornings often find you feeling toxic and sluggish, physical activity can lift you above the haze, toward greater energy and clarity.

Jody, the acupuncturist who had CFS, performs the Five Rites of Rejuvenation, also known as the Five Tibetans, each morning on arising. These five yoga exercises, detailed in Christopher Kilham's book *The Five Tibetans* (Rochester: Healing Arts, 1994), can greatly improve energy, and reportedly help the body to heal from all manner of ills. Start slowly, gradually increasing the number of repetitions you can tolerate until you get to 21 repetitions for each exercise. The more you move, the better you will feel. Efforts in this direction will help strengthen your immune system and your body, reducing fatigue. The stronger the body becomes through mild daily exercise, the easier it will be to resist toxic external stressors.

The Exercise Dilemma

How can you entertain thoughts of expending any extraneous energy on exercise when you have none? There are two schools of thought about whether rest or exercise is most important to recovery. With CFS, some physicians prescribe unlimited rest, advising the avoidance of exercise because it increases physical distress. For some, the stress of exertion makes them feel worse, so studiously avoiding activity that might exacerbate symptoms is the rule. Yet, rest over long periods can be associated with a loss of physical strength. It can also impact the psychological realm as well, as there may be social isolation that comes with ongoing rest. Social isolation can heighten depression.

The other school of thought suggests exercise in moderation, according to individual capabilities. This means doing what feels right, keeping in mind that circumstances may change as your health waxes and wanes. The amount of exercise you can tolerate can vary from day to day. Josh, the nurse with CFS, notes, "There is a point to which I can perform an activity such as walking and still feel well. If I push past that, I pay the price for days to follow. I've had to learn to recognize this point and not go beyond it."

Common sense plays a vital role in exercise. If you have been sedentary for a long time, consult your physician first. It's best to start with an easy, brief activity, gradually increasing the amount of time spent, or the distance, or the vigor of your participation. Perform physical activities in moderation, not going all out at the start so that you lose interest. If you exercise too hard, you may generate an excess of free radicals or become overly exhausted, causing physical decompensation which defeats the whole purpose of the activity.

If you can, devote 15 minutes a day to gentle exercise. Start with something you can do; each week expand the goal a little more. Take a short walk, or a brief bike ride. Maybe the best you can do is walk across the room, that's worth something. Rather than judging yourself for what you cannot do, praise yourself for your efforts.

Gentle exercise can help mobilize your healing resources and will offer tangible demonstration of accomplishment. No matter how small this accomplishment, it can brighten your mood into a more hopeful outlook. Setting your sites on a realistic goal enables you to extract pleasure from performing the most simple exercises. The key to doing exercise on a regular basis is to find something that gives you pleasure; it shouldn't be a chore or you will only be working against yourself.

Moderate physical exercise with simple relaxed movements should be implemented on a daily basis. Initially it may be hard to carve a routine; you can probably think of a million things you'd rather be doing. In time, the more you make yourself get out there, the more you'll come to thirst for and actually enjoy the experience. Those small, self-created islands of sanity clear the way for harmony and balance in the rest of life. Taking time for yourself has a domino effect, creating greater organization and time in other parts of your day. You may even feel bereft if you don't exercise at least every other day; this can become a sacred time you look forward to, an opportunity to nurture yourself.

When selecting a physical activity, don't opt for one that is painful or too rigorous. Choose one you've had previous success with, rather than taking up a new endeavor which might heighten stress. Once you get started, you can alternate between several exercise modes, depending on the weather, your mood, or energy level. Some days you may want to bicycle; in the summer you may prefer to swim. Feel reflective? Try the old standby, a relaxing walk.

Some with EI have found the use of a mini trampoline, also known as a rebounder, to be particularly stimulating to the immune system. Daily use of the trampoline can stimulate the activation of T cells, which help fight foreign invaders. In addition, being able to exercise in the safe confines of the home can prevent toxic exposures.

In a more relaxed state, elusive insights about life have an opportunity to emerge. Problems that have been plaguing you can be resolved through the window of relaxation created by exercise. In this way, exercise can also serve as an outlet for pent-up emotions. Exercise can also offer an opportunity for social community, and some forms of exercise lend themselves to social interaction more than others. Walking on the beach or untrammeled roadways is an excellent opportunity to catch up with EI friends.

Homeopathy

Homeopathy is a therapeutic system of medicine that was developed by Samuel Hahnemann, an 18th-century German physician, based on the "law of similars," which holds that like cures like. This means that a causative substance administered in minute doses will stimulate the body's natural defenses in order to return the person to health.

To effect a cure, the symptoms of disease are not suppressed, instead they are encouraged to surface. The homeopathic remedy neither covers up nor destroys the disease, but stimulates the body to mobilize in order to throw off the harmful agent. This concept can be hard to grasp, as it doesn't follow the principles of modern medicine, which emphasize alleviating and suppressing symptoms.

Also foreign to traditional thinking is the idea that less is better. With homeopathy, the more dilute the dose, the more potent it is. In allopathic medicine the greater the potency of a medication, the larger or stronger the dose. Oddly enough, homeopaths administer small doses, which, in large quantities, would cause the very illness that they are striving to conquer.

Today, over 1200 substances are used as homeopathic remedies, and there are new remedies being discovered regularly. These remedies, regulated by the Food and Drug Administration, are available in pill, powder, or liquid form. People with EI are able to tolerate remedies made with lactose powder or those in distilled water. Growing numbers of these remedies are sold over the counter in health food stores. This dynamic process is becoming more important in light of the emerging medical difficulties that arise from the damage from pollutants and other materials. For some, such as Laura, who have severe EI, homeopathy has been one of the best ways to achieve relief.

The homeopathic practitioner studies the client's symptoms in great detail with the goal of not just alleviating symptoms, but treating the root cause. The practitioner is looking for the remedy that causes symptoms most similar to the physical and emotional symptoms being displayed, keeping in mind that the closer the match, the more precisely targeted and effective the outcome. The practitioner may give the client nosodes, which are substances taken from infected tissue that don't contain the actual disease, but may carry the vibration of the remedy. At times, with acute symptoms, a single dose of the remedy cures the illness, but when the problem is chronic it may take time to achieve a cure.

Since the vibrational qualities of the remedy introduced into the body produce a curative resonance, it is important not to touch the tablet or liquid. To do so alters the vibrational quality of the substance, rendering it ineffective in performing its healing function.

Initially with homeopathy, as with other healing procedures, you may experience an exacerbation of old symptoms. It is difficult to tell if they are symptoms of the current illness, but if your basic underlying constitution seems stronger you are probably on the right track. Intensification of symptoms or the return of old symptoms can mean the remedy is driving out residual viral, fungal, and bacterial forms that have resided in your cells for years. It can be frightening, a test of courage and trust to keep going with the hope that worse is better.

Some classic homeopaths believe that the vibrational frequencies of substances, including prescription medications, can interfere with the positive impact of homeopathic medications. As a result, working with them may require that you stop taking all other medications. Laura is working with a classic homeopath who administers a constitutional remedy that works on healing the whole body. "I like the philosophy that my body is trying to fight for itself. Since I am so allergic to everything, I've found this is the one thing that helps without a lot of unpleasant side effects."

Apex Energetics

Essential to the detoxification process is the need to build the body up first by balancing its chemistry. If the body is not strengthened prior to detoxification, you will only become more ill as toxins are mobilized. Jamie, the therapist with EI and CFS, is particularly pleased with the results of homeopathic remedies made by Apex Energetics, a program that builds the body before detoxifying it. This is a research company offering unique homeopathic remedies (see Appendix II) including a comprehensive program of cellular rebuilding, detoxification, and drainage that allows organs to heal and the body to return to optimal function. Their program is exciting because of their commonsense, multilevel approach to deep cellular healing in which homeopathic remedies work to strengthen and heal the cellular structure first and then proceed through a series of increasingly deeper levels of detoxification.

Like a battery, once the body is repaired at a cellular level it can hold a charge. Before repairing the cellular structure, Jamie says she took all kinds of remedies, vitamins, medications, and supplements and exercised with no positive results. Only when she used Apex products, aimed at cellular repair, did her body have a strong foundation from which to heal.

Undertaking this program requires a lengthy commitment if you hope to see noticeable results. If you are interested in using these products, your physician must contact Apex, as they do not distribute directly to the public. After taking these formulas for 14 months, Jamie says she's no longer engaged in a vicious spiral of bacterial, viral, and yeast infections and she has fewer allergic symptoms.

Radionics

Radionics may be the most unusual, least well known therapy you will hear about; it is mentioned here for information purposes only. The theory behind radionics is based on quantum physics which holds that all matter is composed of small pockets of pure energy known as *quanta*, comprised of atoms that pulsate or resonate at a unique frequency.

Each material object, including the human body, is made up of a combination of atoms that have their own unique, unduplicable frequency. In turn, each atom has a unique resonance. In a way atoms are like snowflakes, each one looks the same, yet each is structurally different. In this same way, each object in existence creates a certain "empathy" between the whole object and each of its separate parts. Every one of the atoms is attuned to the mother ship; the frequency of your entire body has the exact same resonance as a cell of skin that you have shed. This unique frequency is yours alone and has never before existed anywhere in the universe.

Still more astonishing is that there is a permanent affinity between your physical body and, for example, a skin cell that has been shed. Much like radio waves that travel through the air, this affinity forms a link even if the cell that has been shed is shipped thousands of miles away. Miles away this discarded cell can be used as a tuning crystal or transmitter, vibrating it at a specific, beneficial frequency to elicit a healing reaction in the distant human body that it came from. According to holographic principles, each piece taken from the whole contains all of the information of the whole.

Radionics, sometimes referred to as psionics, is a branch of esoteric science that works to psychically diagnose human energy imbalances using instrumentation in the form of a "radionic black box." The "black box" itself consists of a box with several dials, each numerically calibrated. The dials are usually attached to variable resistors which are also connected by wires to a round metallic well that is the location of the "witness."

Radionics operates on the principle of resonance, using a "witness" as a vibrational focus for the radionic practitioner to tune in to. It is possible for a practitioner to examine a drop of blood, a photograph of the individual, his saliva, or lock of hair in order to evaluate the status of the entire body. This sample, known as a "witness," makes it possible for the practitioner to quickly ascertain what the patient is suffering from without ever meeting directly.

Operating a radionics machine is relatively simple. Once diagnosis is achieved, the dials are adjusted at a frequency needed to shift the body back into health. The needed frequency of vibration is broadcast directly to the patient using the radionic device and the vibrational witness. Homeopathic medicines, gems and crystals, flower essences, color sources, and the vibrational frequency of the radionic device itself can be transmitted using these broadcasting techniques.

What isn't so simple is that the technician must be very intuitive in reading and interpreting the information gleaned from the tests in order to properly adjust the machine. The operator tunes in at a sympathetic level with the patient to receive unconscious energetic data in order to sensitively adjust the various dials of the machine. Each dial adjustment reflects a rate of energetic frequency characteristic of the patient who is being remotely tested.

A good radionics practitioner should be able to analyze the deeper levels of illness that are not clinically measurable by traditional medical standards. As with homeopathics, it is the practitioner's practice to gradually heal these unseen layers of illness. Since each layer is interrelated with the next, only when the first layer is repaired can the next level be made whole.

When traditional medicine intervenes, only clinical tests and symptoms are addressed, which means the root cause of illness may not be resolved. Radionics works to uncover the occult causes, which may be emotionally based, or actually belong to someone else, or be miasmic material that is bound up in cellular memory and passed on through generations. Sometimes illness is held in place by past beliefs, repressed emotions, and a life that is spent being out of touch with one's true path. When this is revealed, the practitioner can assist the client to address these factors. And these machines can detect, amplify, and direct human thoughts and emotions in a healing manner.

The typical analytical mind has trouble grasping this concept: the immediate reaction is that it sounds like witchcraft, with unsettling implications. It is common to have trouble accepting or understanding what transpires in the radionics process. Certainly, the American Medical Association says radionics is ridiculous. Dr. Richard Gerber, author of *Vibrational Medicine* (Santa Fe: Bear & Co., 1988), asserts that radionic systems have demonstrated effectiveness as diagnostic and therapeutic tools.[3]

Judy, a 48-year-old health educator who is now well from CFS, was treated through remote radionics for an abscessed tooth that the dentist strongly advised needed root canal work. Since dental interventions had taken such a toll, eroding her overall health, the idea of undergoing another root canal procedure did not appeal to her. Instead she tried radionics. A drop of blood was sent by mail to be used as a "witness" of her overall body state. It was then placed in a radionic device and vibrated at a curative rate. After only a day of treatment, the pain from the abscess subsided, and during the next week the tender sites in her face and mouth disappeared. This was done without leaving her home in California while the practitioner worked with her blood sample in New York.

Over the months, as she became healthier, the blood sample in New York reflected those positive changes. As you become healthier, your changed status is reflected in that old blood sample. This is because, from a vibrational perspective, each portion of the whole continues to reflect the energetic structure of the entire organism.

Reiki

Reiki is one of several forms of hands-on energetic healing that can be a useful tool to heal and energize your body. *Reiki,* pronounced "ray-key," means free passage of universal life force energy, the infinite energy present in all matter that is always available to anyone who wishes to access it.

This healing practice is believed to have originated in Tibet thousands of years ago. What is currently known as Reiki was rediscovered in the 1870s by Dr. Mikao Usui who was the president of a university in Japan. In 1934 Reiki was brought to Hawaii by Mrs. Hawayo Takata who then began to train other healers.

You may not realize it, but you too have a certain amount of healing energy available to you at all times. What Reiki does is energize the body by tapping into its energetic potential, restoring your innate ability to heal. The only requirement is that you give yourself permission for the energy to flow as a healing force in your life. Permitting this flow creates greater balance which is achieved through the harmonizing and balancing of the energy of the chakras.

Chakras are specific nonphysical energy centers that correspond to different parts of the body as well as to different levels of consciousness. The health and activity of the chakras result from the condition of mental, emotional, physical, and spiritual states. On a subtle, nontangible level, examining the chakras offers an accurate guide as to your general state of health. When these centers are open and functioning efficiently, you usually enjoy good health, whereas an imbalance in the chakras is believed to lead to disease.

Anyone can be a Reiki channel; it is not necessary to be a special enlightened being or study for many years. There are different levels of Reiki skill and practice. First and Second Degree Reiki training will enable you to channel Reiki's healing energy to treat yourself and others. It is also possible to perform remote healings, channeling healing energy to someone many miles away. This same energy can be used to treat animals, foods, water, plants, and situational difficulties. With this training you can channel Reiki to a friend while giving them a hug or when sitting quietly thinking about them. Gloria, the CFS activist, discretely runs Reiki energy into herself while attending meetings, so as not to be drained.

What's nice about Reiki is that the healer also feels energized when directing energy toward the client; and the more you channel Reiki energy, the more powerful the flow becomes. It is effortless, simply a matter of allowing. Third Degree work includes personal growth and transformation and can require a commitment to study and practice in order to teach Reiki skills.

David, a former CPA and now a healer in private practice says Reiki treatments healed him from CFS and that he would have died without this intervention. Reiki can help relieve physical pain, speed up the healing process, treat chronic illness, as well as calm emotions. It can be used in life-threatening or acute circumstances as well. You don't have to be physically ill to benefit from Reiki treatment; if your life is out of balance a treatment may offer greater energy and clarity. It's possible to use Reiki any time throughout the day when you are tired or mentally foggy. Some use it to get through allergic reactivity. Like being able to recharge your own batteries, when you run out of energy you can give yourself a lift.

In a Reiki treatment, the Reiki practitioner creates a safe space for the work of healing to occur, but does not actually perform the healing. The Reiki therapist, without using his own energy, acts as a hollow reed through which universal, infinite energy flows. This energy flows through the practitioner into the client when his hands are placed on specific locations on the body, keeping the hands in the same place for a few minutes at each site. With Reiki it isn't possible to direct the energy into a specific area; it contains its own innate intelligence to travel where it is needed.

As the energy flows, you may experience warmth, tingling, sensations of electricity, or energy enhancement. Even if there is no sensation noted, Reiki energy is still being transmitted. If the tingling sensation ceases, it means you are full. Your first Reiki experience may be unnerving; after being without energy it may be overwhelming to have so much energy. Jody, the acupuncturist who is now well from CFS, remembers being deluged with sensation, some pleasant, and some so jangling that all she could do was lay down for several hours following her first treatments.

At times a Reiki treatment can heighten already existing symptoms, as toxins are being mobilized and removed. As blocks are being freed, there may be increased physical or emotional distress. Increased life force energy is helping release the blocks that have previously been suppressed. It is important not to interpret this discomfort as being detrimental and withdraw from the process, as these issues are rising to the surface in order to be healed.

With Reiki and other forms of healing, people experience increased physical energy which enables the body to perform needed repair. Having more physical energy also enables you to think with greater clarity, making it possible to be less disturbed by your body when it careens out of control. Increased mental energy also enables you to attend to living out your higher purpose.

The vibrational quality of this work can enable you to think more clearly in order to function at a more objective level. Being more objective means you have increased awareness so that you are no longer ruled by illness. In this way Reiki provides a bridge to change ways of thinking and perceiving. The more conscious and intuitive you are, the less you will be at the mercy of out-of-control events, and you will now be able to choose how you wish to live.

This practice works well when used with other healing modalities, in particular, with inner-child work. The more permission you give yourself to move through the blocks and disconnections of the inner child, the greater spaciousness is created for love and integration in your life.

Sound Healing

You can heal yourself with sound. Niro Asistant, author of *Why I Survive AIDS* (New York: Simon & Schuster, 1991), healed herself into an HIV-negative state, in part through toning and chanting, a feat unheard of at the time. She believes daily chanting stimulated her pineal and pituitary glands located in her brain, calling healing hormones into action.

Patricia Lynn Mann, former hospital nurse who moved into her bathroom after she became acutely ill with EI, helped heal herself with sound. "The power of vibrational medicine, specifically using sound from the voice and high frequency energy was very powerful for rebalancing my body, settling my emotions, and reprogramming me into a higher level of consciousness and wellness." Today she runs the Center for Sound Healing, teaching classes and conducting private sessions which include the use of healing through sound.[4]

Sound can be a powerful tool to energize the body as it alters its vibrational frequency allowing a subtle but powerful energetic shift to take place. Sound therapists can send sounds into various parts of the body, rearranging and balancing the cells. This vibration of sound can heighten energy, prevent you from being harmed by outside toxins, and lift you out of depressed states. A relaxed, meditative state occurs as your energy shifts, causing sharper perceptions and greater physical energy.

Researchers have been able to verify music's ability to reduce stress, improve recall, and ease pain. You can access the healing power of sound by listening to music. If you want relaxation, look for music that has 60 beats per minute or less; music at this rate will help slow your heart rate. If you are looking to be energized, select music that is uplifting and has a more rapid beat. Al Bumanis, of the National Association for Music Therapy in Silver Springs, Maryland, suggests creating a healing tape using music from the time of your youth.[5]

Experimenting with Sound

Notice how your mood changes when you listen to particular forms of music. What lifts your spirits? How about the song "Amazing Grace"? Does a classical concert, rock music, jazz band, Gregorian choir, Buddhist chant, or church organ do the trick? At times, if you are particularly blue, music can help you to let go, freeing you from burdens and sorrow. Stuck emotions become loosened through sound, allowing for greater clarity and freeing self-expression.

Certain sounds carry healing capabilities, affecting physiological states and rhythms of the body. Melodic sound carries a higher vibration that soothes the mind, energizes the body, fans the emotions, and increases the body–mind link. The thrill of music may come from the release of endorphins, opiate-like chemicals produced by the brain that reduce pain and induce euphoria. The right sound at the right time can bring great joy or energize or relax the body.

How you respond to sound is a matter of much more than personal preference and no two people will share the same experience of its impact. What you ate for breakfast, your posture, the shape of your body, the density of your bones, the shape of your skull all cause a unique resonant experience throughout your body. In addition, your mood, the environment in which you hear the sound, and where you are situated in the room will further cause you to receive sound in a unique way. So what makes you feel good today may do nothing for you tomorrow, and sound that heals you may harm someone else.

One little-known form of sound healing includes the use of piano tuning forks that the practitioner moves over and around your body to clear the chakras. It's simple to learn how to use the forks on yourself or on others. Each chakra requires that a different tuning fork be used, as each chakra matches a specific sound frequency. The vibrational frequency emitted by the fork balances the chakras, aligning the body's energy centers to the optimal vibrational rate. It's hard to describe the sensations that can occur, but a treatment can calm a headache and reduce other discomforts.

Creating Your Own Healing Sounds

You can use sound yourself as a tool for transformation, stirring up and awakening energies that can flood through to heal you. The work you do with sound can move you further than you can imagine toward healing. Music is so much more than mere sounds and words; the experience connects you with the spiritual as well as the unconscious. Songs and chanting are another form of reflection, prayer, and meditation.

Chanting and singing are great exercise if you are sedentary. When you sing or laugh or even cry, you are working your heart muscle, diaphragm, abdominal muscles, and lungs. Engaging in chanting requires no skill, evokes no judgment, and seems to be divinely inspired. The simple act of emitting deep sounds, those groans and sighs that have been locked in your body, can bring powerful, refreshing release.

Don Campbell, director of the Institute for Music, Health, and Education in Boulder, Colorado, believes that "the sounds you make with your own voice can be the most powerful healer."[6] Daily practice, working with the natural free-form sounds that your vocal chords emit, can free up stuck energy and establish a vibration that acts as a protective shield.

Find a private place and try this exercise once a day: sit comfortably with your spine erect and your eyes closed. Practicing loose belly breaths, inhale through your mouth and exhale by humming through your nose with your mouth closed. The humming sound should be loud enough to vibrate through your whole body. Allow yourself to experience the vibration of the sound as it travels through, listening and feeling with your entire being. Try using different tonalities, noticing how each vibration makes you feel After doing this for 10 to 20 minutes, you will notice a flowing movement from the inside to the outside of the body.

When you are done, sit or lie perfectly still, staying awake to note relaxed, expansive sensations. You will notice greater integration, more energy, and greater peacefulness at the same time. In this relaxed state, insights and clarity spring unbidden into awareness. It's important to be silent once sounding is complete; the deep stillness and inner harmony can unlock important information. This form of healing offers an experience that shifts the energy within your body, tuning and balancing it so that your physical and emotional outlook can change.

In addition to focusing your attention inward, humming stimulates the thymus and pituitary glands, both important for the functioning of the immune system. The thymus monitors the production of T cells and the pituitary assists in the elimination of toxins. Humming through your nose also stimulates the pineal gland, opening your "third eye," located in the center of your forehead between the eyebrows. The "third eye" relates to the opening of inner vision enabling you to receive inner guidance.

Sherry combines a soak in the tub with chanting. "Doing both at once heightens the experience. Chanting in the tub is my one great pleasure; it's time away from my husband and kids. Plus the tub offers great acoustical enhancement. Opening up my throat through chanting makes it easier to speak directly and honestly with others when I need to."

Support Groups

You may have understandable reservations about joining a support group if you're too tired or you don't want to hear about anyone else's problems. Investment and alignment in a support group is also an overt declaration of illness; you are openly identifying yourself as being a sick person. This fact may be easy to acknowledge in the privacy of a physician's office or at home among friends, but joining a group whose membership clearly defines themselves as ill can be like coming out of the closet for some, i.e., very threatening.

Couple this declaration with the word *chronic*, which implies the obliteration of the potential to join the ranks of the well, and you may feel as though you are making a lifetime commitment to illness. Openly declaring yourself to be a chronically ill person can become a trap that is hard to leave.

Some worry that their involvement in a support group may cause them to become more attached and obsessed with their illness. "I used to think it was really cruel to shun people who were less well than I am. I now see this as a survival mechanism," says one woman who is reluctant to join a support group because of fears that the suffering of others may have an adverse impact on her health. Another young woman with extreme CFS noted, "If I only have two hours of energy a day, I don't want to spend it obsessing about my health. I want to enjoy my friends and the few moments when I feel okay."

This makes plenty of sense. Venturing into a support group may mean giving illness more than the enormous space it already occupies. Actively focusing on illness makes some feel less capable of attending to the rest of their life. The more attention they give the illness, the more it impairs their ability to function in the world.

On the other hand, openly identifying yourself as a person who is challenged can enable you to be more accepting of your circumstances and empower you to take better care of yourself. Joining a support group can also give you more room in which to live. Successful groups favor avoiding the victim stance which works best if each participant is there to learn and to change. Growth and change cannot occur if group agreement is stacked in favor of helplessness. What is needed is an uplifting experience that calls on the strengths of all group members. The inspired encouragement of a group whose rules require shared goals of self-love and healing can be a potent force for recovery. "I had no idea that other people were struggling with the same issues. In my group I've learned many helpful hints; plus how to advocate for myself. I'm no longer alone or helpless; it's made a big difference," enthuses Elaine about her CFS support group.

Support groups have been known to digress into gripe sessions, invested in staying attached to the negativity of illness. It's easy to fall into the trap of using the experience as a dumping ground for stored-up negative feelings, but pouring out negativity doesn't involve taking responsibility for changing the circumstances of your life. If negative spewing is the agenda, eventually members will feel depleted and defeated and will stop attending.

It can be tricky to encourage open self-expression, as there can be a fine line between honesty and the opportunity to wallow in self-defeating pity. This tendency can be handled skillfully by group agreement to keep the emphasis on positive feelings and experiences, without denying true feelings.

It is natural to want to be with people who are moving toward life, even in the midst of ongoing illness. Gloria, 50 years old and recovered from CFS, left her original support group to join the Center for Attitudinal Healing. It's been a perfect match: her involvement with this organization has brought her deep wellness and healing.

A successful group is created when there is a mutual agreement to keep the issues on a positive constructive focus, optimizing participants' strengths. Holding this as a common goal makes it possible to unlearn obsessive negative thinking. In turn, this allows healing positive experiences to unfold. This doesn't mean that difficulties cannot be addressed; it just means that the emphasis should be toward seeking the highest and best resolution of problems.

A dynamic group enables you to learn of new developments in medical science. People with EI and CFS tend to have a tremendous thirst for information and the group setting offers a great opportunity for sharing to unfold. Emotions, frustrations, and technical information are shared, as well as interventions that have met with success.

Involvement in a group offers the opportunity to meet others who have adjusted without losing themselves to the illness, which can be of particular value for those who are newly sick. Months of fact finding efforts can be saved by accessing the collective wisdom of the group. Groups can be peopled with those who have been ill for years as well as those who have just received a diagnosis. It can be rewarding to reach out to the newly diagnosed who may be frantically searching for relief.

There can also be comfort and inspiration found in hearing of the sensible actions and progress of the long-timers. In addition, coming in contact with people who understand your struggles can be an incredible relief. This sense of commun-ion can make an enormous difference in helping you to cope with experiences you have previously tried to deal with alone. Meeting people who are struggling with the same problems or who are worse off can put your own problems into perspective. Setbacks no longer mark the end of the world and naming your fears can soothe you into greater clarity.

You've undoubtedly tried to go it alone because the illness forced you into isolation. Isolation may have made it difficult to find mirrors that offer healing information. Your support group will allow you to make these comparisons. How well are you coping? If you're struggling, why is that? What else can you do to improve? Are you as well as the next person? Do you have as positive an attitude? These and more questions will surface.

Coming together can make ripples too. The downside of group involvement is the tendency to use shared information to feel superior. Elaine confided in a CFS support group, "Time and again I've caught myself running critical dialogues in my head; thinking, 'Doesn't she know how negative she sounds?' Sometimes I feel smug when I notice how attached other people are to their illness, but then I wonder about myself."

At times, shared details surrounding the illness sound as if they are proud, treasured wounds being held out for all to admire. Observing what seems to be another treasuring her illness may make you uncomfortable, yet grateful. Secretly, her attachment may remind you of your own. A support group isn't a contest. Each participant comes to heal in her own unique time and manner; there should be no judgment and no blame. The way of another may not be your way, but her way is necessary for her journey.

Involvement in a group allows the opportunity to help each other find larger containers for our lives. The image of multitudes of people standing on an infinite stairway comes to mind. Individuals on the steps ahead reach down, assisting you to climb up beside them, closer to the light. The people behind you receive a hand-up as you reach down to assist them to move upward to a higher level as well. No sense in butting in line, moving ahead faster than you are able; no sense in feeling superior to someone who is behind you. There can be no judgment as to who stands behind you because there are always multitudes of others who stand ahead. Understanding our interrelatedness is both humbling and exhilarating.

An important technical detail in establishing a support group is finding a safe place to meet. One EI support group devoted their entire first meeting to finding a toxin-free room in their doctor's office. In the end, they chose the waiting room after they'd sniffed their way through every room, systematically exploring and ultimately declaring each space to be unsuitable for the needs of the most reactive.

When they finally got settled, one woman began sniffing anew, eventually sniffing other participants. She then announced she could not stay; the scent of hand lotion belonging to one of the other women was driving her wild. Though the others breathed sighs of relief that they hadn't offended anyone with their laundry detergent, skin cream, or shampoo, the woman wearing the lotion never returned.

Creating a Safe Environment

What most people come to a support group for is honest support and encouragement. The above-mentioned group did not start in such a way as to foster openness and safe self-disclosure. The depth of group disclosure depends on the tone that is set for safety and trust and they certainly started out on the wrong foot.

It is important not to harm others with your sensitivities. You probably know firsthand how painful it is to internalize criticism and judgment resulting from these illnesses. A safe place must be established so that people can feel comfortable and protected in sharing their deeper selves. If this cannot occur within the confines of the group, it's a waste of time. Elaine attended one group in which the participants discussed the damage done in a different CFS support group the week before. Apparently, one participant was verbally abusive toward another and the facilitator did not intervene to relieve the situation. As a consequence, other group members did not feel safe and decided not to return.

Many groups are set up and run by well-meaning people who have little idea of how to facilitate a support group. It is essential in forming a group to know something about group dynamics, or to seek the wisdom of someone who is experienced in this process. Even with the best of intentions, damage can be done when there is no one with skills to handle difficult situations. There must be an agreement as to the parameters of acceptable behavior. Typically the person who forms the group, serves as the unofficial monitor to maintain safety and order should difficulties arise.

The main thing that a good support group offers is someone to listen. Listening is helping. The act of listening implies, "We're all in this together; we're on each other's side." There is great comfort in having your feelings acknowledged and confiding is good for your health. Verbal release can help increase your perspective. It's not always necessary to delve into details or take on the suffering of another. It's not necessary to give advice or to try to fix someone. Giving advice can shut down the flow of expression, as it implies inadequacy.

The sense of acceptance that comes from feeling heard is enough. Listening is an acquired talent that forces you to shush the busy chattering in your own head. You are probably in the habit of listening with half an ear while discreetly conjuring up a smart response to the extent that you fail to hear what's being said. Quieting down your own mental noise enables greater empathy and understanding. Then when it's your turn to speak, you are more likely to receive the same respect.

Steps to Organize a Self-Help Group

CFS and EI support groups are numerous and diverse, and you may decide to start one in your area. The following are suggested steps to take to successfully organize a group:

1. Define the target population, as well as loosely define the general purpose of the group. This purpose should be fluid, as it will be reshaped to meet the changing needs of the group.
2. Recruit members by putting out the word through physicians, therapists, acupuncturists, traditional and nontraditional practitioners, and those who are ill. Post notices at strategic locations such as medical offices where people with EI and CFS are treated. Next, establish a screening process to determine who should participate.
3. Find a safe location for the first meeting. This may be a major obstacle for those with EI; so find out ahead of time about individual restrictions. Try to locate a place you can use for free, as the added expense may prove to be a barrier to participation for some.
4. Conduct the first meeting with the facilitator serving as host, assisting participants to feel welcome. The behavior of the facilitator will be crucial in setting the tone of the group, modeling effective ways to initiate self-help and showing how to extend mutual aid.
5. During the first meeting, identify issues and expectations which will help shape the group's direction and confirm the group goals and purpose. Determine how the leadership role will be handled, perhaps the role of group facilitator will change each week.
6. As a group, establish a few simple expectations, putting this in print for the next meeting. Expectations might include: no perfumes or scents, no advice giving, and an expectation that confidentiality will be maintained.
7. The facilitator should be responsible for making sure each person has adequate time to speak. Redirecting conversation can keep certain participants from monopolizing the time. The leader should also help create a safe, comfortable atmosphere.
8. General goals that have been identified may change as the group develops over time. These goals for the group are different than the predetermined code of expectations.
9. Decide on a group format. Attitudinal healing is a great model for self-help groups. Some groups have a guest lecturer once a month who covers educational developments.
10. The group organizer should gradually withdraw from the leadership function, allowing others to assume greater responsibility once the group takes on a life of its own.

Summary

You may want to explore some of the interventions mentioned in this chapter. Acupuncture and homeopathy may be most familiar, but radionics, Reiki, healing with sound, and Bio-Magnetics may open up a world of greater possibilities. Exercise in some form can be accessible to you at any time. If you are interested in joining a local support group, ask your physician, or your friends who have been ill, and be prepared to open up your life.

Endnotes

[1] Richard Gerber, *Vibrational Medicine* (Santa Fe: Bear & Co., 1988) 194.

[2] For further information contact Amini Peller, cranial-sacral therapist, 2150 White Oak Way, San Carlos, CA 94070, (415) 595-5660.

[3] Gerber, 222–237.

[4] For information about her work, contact Patricia Lynn Mann, RN, MSN, Center for Sound Healing, P.O. Box 2157, Carmel Valley, CA 93924, (408) 659-3031.

[5] Michael Castleman, "The Healing Power of Music," *Natural Health* Sept.–Oct. 1994: 71.

[6] For more information, contact Don Campbell at The Institute for Music, Health, and Education, P.O. Box 4179, Boulder, CO 80306, (800) 490-4968.

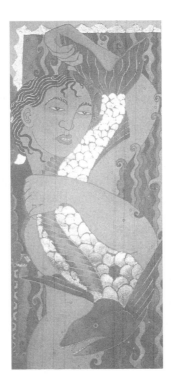

*Chapter
Eight*

*Healing
through
Physical
Self-Protection*

*t*his chapter is about finding remedies and treatments you can perform that will help you make a shift toward improved health. Being able to intervene on your own behalf can be a potent step in moving from being a victim, to empowerment. In order to produce results you must allow your life to change: loosening your hold on the ideal body state and freeing up your mental and emotional life as well. Reprogramming yourself will create resourceful states conducive of recovery which will help build immune resistance.

Selima, the 42-year-old who is now mostly well from EI and CFS, worked with a health practitioner who offered an important source of support. In addition to frequent phone contact, the practitioner helped screen out inappropriate interventions which might have offered a pleasant diversion, but ultimately would have distracted her from her goal. The day came when she outgrew this source of guidance and she began to discriminate as to what was best for herself. This meant stepping out on her own and taking charge of her own path toward healing. Recovery, for Selima, now means maintaining a balance. "Listening to my body. Going to bed as often as needed. Learning to discern what is healthy and knowing when to relax and slow down."

Having a sense of control can go a long way toward facilitating recovery. The only prerequisite to intervening on your own behalf is that you have a healthy curiosity and interest in learning how to help yourself and that you are willing to experiment to discover what works for you. Armed with helpful interventions, you can act as your own advisor, selecting what's best. Some self-help practices may seem too far-out or too risky to suit your personal program; yet there may be other exercises which will resonate.

It will take trial and error to find the interventions that work best. A particular intervention may not help in one situation, but may provide great relief in another. As your needs change you may adapt your practice, employing different interventions in combination. The main objective is to have a few tools to get through reactions and general discomfort without prolonged suffering.

If you are not suffering from allergic sensitivities, you may wonder why you should make an effort to detoxify your body or clean the external environment. The fewer demands there are on your immune system, the easier it is to attend to the job of getting well. Avoiding exposures to outgassed fumes, despite your conviction that this is not a problem, can, in fact, increase your overall health.

It can be invaluable to know that you can master external circumstances. Examine what has worked for you in the past. By sharing this information with others, you may both reduce their suffering and come to learn other pointers on how to achieve relief.

Breathing into Life

What a surprise to discover how few of us really know how to breathe properly! Most likely you consider yourself to be an expert on the subject, yet you probably have no awareness that you could really excel at this activity.

It may be difficult to understand why proper breathing is so important. You take air into your body—so what, no big deal! However, proper breathing is the single most effective intervention you can perform on your behalf to achieve relief. It can help energize you, get you through episodes of reactivity, increase relaxation, and improve mental clarity when experiencing brain-fogging.

Oxygen fuels the fire of life. And it is breathing that supplies oxygen and cleanses the system. When you exhale, toxins are eliminated by your lungs and the lymphatic system. So you see, it is a big deal to breathe deeply and fully.

Inhale right now, noticing how you do this. At first glance, an inhalation most likely includes hunching your shoulders, tensing your body, and only filling your lungs. Don't be embarrassed; few of us are expert at breathing.

Though breathing primarily involves the lungs and the action happens in the chest, it also includes the stomach and ultimately every pore and cell of your being. When you breathe properly, your lower diaphragm should contract and descend, making greater room for your lungs to expand. Your abdomen should protrude when the lungs become filled.

Most people, being self-conscious about their appearance, think their abdomen should be sucked in when they inhale. Breathing properly, from the bottom up, the

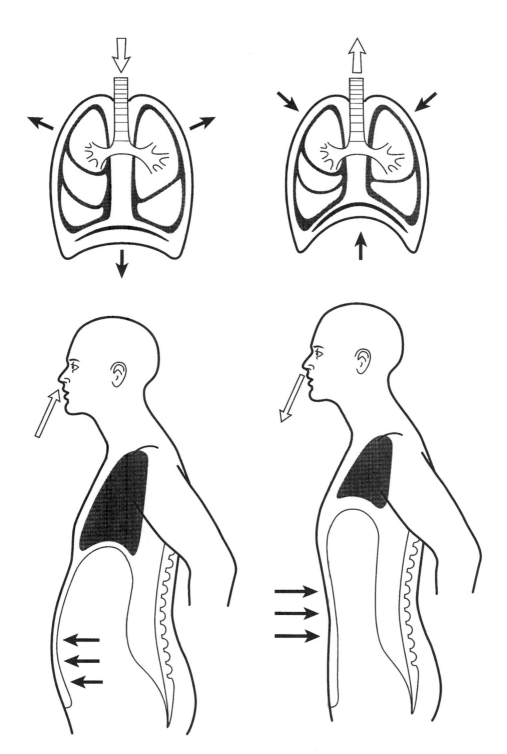

The diaphragm during healthy inhalation and exhalation.

inhalation should cause your stomach to push out. This permits the air to fill every crevice of your lungs, expanding to oxygenate the rest of your body while strengthening abdominal muscles at the same time. Breathing this way you may not look so attractive but you will begin to feel better.

Throughout the day take time to notice how proficient you are at breathing, allowing yourself to breathe deeply and comfortably. Breathing through your nose keeps the charge of energy in check, increasing control and slowing your metabolism. Breathing through your mouth increases the charge of energy and facilitates the discharge of emotions.

When tired, discouraged, or reactive, you can change your entire outlook by redirecting attention onto your breath. Notice the tension locked in various parts of your body and consciously send the breath in to relax these areas. Note the tension in your chest. Turn your attention to your jaw muscles and breath into these areas with freeing release. Notice all of the areas of constriction and withholding. Every time you exhale your body is more relaxed and awake.

Tension often blocks the movement of the breath. By allowing yourself to breathe properly you will bring vitality into these blocked areas. When breathing with this sort of attention, notice your breath warming you, feel your cells wake up during the act of inspiration. Your hands may tingle as you do this.

The breath is considered to be the bridge between the conscious and the unconscious. Noticing the breath enables you to be more connected and clear about your own needs, slowing you down in order to witness your life. Spiritual practices often include mindfulness of the breath or practices that attend to breathing. The physical body and the spiritual self have an easier time becoming acquainted when you breathe properly, bringing your attention to the moment, allowing you to fully experience your body.

Alternate Nostril Breathing

Elaine, who has EI and CFS, reports that the following exercise has an immediate energizing, relaxing, and warming effect on her body. Start by finding a quiet place and sitting comfortably. Using your dominant hand, place the thumb of that hand on one side of your nose and your middle finger on the other side of your nose. You may wish to rest your forefinger on your forehead, making a tripod. When you are ready, breathe out and back in on one side, then close that nostril and switch to the other side breathing out and then back in, always switching nostrils before the outbreath.

As you do this, notice the sensation of the air moving in and out of your nostril, keeping your stomach muscles relaxed as you breathe slowly and deeply. Practice this for 3 minutes and then switch to your nondominant hand, alternately closing each nostril. Switching hands is believed to balance the right and left hemispheres of the brain, bringing about balance.

Sinus Irrigation

Since many people with EI and CFS have sinusitis symptoms, it can be difficult to breathe properly; so all of these breathing exercises will be of no benefit until you heal your sinuses. The rationale for healing the sinuses is that allergens, irritants, and vasomotor rhinitis cause the production of inflammatory mediators in the nose. This leads to the blockage of sinus passages and problems with absorbency, which in turn result in many systemic symptoms. Treating sinusitis problems can improve these systemic symptoms.

Dr. Jim Jones asserts that the preferred therapy to resolve sinusitis is the irrigation of the nasal passages, mixing 8 ounces of distilled water, 1/2 teaspoon of sea salt, and a pinch of baking soda which acts as a buffer.[1] Using a bulb syringe or Neti-pot, the nasal passages can be rinsed twice a day to help you to breathe with greater ease. Sherry, who has EI, also has chronic sinusitis and advocates the use of Bi Yan Pian, a Chinese medicine found in health stores, to help resolve sinus pain, infection, and inflammation.

Healing Energy

Everything in the universe is energy. Energy vibrates through you, and is always available with the potential to make you feel completely awake and aware. As with your breath, when your energy flows in a natural balance, health flourishes. In order to become well you can learn to direct your energy in ways that allow it to flow freely. One simple way to direct this energy is to say yes to life.

Energy gives you the force to take action and the power to produce results. Energy is life force, a potent gift to respect and use to change the direction of your existence. What these illnesses are about is feeling incapable of summoning enough energy to proceed with life in order to produce desired results. Yet, you can learn how to access and sustain this vibrant, healing source in order to create greater health.

It's easy to recognize forms of physical energy, but there are more subtle forms that are little understood. Even when you aren't able to see these energetic sources, it is possible to feel them. For example, emotions are a form of energy that can affect you as well as those near you.

Energy as Life Force

An astonishing path opens when you give consideration to the idea that subtle energies are real. In the same way that unseen, subtle energies, such as electromagnetic radiation and toxic chemicals, have an adverse influence on health, it's possible to harness other unlimited, benign energies toward greater self-support. One example is Therapeutic Touch, a form of hands-on healing; studies have shown that healer's energies can increase a patient's hemoglobin levels, confirming the benefits of subtle energetic healing.[2]

Although you may ignore your relationship to the vast array of energy forms, you are nonetheless affected by them. There are many kinds of energy that revitalize and instill life-force. There are subtle energies that surround and emanate from your body. When these energies are in balance you experience health; when they are disturbed you become sick.

The energy of the earth is another form that is available to you continuously. Permitting yourself to feel the energy of the earth flow through your body will increase your physical energy as well as mental clarity. Learning to experience the flow of this energy can be nourishing and life-giving and can be easily channeled with practice. You need not be physically ill to access this powerful force.

Grounding with Earth Energy

Grounding is the process of connecting with the earth and enjoying the resulting free flow of abundant energy. Grounding means directing your attention inward, into your body and being in the present to bring energies into calm harmonious balance within. When you are grounded, it is easier to pay attention and focus and this can make an enormous difference in how you feel.

To connect with the earth, stand with your feet flat on the floor, placing them wide apart, with your knees slightly bent. Each time you inhale, imagine energy flowing into your body, up through the bottoms of your feet. As you do this, allow your body to relax, noticing the energetic sensations in the soles of your feet and in your legs. Next, with your mind's eye visualize your feet sinking into the floor, through the ground, deep into the earth.

It helps to imagine your feet as tree roots, growing down into the earth, traveling through the hard rock of its crust, traveling into the molten core. When your imagination reaches the earth's center, visualize your feet anchored by a firmly placed pipe or a ship's anchor. Anchoring yourself in this way will keep you connected to the energetic flow, yet enable you to move freely.

Once you establish this connection, return your attention to the energetic sensations traveling into the bottoms of your feet, up your legs. These sensations may feel like heat, tickling, movement, or waves of light, or whatever you notice. Gradually permit the energy to move up farther into your body until it flows into every crevice and pore of your being. Allow the energy to fill your heart and to travel into your arms and fingertips. As the energy flows from your hands you may note tingling sensations that signal that your body is being awakened and vitalized.

You can use this procedure when tired, allergic, or in order to achieve greater mental clarity. Laura, who has EI, uses this technique when she's having an allergic reaction. It keeps her from becoming anxious and heightening the discomfort. Only taking a few seconds to ground, sometimes she avoids reactivity altogether. The more you practice, the stronger the energy flow will become. Even when you don't feel energetic sensations, they are flowing all the same.

Your Healing Hands

As an extension of the grounding exercise, you may wish to direct healing energy into specific areas of your body. First, make yourself comfortable by lying or sitting in a quiet place where you won't be interrupted. From here you can move into the grounding exercise, slowly relaxing and watching the rise and fall of your breath.

Once you feel relaxed, gently bring your attention to an area of tension and discomfort. When you find such a constriction, place your hands, one on top of the other, over that part.

Placing your hands in this way directs the energy to flow out through your hands, channeling it back into your body. As you lie or sit there quietly, you may notice tingling sensations or warmth flowing from your hands into the target region. If you don't notice anything, that's okay. Continue to breathe and notice any changes as you send healing energy into that part of the body.

Just watch and take notice; you need do nothing except allow the process to occur. You may want to move your hands somewhere else; let your intuition guide you. Your hands may be placed simultaneously on different areas of the body. Jamie notes feelings of increased energy running under the skin surface between her hands when she does this. Gloria, the CFS activist and mother, performs this exercise discreetly and frequently throughout the day; placing her hands on an area in need while sitting in meetings.

During this experience you may unexpectedly free-up blocked emotions that have been locked in your body. If this happens, use your newfound understanding of how to breathe properly to move into them. Part of your healing may include permitting these feelings to surface so as to be fully felt. Remember, you are in charge and can call a halt if you feel overwhelmed by the emotional release.

There are growing numbers of hands-on energetic healers and schools that teach people to become healers. The School for Enlightenment and Healing in San Diego, California, directed by Michael Mamas, trains people to perform hands-on and remote healings (see Appendix II). "Hands-on healing helps break the negative electrical pulse which then frees the physiology to create a tone that is more innately correct for the individual." Michael Mamas notes, "Hands-on healing work is about reclaiming that innate intelligence."

Quick Fixes for Increased Energy

The hallmark of CFS is chronic, debilitating fatigue that interferes with the ability to perform normal, everyday activities. Rationing limited energy can make it possible to get through the day. This means constantly reevaluating whether an activity is truly important to you and forgoing all others that you can do without.

Judy, in recovery from CFS, feels better when she pays attention to the messages her body sends and moves in concert with its demands. When she forces herself to get out of bed before her body is ready, she pays dearly with increased physical discomfort. She feels best if she takes time to meditate and to organize her day before getting up.

Theresa, who has severe chemical sensitivities, helped herself when she purchased an answering machine to give her greater control over fatiguing, unwelcome phone calls. By paying attention to the energy levels expressed by your body you can pace and prioritize, deciding what is most important to accomplish and moving at a speed you can tolerate. For some, life then becomes pretty basic;

strength is saved for mundane survival activities.

As you become stronger, it is easy to overdo; with increased energy, you may try to take advantage, frantically attempting to accomplish long-postponed tasks. This can propel you headlong into a relapse. As you learn greater balance, you may discover how important it is to apply your limited energies toward self-nurturing. You may want to set aside time on a daily basis for activities that offer self-nourishment. This doesn't mean catching up on chores, but doing something that renews and excites you. If you do this, you may have more energy when you need to perform less exciting tasks.

In order to get the ball rolling, you may need to be creative. To save energy for activities that you enjoy, you may decide to hire someone to help with the housework. Or you may enlist the assistance of friends, or come up with energy-saving tactics such as those Theresa and Judy have devised. Even better, you may want to consider the following self-nurturing interventions that may provide you with increased energy:

- *Yoga:* Yoga stretches offer a quick way to recharge when you are at a low ebb. This activity is the ideal low-impact exercise for those with EI and CFS, gently stretching muscles and increasing circulation. It also increases flexibility, increases strength, tone, and endurance. Ease into stretches gently and you will note rapid improvement. If any stretch is painful, don't do it.

  Yoga benefits the immune system, aids digestion, assists lymphatic drainage, and prompts an overall sense of well-being and mental clarity. Added attention to the breath can deepen the experience. Ten minutes of daily yoga stretches can help strengthen and support the flow of subtle energies. If you don't know what to do, get a book from the library or attend classes. For beginners, Selima recommends Howard Kent's book, *Yoga Made Easy* (Allentown: People's Medical Society, 1994).

- *Bioenergetics:* Take a pillow and pound on it with your fists. This works best if you stand with knees bent and feet flat on the floor at the edge of a bed. You may wish to stomp on the floor with your feet or make loud noises as you pound on the pillow with your hands. In a matter of minutes, the pent-up feelings that may have been trapped in your body can be released.

  Trapped feelings of sorrow, fear, and anger are denied expressions of your life force that become diverted into muscular and emotional armoring, depleting and devitalizing your entire being. When feelings are not safely expressed, energy is diverted inward, creating disease. When trapped energy is released, integration takes place on all levels, causing increased aliveness and awareness. For those who think they don't have any energy to spare, try it anyway. When you stop, notice how you feel. Many report feeling energized with this simple physical release.

- *Breathing to vitalize:* As previously noted, the most immediate way to build up energy in the body is to increase oxygenation by breathing more deeply and fully. Increased oxygenation to the cells then helps the body heal and improves circulation.

In this exercise, sitting comfortably, breathe deeply into your belly. When you do this, your hands and fingers may tingle and vibrate. As you inhale, hold your breath four counts, then exhale. After you exhale, hold that empty state for four more counts, repeating this cycle four times. After the fourth inhalation hold your breath 15 to 20 counts. Then begin the cycle again, repeating it ten more times.

Remember to breathe evenly and slowly, and avoid holding your breath by closing your throat. As you become more experienced with this exercise, you will not need to concentrate so hard on counting. Notice how the energy flows, as you feel relaxed, more awake, and invigorated. When you are tired or having difficulty concentrating, do this exercise and inevitably your energy will increase.

- *Increased cranial circulation:* The gravitational field of the earth is a force that compresses and holds everything together in its particular form. Most of your life is spent in an unconscious relationship with the effects of gravity, and most of your waking hours are naturally spent in a vertical position, which subjects you to gravitational stress. Though you cannot alter the direction of gravity's pull, you can alter the direction of your body as it is exposed to this force.

   You can alleviate the impact of gravity by periodically elevating your feet above your head, either in a yoga posture, standing on your head, or by lying on a bed and hanging your head over the side. Yoga exercises are helpful, as they generally counteract gravity in ways that allow energy to flow through the body in different angles and directions that defy it. Some people use slant boards or other inversion devices to counteract gravity's pull. Jody cannot achieve these postures, but when she needs a quick burst of energy she bends over at the waist while standing so that blood flows into her head.

   Holding any of these positions as long as you are comfortable can help increase mental clarity. Inversion postures increase circulation and improve oxygenation to the brain, which facilitates mental function as well as reducing fatigue. Reducing the pull of gravity counteracts accumulated compression of bones, organs, and musculature. Lymphatic flow is stimulated, which increases drainage into the main thoracic duct, preventing toxic buildup. Inversion postures also help stimulate the pituitary, considered to be the master gland of the hormonal system, as it regulates the activities of all metabolic processes. When the pituitary gland becomes revitalized all other glands are stimulated.

- *Movement:* Movement through dance allows the expression, rather than repression, of feelings. Permitting your body to manifest what you are feeling in a complete way makes it difficult to suppress emotions. Healing energy flows through the body with greater ease the more you are in touch with your feelings.

   In the privacy of your home, put on a favorite record. Allow the words and the sounds to move through as your body connects energetically with the notes. Move in any way you like; nobody is watching, no one is judging. If it's difficult for you to move, visualizing yourself dancing and spinning freely can have beneficial effects.

Creating a Safe Zone

The more toxin-free your home, the faster your recovery will be. Cleaning up your home environment will have a positive impact on your health. The best means of reducing toxic exposures is to create a safe zone, a place you can retreat to in times of need. By keeping this environment as chemical and allergen free as possible; you can enter this space when your toxic load is high, allowing your body to repair and regroup. Since a third of your life may be spent in the bedroom, this is the logical spot to set up a safe zone.

The central furnishing of a safe bedroom should be an old innerspring mattress, one made before fireproofing laws were in effect. Some safe rooms contain nothing but a bed, as anything else carries or attracts allergens. Over time, your mattress may have become damp and moldy, becoming an excellent breeding ground for mold, dust, and dust mites.

If you decide to throw out the old mattress, be careful to avoid the new treated ones. Ideally, your new mattress should be made of untreated cotton, which can be hard to find. If you cannot find an old mattress or an untreated cotton one, encase the mattress in cotton barrier cloth to protect from outgassing fumes.[3]

Bed sheets and blankets should be undyed cotton or wool. New bed linens should be washed repeatedly to remove formaldehyde, pesticides, bleach, dye, or fixative residues found on new materials. If you are more sensitive, you may need to wash sheets daily. Frequent cleaning of sheets as well as cleaning the room itself will keep allergens to a minimum.

All furniture should be fully outgassed. This works best using old pieces, or those made of hardwood, metal, or glass. Using homemade furnishings allows you to control what ingredients go into finishing the piece. Floors should be bare, though you may choose to put down washable cotton area rugs.

Depending on your level of tolerance, the room should be devoid of books, knickknacks, and plastic materials, such as trash cans, as these objects gather dust and outgas damaging fumes. Ideally, all clothes should be removed from bedroom closets. If this is not possible, keep closet doors closed because clothes gather mold and dust and hold detergent residue that can cause reactivity. Laura, who has Crohn's, severe EI, and CFS, jokes, "My bedroom is so bare it looks like nobody lives there. I do well if it's completely clean, but if I get sloppy the first thing I notice is that I wake up tired, a sure sign I'm toxic."

Electrical devices like digital clocks should be situated away from the bed. An air purifier may assist you to heal and reduce the toxic load. Some elect to cover the heat register to prevent air that has been heated by a natural gas furnace from circulating. Closing air vents prevents and controls dust. Water-heated radiators or electric heaters are usually the least bothersome sources of heat, as there are no troublesome fumes. Sleeping with the windows open will keep the room free of gas and other odors, enabling you to feel more clear and revitalized after sleep.

Damage Control

It is of no benefit to become agitated and overwhelmed at the first hint of reactivity. This doesn't mean that you should not protect your health, but you need to be aware of how much energy you waste trying to control fatigue and reactivity. You may think that shutting down will prevent further damage, but on the contrary, it often heightens a reaction.

When you notice that you are having a reaction, first and foremost, keep breathing. Your inclination may be to hold your breath, thinking this will minimize the entrance of toxins into your body. This only closes down the healing energy your body needs to repair itself; instead, try to relax. Closing down occurs when you aren't able to separate the good healing energy from the bad. By simply allowing the emotions, such as fear and anger, to surface—allowing the reaction to take place—the experience will pass more quickly. During this time, there are things you can do to control and reduce reactivity.

The guiding principle in getting through a reaction is to aid the allergen to leave the body as quickly as possible before the reaction gets going full force. When you first notice an allergic reaction, leave the environment you are in. If you cannot leave, put on a mask and try to identify the source of the exposure. Coconut shell charcoal masks are excellent at filtering fumes.[4] If you don't have a protective mask, breathe through your mouth, rather than your nose. This helps reduce discomfort, as your mouth has fewer sensory receptors than your nose.

When you have identified the source of reactivity, isolate it away from contact. Once this is done, Laura says she immediately ingests an appropriate dose of calcium ascorbate. "E-mergen-C" produced by Alacer Corporation is a product that works well for her. This supplement also contains calcium, potassium, and magnesium and functions as a free radical scavenger, acting to quickly reduce allergic reactivity.

Alkali salts, composed of two parts sodium bicarbonate and one part potassium bicarbonate, are used by some to offset food and chemical exposures. These salts should be taken with caution by people who must monitor their sodium intake. Laura also shortens acute reactions by taking *tri-salts*, which contain buffering compounds of magnesium, potassium, and calcium, or *Alka-Seltzer Gold*, or by taking one teaspoon of baking soda in a half cup of water. She also takes Rescue Remedy, a homeopathic flower remedy that reduces the impact of stress when she is reactive. This substance, created in the 1930s by British physician Dr. Edward Bach, is commonly sold in health food stores.

Drinking several glasses of purified water helps flush toxins through the body more rapidly, and can also help induce a bowel movement. Remember, the bowel is a primary route for the exit of toxic substances, so moving your bowel helps reduce the toxic load. In addition to drinking water, the toxic burden can be relieved by consuming organic prunes, raw garlic, high doses of calcium ascorbate, or by taking a natural laxative such as psyllium husks, a natural fiber that adds bulk to the intestines.

When overloaded with toxins, you will feel better faster if you eat lightly or fast until the symptoms clear. The body thus can focus on resting and repair rather than having to also summon the energy to digest incoming food. Intake of foods, particularly those that are refined, can increase the total load, as well as prolong and intensify allergic reactions.

Mild exercise and accompanying perspiration helps increase metabolism, hastening the removal of offending antigens from the body. Scrubbing your skin with a loofah, a natural vegetable brush, helps remove dead skin cells, and increases the excretion of cellular waste. Taking a long hot bath to which you have added two cups of apple cider vinegar further aids in removal of toxins through perspiration and by changing the pH to a more alkaline level.

A bath also helps relax all systems. Once in the tub, taking deep breaths will increase oxygenation, facilitating the excretion of toxic waste. After the bath, wrap your entire body, including your head, in towels and allow yourself to continue to perspire. Laura believes that this helps pull heavy metals and other toxins out of her system.

Yawning is also useful, as it helps you relax and quickly induces the alpha state in which healing is enhanced. To help her get through more acute reactions, Laura keeps an oxygen canister in her car at all times. Adding oxygen to the bloodstream helps burn up toxins. Under the direction of a physician, epinephrine can be used to mitigate and control severe reactions.

If you are still uncomfortable, a nap allows the body to heal while you rest. Sleep also permits you to escape discomfort; you may want to "check out" during the worst of your reactivity.

Incomplete Detoxification

Even when you strictly control your environment, reduce stressors, and minimize chemical exposures, you may not be getting well. You may be doing everything by the book: following doctor's orders, adhering to a strict diet, resting copiously, yet reactions and disturbing symptoms may continue despite your best efforts toward self-protection. If this is the case, it can be frustrating and discouraging to try to figure out what to do next. Still worse, it's hard to understand why you may not be improving when others improve more rapidly. This mystery can be partially solved when you understand that you may have a problem with "internal pollution" as well as external environmental pollution.

Besides the accumulation of poisons from chemicals, the bio-accumulation of toxic residue can include vaccinations, pills, and drugs, and inherited toxic information. The intracellular system of connective tissue is intended to function to transport oxygen nutrients and waste between the cells and capillaries. This system can become plugged up and rigid because of the presence of toxins and metabolic waste, leading to reduced cellular oxygenation as well as impaired homeostatic capability.

The body is generally able to excrete water-soluble chemicals acquired through toxic exposures. However, saturated fats introduced through the diet can adversely affect the membranes of macrophages and other phagocytes, which are the large scavenger cells that patrol the bloodstream looking for foreign objects and pathogens. These large white blood cells use their sensitive membranes to bump into objects to determine if they are invaders. When these cells detect an invader or a diseased cell, they destroy it or mark it with an antigen, signaling the immune system to go into action.

Saturated fats coat the membranes of these phagocytes, causing them to lose their sensitivity as well as ability to detect invaders. Lacking this sensitivity, the cells cannot mobilize to fight viral and bacterial invaders. Once these fats are eaten, they oxidize or become rancid; as they decay, they lose electrons and form free radicals. As previously noted, when an atom loses one or more electrons, it takes electrons from neighboring atoms, causing a chain reaction that destabilizes molecules in the tissue.

The reason people often feel terrible when they lose weight is that they are losing fat, which in turn increases free radical activity. Typically, fat cells hold insecticides and heavy metals. When weight is lost, toxins are free to circulate through the bloodstream, causing an increase in symptoms. The success of the weight loss is often offset by the misery resulting from the presence of poisons in the blood, which, in turn, heightens allergic-food cravings and overall reactivity.

Fat is capable of becoming mobile through exercise, stress, increased body temperature, and physical illness as well as fasting. When the body experiences any form of stress, stored fat can be released into the bloodstream, carrying the toxins back into the system. If they are not excreted, these toxins circulate in the body and are later returned to the fatty tissue. The episodic release of fat-soluble toxins through the above-mentioned vectors may explain the ongoing reactivity you experience even when the internal and external environments are scrupulously clean.

As mentioned, toxic chemicals are stored in the fatty tissue of the body. In addition, endogenous toxins, which are the by-product of the metabolism and the defense functions of the body, accumulate in the tissues, specifically the connective tissue around blood vessels, joints, ligaments, and muscles. Understanding the characteristics of fat-soluble toxins as well as endogenous toxins may provide a clue for those who do everything right, attending to their program, yet still experience acute symptoms.

It is difficult to excrete fat-soluble toxins that accumulate in the fatty tissue of the body. The late Dr. Theron Randolph, past president of the Human Ecology Research Foundation, called this *bio-accumulation*, in which fat-soluble toxic chemicals stay locked in fatty tissue. Yet, there is an avenue to mobilize and assist these fat-stored toxic substances out of the body. Medical clinics such as the Environmental Health Center of Dallas have protocols that assist the mobilization and excretion of toxins under carefully controlled conditions. These programs offer individualized care to help mobilize fats, facilitating and maximizing the excretion process while maintaining proper biochemical and nutritional status. In this way chemicals stuck in the fat cells are mobilized, leaving the body by increasing circulation.

The mobilization of fats is assisted through cardiovascular exercise and closely monitored doses of vitamin B_3, known as nicotinic acid or niacin, along with ingestion of polyunsaturated oils, which enhance the mobilization of fats. Vitamin B_3 is known to initially block the mobilization of free fatty acids, but subsequently causes a profound mobilization of these fatty acids into the blood. Vitamin B_3 is involved in many metabolic reactions, particularly those that impact the release of energy from carbohydrates, the maintenance of a healthy digestive tract and nervous system, and healthy skin. Precise adjustment of the dosage of niacin is critical to avoid the flooding of toxins into the blood.

Exercise plus the niacin regimen increases blood circulation, assisting in the elimination of toxins. Excretion is enhanced through the skin, via sauna treatments under controlled temperatures. Along the way, water, potassium, and salts are administered to replace those lost through perspiration. Nutrients are also supplied in strict proportion to the dose of niacin.

During the physical therapy portion of the program, the chemicals stored in the fatty tissue are released into the bloodstream and excreted, rather than being allowed to be reabsorbed. The subsequent mobilization of these toxic chemicals may cause an exacerbation of symptoms, but this is a transitory state, and one can look forward to improved health.

Theresa, who continued to exhibit unexplained symptoms of reactivity not related to external agents, undertook this program and experienced excellent results. It can also benefit those who have high levels of toxic chemicals, reducing the total load of those who have undergone acute or chronic exposures. During the program, Theresa had to follow the exact protocol, get adequate sleep, and maintain her regular strict diet. She was there 40 days, although the length of treatment varies depending on the toxicity of the individual, averaging about 25 days.

Under the guidance of your health practitioner, the general concepts of mobilization of fat-soluble toxins can be applied to your own personal healing program. This information offers clues as to how you can promote physiological elimination of waste through enhanced circulation, excretion and avoidance of fat-soluble foods that bind with fatty tissue.

Skin Care

Toxins are absorbed not only through your nose and intestines, but also through your skin. Inhalation takes place through your skin as part of the normal respiratory process. If your skin cannot breathe properly, the transfer of essential nutrients will not occur. The more toxic your environment, the more crucial it is to maximize skin hygiene, which is tremendously important to the removal of toxic matter. There are several simple things you can do to enhance the respiratory capability of your skin.

The skin is an organ of respiration and elimination, and brushing it keeps the pores clear, which assists in detoxification. Scrubbing your skin with a natural bristle bath brush or dry loofah, a natural abrasive vegetable sponge, on a daily basis removes dead cells so your pores can take in the oxygen the skin needs. Elaine finds this particularly useful when seeking relief from a toxic headache. Moving the brush in a circular motion toward the heart also enhances circulation to the extremities, drawing the flow of blood away from your head.

As you scrub, you have the chance to draw your attention in a loving manner to all parts of your body, taking time to nurture yourself. How about taking time to brush your skin awake in the morning instead of drinking a cup of coffee? Rubbing the loofah all over will cause you to feel alert and more awake.

When feeling tired, the loofah can energize you past the fatigue and tension, often releasing blocked energy. In addition, this process increases skin elasticity and helps break down cellulite. To further facilitate this release you may wish to refer to the next section. Combining the loofah scrub with a detox bath and deep breathing can heighten relaxation and bring energizing relief from discomfort.

Detox Baths

Your relationship to water has a powerful influence over your mental and physical well-being. The majority of your body is comprised of water so your affinity for it is based on survival as well as nurturance. Water cleanses toxins from the blood and tissues and carries them out through the kidneys, lungs, bowel, and skin. Water heals wounds by stimulating circulation, which drains away bacteria, dead cells, and pus, permitting the process of tissue repair to take place in a clean environment.

The body depends on water for digestion, elimination, circulation, and the movement of nutrients and toxins. Drinking eight glasses of purified water daily replenishes you and keeps the waters of life flowing. Flushing the system moves toxins that would otherwise accumulate in the fat cells, muscles, and joints. This doesn't mean drinking coffee or sodas, though, as these water-based drinks have a dehydrating effect.

Many of us are at our happiest when around water. So when you feel poorly, you may seek remedies that have some relationship to water. You may use water as a means of cleansing yourself, physically, emotionally, and spiritually. When you're hot, tired, or irritable, cooling off in the shower or in a lake or pool restores you. Cold water awakens and vitalizes and hot water relaxes and penetrates into your core.

Have you noticed that it's nearly impossible to remain tense in hot water? Though not always used humanely, hydrotherapy was once used in mental hospitals to facilitate the relaxation of inmates. They had the right idea, but forced relaxation is self-defeating. When used properly, it can be a benevolent healing force. Temporarily overheating the body stimulates the immune system, increasing the number and mobility of white blood cells.

Allowing your body to soak and sweat by sitting in a tub, sauna, or steam room will increase relaxation, improve circulation, as well as help eliminate pollutants. Hyperthermia is safe for most adults, but those who are pregnant, or who suffer from high blood pressure, or diabetes should seek their physician's approval before starting these baths.

In addition to being relaxing, the heat of a tub bath may also cause the release of endorphins and boost immunity. Perspiration generally reduces the acuity of symptoms because it relaxes the body and reduces the toxic load. In addition, with CFS, the process of perspiring can greatly reduce night sweats that interfere with sleep.

Spending time in the bathtub offers one of the easiest, least expensive ways to rejuvenate and detoxify and achieve symptomatic relief. Tub soaks work best if you submerge as much of your body as possible in water for 20 to 60 minutes. Drinking water during and after the bath helps prevent dehydration, fatigue, and muscle weakness. The benefits of this experience can be further enhanced by taking a nap or meditating immediately afterwards.

When you take a bath, you may place an inflatable pillow or towel under your head. If you wish, take your bath by candlelight. Some prefer to read, chant, listen to music, practice breath-work, or meditate. Sherry, who has EI, climbs into her enormous Japanese bath and does Reiki on herself, heightening the positive effects. Soak for at least 20 minutes: the longer you remain, the more effective the results. Be sure to shower afterwards to remove toxins that may cling to the skin; if you don't, they can be reabsorbed. The following are several types of healing baths.

Apple Cider Vinegar Baths

The apple cider vinegar bath aids in general systemic detoxification. The vinegar helps alleviate itchy skin and soothes sore muscles. In addition, vinegar helps balance the pH of the hair and skin and helps kill fungal overgrowth. Pour 1 to 4 cups of pure, unprocessed apple cider vinegar in a tub filled with hot water. The ideal temperature is about 96 to 98 degrees, though some prefer hotter.

Sea Salt and Baking Soda Soaks

The combination of sea salt and baking soda in a bath assists the body to detoxify from heavy metals and radiation exposure. Like vinegar, baking soda helps restore the skin's acid balance. Though vinegar is acidic, and baking soda is strongly alkali, both relieve itchy skin. This is Laura's favorite soak, greatly improving her sense of well-being.

She places 1 pound of sea salt and 1 pound of baking soda in hot water. Rock salt and ordinary table salt are depleted of minerals and thus are less effective ingredients in a soak. With this soak, you will perspire more than usual so be careful when getting out of the tub; stand up slowly to avoid becoming dizzy.

Our bodies are continuously exposed to x-rays and radioactive substances, which have damaging, cumulative effects. When Jamie's brother underwent radiation and chemotherapy for cancer, he was advised by his radiologist to perform this soak. It is thought that these baths help draw radioactive matter out of the tissue.

Epsom Salt Soaks

Heavy exposure to auto exhaust calls for an Epsom salt bath to help remove the residue. Epsom salt baths also help detoxify other heavy metals, including mercury, lead, aluminum, and arsenic. All of these substances are poisons that interfere with the balance of health. This soak is taken by pouring 1 pound or more of the salt in the tub with the water up to your chin, soaking for at least 20 minutes.

Powdered Ginger Soaks

Add between 1 teaspoon and 1 tablespoon of powdered ginger into the bath. This will ease sore, aching muscles and help warm the body. Start with a smaller amount of ginger at first, becoming accustomed to its warming effects. This is a good soak for those who have trouble with body temperature and for those fighting off the flu.

Following any of these baths you can enhance the mobilization of toxins if you don't dry off, but instead wrap your body in towels from head to toe when you get out of the tub and then lie down. The insulation of the towels creates its own steam bath, allowing you to relax while perspiring profusely which enables more damaging materials to leave your system. This procedure is much like the treatments that health spas offer, without the expense.

If you are particularly daring, you may want to shower in cold water after the soak, which will cause your pores to slam shut. So long as you don't have cardiac problems, cold water is invigorating and good for the heart, causing the muscle to contract more forcibly. Alternating between hot and cold water also increases circulation and reduces swelling, inflammation, and pain.

The healing qualities of these experiences are heightened by the fact that you are taking care of yourself. The act of self-nurturing is an invitation to healing and gives you a growing a sense of control, which is one of the keys to increased wellness.

One word of caution: Our skin readily absorbs toxins such as chlorine, chloroform, and trichlorethylene (associated with cancer, heart disease, and other illnesses) from tap water. Scientists now believe hot showers and baths are the most common source of exposure to these toxins. For this reason, the use of a filter to remove chlorine from the water is recommended, or such soaks might be toxifying rather than detoxifying.

Naps and Sleep

Sleep is a powerful healer. We seek refuge and release in sleep when all other interventions fail to bring relief. There is a biochemical link between deep sleep and the function of cells of the immune system. A variety of chemicals trigger slow-wave sleep and activate the immune system.[5] The most frequently noted sleep abnormalities in CFS include: awake-type brain waves which intrude into deep sleep and a high number of nocturnal awakenings.[6]

With sleep, the body is able to repair and rest, enabling damaged tissue or toxic organs to rejuvenate. Achieving normal, restful sleep is a serious problem for those with EI and CFS and may be one of the most important symptoms to manage, because good rest is needed for the body to be able to repair itself and because of the overall impact fatigue has on the rest of your life.

Theresa, who has EI, says that when she has been exposed to toxic fumes, she may go without sleep for days. Even when utterly exhausted, many with CFS are only able to sleep a few hours at a time, often awakening at night for no apparent reason. And nearly all people with CFS wake up unrefreshed in the morning. Though the illness requires that you devote much time to rest, quality sleep can be elusive, causing ongoing exhaustion. Despite the difficulties CFS victims have in achieving refreshed sleep, naps and rest can alleviate pain and discomfort.

Let's talk about naps first. It is difficult to openly declare a fondness for naps. You may hear others furtively describe their napping habits, lest they be considered lazy or unproductive. Don't be ashamed if you are in the habit of napping. Many people think naps spoil their ability to sleep at night; yet naps offer the perfect opportunity for those with EI and CFS to achieve relief. Josh, the oncology nurse with CFS, says naps help relieve his joint and muscle pain better than taking painkilling medications. Naps offer temporary, blessed release from grave discomfort, releasing you into oblivion and removing you from the scene. This kind of sanctuary also gives your awareness a rest so you can come back to reality refueled and nourished.

CFS disturbs sleep patterns, making it necessary to nap to get through the day. Rest and sleep as much as you need to. If you are having extreme problems, you may need to further accommodate your body's preferred sleep pattern, rather than forcing yourself to adhere to a conventional schedule. Eventually, as you become stronger you may need to force yourself to normalize your sleep habits by staying awake during the day and allowing only brief rest periods.

When you do sleep, the quality of the experience may not be very satisfying. Lying awake for hours at a time trying to achieve rest can be as disturbing as the fatigue itself. Sleep that is disturbed affects immune function and can produce symptoms similar to CFS, as unrefreshed sleep heightens pain and psychological disturbance.

Traditional medicine offers tranquilizers such as Xanax and Valium for short-term relief. However, the *standard dose* of antidepressant medication often leaves persons with EI and CFS more fatigued and depressed than helped. *Small doses* of an antidepressant can improve sleep and reduce pain. Examples of useful antidepressants include Sinequan, Elavil, Pamelor, and Prozac.

Melatonin, a hormone secreted by the pineal gland, has been noted to be of benefit in treating sleeping difficulties. The body produces melatonin in a rhythmic fashion, less during the day and more at night. The secretion of melatonin is believed to be driven by the body's circadian pacemaker in the hypothalamus. Since melatonin plays a role in regulating the sleep–wake cycle, it has been of benefit for those with sleep disturbances.

Sleep supportive interventions may include adjusting your body temperature through exercise and hot baths before retiring, as a drop in body temperature can facilitate sleep. You may also want to adjust the room temperature and noise level of the surrounding area to heighten relaxation. Some foods such as carbohydrates can bring on sleepiness and relaxation. A little warm milk or an herbal tea can help too. Other measures to promote sleep include herbs such as valerian, passion flower, skullcap, hops, and kava; the amino acid L-tryptophan (now available by prescription); magnesium; and homeopathic remedies.

Elaine says, "The fastest way for me to get to sleep is to read a really boring, technical book, one that I have to pay attention to. That puts me out." If you still cannot sleep, get out of bed and use the time to do something you wouldn't otherwise do. These efforts to force yourself to stay awake can make you drowsy.

The brain requires sleep to relax and restore itself. Meditation, progressive relaxation, and attention to the breath have a calming effect on the mind, reducing the level of neurological overstimulation. While these efforts may not induce sleep, they offer a certain degree of quality rest.

Josh says, "When at my worst, overwhelmed with discomfort that nothing could alleviate, sleep always brought relief." Most of the time it is possible to sleep and wake up renewed, with symptoms reduced or gone. Sometimes it's even hard to recall how awful you felt. Being able to retreat from discomfort is a helpful opportunity that allows the body to be recharged.

Restoration of Healthy Flora of the Gastrointestinal Tract

Your body hosts over 100 trillion bacteria, most of which are necessary to sustain health. The sheer number of intestinal microflora enables you to adapt to the diversity of matter that it may encounter in order to respond to changes in diet, environmental microorganisms, and climate. The presence of beneficial bacteria in the intestines aids digestion, synthesizes vitamins, and inhibits the growth of disease-promoting pathogenic bacteria.

A potent means of maintaining overall health is to keep the environment of the bowel properly balanced. In the healthy body, *Candida albicans* and acidophilus compete for space in the digestive tract. This competition helps keep candida from taking over and getting out of control. Factors that influence the resident flora include: antibiotics, alcohol, refined foods including sugar, excessive intake of red meat, pesticide and herbicide residues found in fruits and vegetables, and chemicals such as chlorine found in drinking water. Some raw vegetables also contain natural compounds that can inhibit the implanting of microflora.

Antibiotics tend to be overused and have damaging effects, primarily altering the intestinal flora. When you take antibiotics you successfully kill off harmful bacteria; at the same time this alters the intestinal environment, removing healthy bacteria as well. Once the walls of the intestines are stripped of healthy organisms, candida, staphylococci, and *Clostridium difficile* can proliferate, leading to sepsis, infection, diarrhea, and colitis. To prevent candida overgrowth, probiotics such as *Lactobacillus acidophilus* can be taken several days before ending an antibiotic regimen.

Asking your body to subsist on foods that it cannot digest causes changes in microflora to the extent that it cannot produce enzymes that help extract nutrients from food. Eating certain cultured, fermented foods can help increase digestive capability. Adding microflora to the diet helps boosts the immune system, inhibits the growth of pathogens, detoxifies and protects against toxins, and synthesizes vitamins.

Procedure for Restoring Intestinal Flora

The following procedure, used by Jamie to help resolve chronic candida problems, aids in restoring and maintaining intestinal balance. She says it should be followed for five consecutive days. During this time do not drink milk or eat meat, sugar, sugar substitutes, or honey. After this, she suggests restricting intake of sugar, processed foods, and alcohol for several months.

1. Take one capsule of a potent combination of acidophilus and *Bacillus laterosporus* supplement on an empty stomach before bed and before breakfast. Taken in combination, they replenish the lower and upper digestive tract.
2. Next take two tablespoons of lemon juice with a glass of water three times a day: after dinner, before bed, and before breakfast.
3. At the same time take:

    a. Two capsules of "oil of garlic"
    b. One tablet of zinc 30 mg
    c. Two grams of vitamin C (ascorbic acid or sodium ascorbate)

4. Twice a day, between the above scheduled times, drink two tablespoons of lemon juice in a small glass of water, accompanied by a small serving of plain unsugared, unflavored yogurt. (According to Jamie, Alta-Dena, Mountain High, or Brown Cow are best.)
5. On a daily basis, drink food-grade, whole-leaf aloe vera juice, which cleanses the digestive tract and reduces inflammation, permitting the damaged tissue of the bowel to repair.

When you first take acidophilus, you may note increased gas, which signifies that the healthy flora is regaining dominance over pathogenic microorganisms. Ongoing efforts to sustain the flora of the bowel by taking lactobacillus-acidophilus and aloe vera juice, as well as efforts to reduce the total yeast population may be necessary. Elaine reports that the brands Flora Balance and Lateroflora helped resolve her bowel and digestive problems. The benefits of healing the bowel include a reduction of allergic reactions, resolution of gastrointestinal symptoms, and often the ability to reintroduce some foods that previously caused allergic reactions.

Liver Detoxification

The liver detoxifies all potentially harmful substances in the body, extracting poisons and thereby enabling all other organs to function efficiently. Because of its essential role in detoxification, it is important that the liver function at optimal levels. If your energy is at a low ebb, it may mean your liver is having trouble doing its job. Liver detoxification can optimize its capabilities, improving overall health and giving you more energy.

One such intervention adapted below is "The Liver Flush," recommended by Christopher Hobbs, herbalist and botanist, in his book *Natural Liver Therapy* (Capitola: Botanica Press, 1995). This procedure can be undertaken at the change of each season for 10 days or as often as desired. It stimulates the elimination of wastes from the body, increases the flow of bile, and improves overall liver function. This flush also helps purify the blood and lymph.

The Liver Flush

1. Mix fresh-squeezed citrus juices together to make 1 cup of liquid. Orange and grapefruit work well, but always include lemon or lime. The more sour the taste, the more cleansing and activating the mixture. You may want to dilute to taste with distilled water.

2. Add 1–2 cloves of fresh-squeezed garlic, along with a small amount of fresh-squeezed ginger juice, obtained by grating ginger on a cheese grater and pressing the fibers in a garlic press.

3. Add 1 tablespoon of quality olive oil, shake well, and drink.

4. Follow the flush with 2 cups of cleansing tea such as Polari-Tea or premade Puri-Tea.

5. Polari-Tea is made with equal parts of fennel, fenugreek, flax, and peppermint, along with one-quarter part licorice and one-quarter part burdock root, simmered for 20 minutes and steeped for 10. These herbs can be purchased at herb and health food stores.

6. Drink this flush in the morning and don't eat any other food for 1 hour.

To amplify the cleansing action, you may wish to fast, drinking fresh fruit and vegetable juices. Christopher Hobbs also mentions taking an enema of one-half a lemon mixed with one quart of tepid distilled water, retaining it for 10 to 15 minutes if possible. Lemon juice is an excellent cleanser because citric acid in the juice binds with and removes heavy metals and toxic matter accumulated in the body. Hobbs's excellent book also mentions "The Gallbladder Flush," a technique for those who have had previous experience with cleansing programs and want to remove deeper levels of waste stored in liver cells, the gallbladder, and other tissue.

Summary

This chapter offers helpful information on new options in coping with your health, including tools that may allow you to get adequate rest, ways that you can energize your body, and several pointers that can optimize the detoxification and healing process. Key to health is assisting your body in the process of mobilizing and releasing toxins and protecting it from further harm.

Endnotes

[1]Kimberly Kenney, ed., "Breathing," *The CFIDS Chronicle* Winter 1995: 31.

[2]Richard Gerber, *Vibrational Healing* (Santa Fe: Bear & Co., 1988) 306–324.

[3]For barrier cloth and less toxic household products, contact Allergy Resources, P.O. Box 444, Gussey, CO 80820, (800) USE-FLAX.

[4]For information regarding custom-made face masks, contact Sandra DenBraber, RN, 144 Ray St., Arlington, TX 76010, (817) 860-9299.

[5]R. Ornstein and A. Sobel, *Healthy Pleasures* (Reading: Addison–Wesley, 1990) 121.

[6]"Is Your Central Nervous System Over-Reacting?" *Fibromyalgia Network* Apr. 1995: 4–5.

Part
Three

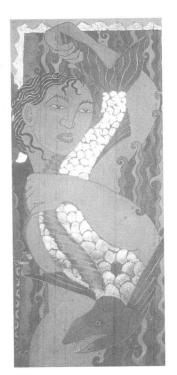

What Helps

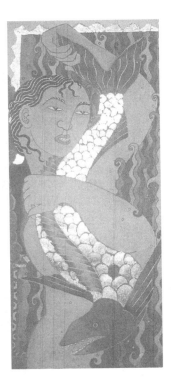

Chapter
Nine

Dietary Habits

*t*here are growing concerns about the quality of our food supply. Foods are treated with synthetic chemicals of all kinds. Over a billion pounds of pesticides, containing over 600 EPA-registered ingredients, is sprayed on U.S. food crops each year.[1]

Studies show that 95 to 99% of all toxic chemicals in the American diet comes from meat, fish, dairy products, and eggs.[2] Because animal flesh is high on the food chain, it often contains high levels of contaminants such as pesticides and herbicides that have been consumed by the animal. Animal flesh is also contaminated by a variety of drugs such as hormones, stimulants, and antibiotics used to speed growth and combat infectious diseases.

Meat is also typically hard to digest; as a result, it does not supply you with much energy, but rather drains you by forcing your digestive system to work extra hard. A dietary intake that is high in protein burdens the liver, GI tract, and kidneys. Dairy products, also high on the food chain, may contain unsafe levels of environmental contaminants,[3] and are a significant source of allergic reactivity.

Then, there's the problem every community is struggling with: what to do with toxic sewage sludge. John Stauber, coauthor of *Toxic Sludge is Good for You*

(Monroe: Common Courage, 1995), notes, "Rather than deal with sludge as a toxic waste, the sewage industry and the EPA for the last fifteen years have gotten behind a P.R. campaign to simply rename it bio-solids and promote spreading it on food crops. Unfortunately the EPA which is supposed to be protecting the environment and the health of citizens living in the environment is working hand-in-hand with the sewage industry to promote sewage-sludge fertilizer."[4] What's in toxic sludge? It's a semisolid mixture of viral, bacterial, protozoal, and parasite-laden waste material which also includes heavy metals, pesticides, and polychlorinated biphenyls (PCBs). This waste-ridden material, when used as fertilizer, seeps into and becomes a part of the food you eat.

The food industry is also trying to figure out how to remove the enzymes from foods such as fruits and vegetables in order to increase their shelf life.[5] If you recall, consuming foods depleted of enzymes requires your body to render its finite enzyme stores to the digestive process, thereby taxing your health. You may wonder how it is that foods are being altered and how these harmful substances are knowingly allowed into our food and water supply. Large industries hold tremendous persuasive sway with government sources and their lobbyists and public relations firms are able to sell products such as cigarettes to the public despite known health risks.

Understanding the cause-and-effect relationship between diet and disease will hopefully compel you to make dietary changes. When you make these changes, you will most likely not be able to look to your physician for supportive information. Physicians seldom emphasize nutrition as an essential aspect of medical care; on the average they receive less than three hours of nutritional training during their four years of medical school.[6]

The presence of food additives and food contaminants has become a significant source of concern for the immune-compromised individual. For those who are struggling to boost their immune system, it is necessary to understand the sources of chemical contamination in the food you eat. The purpose of this chapter is to explore what you can do to counteract the impact of these harmful substances in foods.

Healthy Dietary Habits

Everything you eat has ramifications in every aspect of your life. Mental and spiritual awareness has its seeds firmly planted in the healthfulness of the food you consume and when your body is healthy there is no limit to what you can accomplish with your life. There is so much about the workings of your body that you probably take for granted until you lose your health. Cleaning up your diet may be the single most important thing you can do to help yourself get well. In addition, it is the primary factor you can actively control in order to influence your health.

Life-Taking Foods

Ingestion of foods high in fat such as potato chips and fried fish can impair immune function. These foods, being empty calories, create nutritional imbalance and can set the stage for illness. It is also more difficult to digest healthy foods after you have consumed devitalized ones. Convenience and flavor may be more important than nutritional considerations, at least until you become sick.

A diet high in saturated fats causes these substances to accumulate in the cell membranes, making the cells rigid and less permeable to oxygen. Eating excessive fat causes the body to store toxins, which diminishes immune function and accelerates aging. This storage of fat can be a source of chronic fatigue, as the body holds unnecessary excess weight and fat-soluble toxins remain trapped in the tissues. Excessive intake of cholesterol and fatty foods also leads to heightened rancidity and can cause the production of an excess of free radicals.

It can be a challenge to avoid eating simple sugars, such as white refined sugar, brown sugar, honey, corn syrup, and fruit juices; it is a hidden ingredient in most processed foods. Sugar is good for the food industry because it stimulates the appetite, causing you to want to eat more, even when you are full. Simple sugar also encourages the growth of streptococcal bacteria and leads to elevated blood fats in some people.[7] Foods high in sugar, such as ice cream and candy bars, also promote mucus, making you more susceptible to viral and bacterial invasion.

The most frequently used noncaloric additive is salt, an important mineral that, if taken in too large an amount can have an adverse impact on blood pressure, and tax the kidneys and heart. Sulfites, commonly used to prevent discoloration and spoilage, and monosodium glutamate (MSG), found in a large number of foods, can prompt allergic reactivity, and may be primary culprits in attention-deficit disorders. There are also reports that MSG may cause brain damage.[8] Tartazine, or Yellow dye No. 5, is a coloring agent that is known to cause itching, and asthma in people who are sensitive, and is found in sodas, ice creams, desserts, salad dressings, and other products.

One of the newest concerns is about the deliberate irradiation of foods. Irradiation of foods is what is being done with nuclear waste because the country does not know where to store these materials,[9] and foods exposed to these wastes will absorb them.

The effects of these foods, additives, and chemicals on the body are just now being understood. The US Public Interest Research Group warns, "Sixty-nine different pesticides linked to cancer are legally allowed on food, thirty-two of these are not detectable by FDA's routine monitoring methods, and thirty carcinogens are among 118 pesticides found in food by the FDA in their 1988 food monitoring."[10]

Unsuspectingly, you have probably trusted farmers, industry, and the government to market foods that sustain life, when in fact much of our traditional diet is replete with life-taking substances. Aside from processed, canned, packaged, and frozen foods, many farm-grown, "natural" products have been sprayed with or grown in toxic materials.

So much of what we eat has been stripped of nutrients. In the interest of selling foods that stimulate and thrill the senses, most processed foods are low in nutrition and high in calories and salt. Small wonder it is so hard to recover from EI and CFS with a steady diet of devitalized foods. When you are sick, continuing to eat processed refined foods means putting lifeless matter into your body and forcing it to work harder, as it takes more energy to digest, metabolize, and process these substances. The intake of refined food also reduces the quality and amount of body-building materials necessary for your body to heal. Not only do they deplete you of vital nutrients, but they also fill you with damaging substances such as antibiotics, pesticides, and fumigants.

Many processed foods—frozen, canned, preserved, and those filled with synthetic ingredients—are considered to be the standard, normal fare. After having been raised on synthetic foods, fresh, whole foods may seem strange to the average person. Fortunately there is a growing awareness of the need for foods that are organic and chemically clean.

Excessive quantities of refined carbohydrates are stored in the body as fat whereas healthy carbohydrates make up nearly our entire source of energy. A diet high in complex carbohydrates, including fruits, grains, and vegetables, can be easily translated by the body into energy. Complex carbohydrates should be your primary source of calories.

Foods that Give Life

Ordinarily, people are pleased with themselves if they eat an occasional fresh vegetable or fruit. Rarely do they suspect that those foods cause any problems, but the pesticides found on them can be causing harm. With EI and CFS there is often a swift and clear correlation between ingestion of unhealthy foods, reactive symptoms, and energy loss. Still, it may take time to realize how far out of balance your body is if you are able to get away with eating whatever you want.

By reeducating your taste buds you can enjoy a diet that is lower on the food chain and more supportive of your overall health. The more you are able to trace your fatigue and allergic reactivity to the processed and pesticide-coated foods you consume, the easier it will be to change your dietary habits. The more you work at conscious, conscientious consumption, the more you will notice improved health as you make the transition into a mostly vegetarian diet.

Making changes all at once will be a traumatic shift that can be doomed to fail. You cannot undo a lifetime of habit all at once. Setting a personal goal to educate yourself about the foods you are consuming will make it difficult to continue making selections solely for convenience or financial savings. Don't rely on the media to tell you what is good for you, because what you are told is often in direct contradiction with reality. Look further, even when you are told that a food is natural or organic.

Set a goal in the first 6 months to stop eating dairy products. Next, make the transition away from meats. Notice what foods make you feel whole and alive. If you are too sick to eat most foods, you may need to make abrupt changes. Over time, if you go back to old habits, what you eat may have a swift, ruthless effect on your health.

Food is the fuel of life that can give you vibrant health. When you eat live foods, you absorb those positive qualities. A good rule of thumb in deciding what to eat is: the more recently the food has been alive, the more life-giving nutrients it will have to fuel your body. Foods that have been cooked, purified, processed, packaged, or canned are essentially dead. The longer their shelf life, the more dead they are.

Develop the habit of reading the labels on all processed foods and think twice about eating anything that has a list of ingredients. Allergic sensitivities are often the result of reactivity to the preservatives and "extras" in foods. An organic apple or carrot doesn't come with a list; you know what you are putting into your body.

The late Dr. Theron Randolph, an EI specialist, advises that people with chemical sensitivities eat only organically grown uncontaminated foods.[11] Organic foods grown without hormones and pesticides are ideal because they are as whole and alive as possible. These foods tend to be expensive, but they have little chemical contamination and will help lower your body's chemical burden.

While eating organic foods is a good idea, be aware that some organic farmers use insecticides, some of which are required by law.[12] Only farms and produce stores offering truly organically grown foods are considered safe; but the best way to know if foods are organically grown is to grow them yourself. At farmers markets springing up all around the country, the foods grown locally by small farmers have a better chance of being "safe."

Eat as purely as possible. Uncooked raw foods are ideal, as they contain the most nutrition. When you steam, bake, broil, fry, stew, or microwave foods, most of the enzymes are destroyed. However, raw foods can be difficult to digest and tend to make the body cold. Some foods are more easily digested and give you more energy if they are lightly steamed. Steaming foods accentuates the delicate, subtle flavors and is the best way to cook, as water-soluble vitamins and minerals are retained.

Microwave safety has yet to be verified, but there are concerns regarding the frequency of leakage around the door seal. Some physicians are discouraging patients from microwave use because of evidence of nutritional deterioration, citing that the healthful qualities of the foods are destroyed. Microwaveable plastic wrap can leach chemicals into food. Aluminum, copper, and Teflon cookware should also be avoided because these materials leach into the food.

Diet and Acid–Alkaline Balance

Illness often happens when the body is too toxic, and therefore too acidic. It is necessary to restore the acid/alkaline, pH balance in order to rebalance your internal chemistry. Consuming foods that make the body alkaline results in the optimal pH for body function and for beneficial bacteria in the bowel to flourish.

The acid–alkaline balance of the body is measured by the pH, or presence of hydrogen ions. The pH of an area of the body varies according to whether a fluid such as the blood or a particular digestive enzyme is present. Maintaining the proper pH is very important to your health. If a pH level is abnormal, digestive enzymes are inactivated, food is not digested properly, and allergic reactions result.

Foods are categorized as to whether they are *acid-forming* or *alkaline-forming*, terms referring to the pH in the body after digestion of the particular food. Foods that contain a predominance of acid elements, such as sulfur, phosphorus, choline, and iodine, are acid-forming. Foods that contain large amounts of sodium, potassium, calcium, magnesium, and iron are considered to be alkaline-producing. Acid-forming foods are not the same as those that contain acid, such as citrus fruits.

The serum pH is slightly alkaline, 7.4, and should be kept constant. The closer your body is to this optimal value, the more oxygenated it is. The more alkaline the body, the less likely that candida, viruses, and bacteria will grow. An acid state is commonly caused by a diet high in protein.

The best way to control pH is through diet. Optimally 80% of your diet should include alkaline foods such as fruits and vegetables, and 20% should be made up of acid foods such as grains, seeds, and nuts instead of meat, dairy, and egg products.[13] If the diet consists of too many acid foods such as dairy, meat, beans, fats, poultry, cooked grains, and protein, the body becomes too acid. If you eat too many alkaline foods such as fruits and vegetables, the body becomes too alkaline.

If your pH is too acid, add more vegetables and raw fruits and decrease the amount of protein and fats. If it is too alkaline, your ability to digest proteins may be impaired, or you may not be eating enough protein. Ultimately you must find the proper balance that allows you to feel most comfortable. Some people with parasite and candida problems have found monitoring of pH to be helpful in restoring health. Testing the pH of urine and saliva is a simple process that can serve as indicators of your acid–base balance.

Healing Diets

At one time there were no foods Selima, who is recovering from EI, could eat without becoming reactive. Despite her efforts to eliminate offending foods, the more restrictive her diet, the more sensitive and vigilant her immune response became. Mealtimes were a trial, and eating left her nauseated, bloated, and depleted. Consuming small quantities of new foods not previously a part of her diet helped reduce reactivity because her body had not built up allergic responsiveness.

Even today she can only eat organic foods and she still has problems. If she has millet cereal in the morning and later has even a mouthful more, she becomes ill. As a rule, she cannot eat the same food until several days have passed and cannot combine two different foods in the same meal. Lunch may consist of a bowl of steamed beets. If she tries to mix broccoli with the beets, she risks a severe reaction. There's no leeway for her to cheat.

At first when you clean up your diet, you will have trouble cheating. Eating any reactive food may cause old symptoms to return. When you are more acutely ill, the line between health and reactivity is narrowly circumscribed; as you become healthier, the boundary becomes more liberal. In time you may be able to get away with more dietary transgressions, but it is deceptively easy to slide back into old eating habits.

As you become healthier, you may be able to tolerate less healthy foods, occasionally splurging without distress. But, making this a habit will cause you to lose energy and mental acuity. If you do splurge, enjoy every minute of it; self-criticism while eating a "no-no" may cause as much damage as the food itself.

Going back to eating "normal" foods may pose new, unexpected difficulties: your digestive system may be so cleaned out by pure foods that everything else may be seen as a foreign invader. The immune system then mobilizes to fight off these foods the same way it would react to a bacterial or viral invasion. Even organic foods can receive an unfriendly reception. Ongoing reactivity of this sort depletes your body when it is constantly fighting off the very thing it needs to repair and mend.

Josh adheres to "the Zone" diet outlined in Barry Sears's book, *Enter the Zone* (New York: Regan, 1995). This diet, good for those with autoimmune disease and chronic fatigue, advocates a Zone-favorable diet that involves calculating your specific body requirements for proteins, carbohydrates, and fats, maintaining them in a constant ratio. The Zone-favorable diet only restricts high-density, high-glycemic carbohydrates such as breads, pasta, rice, grains, and other starches; along with protein sources rich in arachidonic acid, an unhealthy dietary fat found in egg yolks, fatty red meat, and organ meats.

Remaining within "the Zone" is not about adhering to strict dietary limits, but rather about controlling hormonal responses and insulin levels. Every time you eat, you begin a flooding of hormone activation. This diet can help you control this activation. "Within a week of undertaking the Zone diet I felt an enormous increase in energy," notes Josh. You can also access technical support by phone if you have any questions or difficulties with the diet.[14]

When you have multiple food sensitivities, you may need to restrict your diet; yet there is currently no general, all-purpose diet identified as being better than another. Dietary restrictions can be an austere but necessary step to accelerate your healing. Two diets effective in treating allergies are the *elimination* and *rotary diversified* diets, examined next.

Elimination Diet

The elimination diet is the most accurate, least expensive way to determine if a food is causing allergic symptoms. This diet consists of foods that are the least likely to cause allergic reactions and should emphasize brown rice, sweet potatoes, winter squash, and grains such as millet, items not typically consumed. Cooked peaches, cranberries, apricots, papaya, plums, prunes, and cherries can be eaten freely, but no citrus fruits are allowed. Cooking these fruits alters the proteins, making them less likely to cause allergic reactivity. Cooked beets, greens such as chard and kale, summer squash, carrots, artichokes, celery, string beans, asparagus, spinach, and lettuce are permitted. All spices are excluded and purified or spring water is the only beverage permitted.

After restricting your dietary intake for 7 days, your sensitivity to foods should be reduced. Then gradually reintroduce foods, one at a time, on an empty stomach to determine which cause allergic reactions. Each reintroduced food should be consumed in large amounts three times a day for 2 days. If you do not have a reaction, you can consider that food safe. Reactions usually occur within a few hours of ingestion, but some don't show up for several days. Each food should be tested individually; don't add two foods at once.

If you do have an allergic reaction to a particular food, you must wait 4 days before testing the next food, allowing that substance to clear out of your system. Start with foods in a particular food group, such as vegetables, then move to fruits, and later onto grains. Once you clarify sources of reactivity, you can eliminate or restrict intake. Since your body is no longer busy reacting, it can attend to rest and repair.

The Rotary Diversified Diet

People who get well learn to diversify their diet, which means eating foods other than repeated favorites. Most likely, the foods you seldom eat are the ones that are the safest for you, because you haven't built up antibodies that call the immune system into action. Clinical ecologists recommend the rotary diet to help eliminate and prevent food allergies and addictions.

With this diet the same food is consumed no more than one day out of four. Since it takes up to 4 days to clear a food out of the intestinal tract, this allows a long enough interval to reduce toxic overload. In this way, the body can fully recover from the impact of a food before it is ingested again. You may have to completely eliminate foods that cause the most allergic reactivity, usually the ones you think you can't live without.

Initially, the foods you eat should be ones that don't cause troublesome reactions. If you are allergic to one food family, odds are you'll have problems with foods in the same family. Food families include: fruits, vegetables, specific grains, nuts, seeds, meat, fish, or fowl. For example, if you react to walnuts, it is more likely that you will be reactive to foods in the nut family.

On this diet eat three meals a day, ingesting as much as desired. If you follow a 4-day rotation, you can eat a particular food on Monday and then eat it again on Friday. Most people regain tolerance for foods after a period of avoidance, yet the greater the reaction to the food, the longer this can take. Until there is greater tolerance, it may be advised to avoid the food completely. Once the diet is stabilized, you can gradually add new foods. This diet is helpful in reducing reactivity and preventing new allergic reactions and the variety offered by rotation helps reduce the strain on the immune and enzyme detoxification systems.

Whole Live Foods

Consuming raw foods may enable you to feel more energetic and productive. When you consume fresh foods, your digestive system extracts the healthy juices from the fiber; the life force from these enzyme-filled foods offers greater life energy to each atom of your body so that it can repel disease. The best sources of live foods are raw vegetables, fresh fruits, germinated seeds and nuts, grains, sea vegetables, and freshly made juices. It should be noted that a diet completely filled with raw foods may not necessarily be best for everyone; but once you get in the raw food habit, you may notice positive effects.

Other food sources that should be considered for your diet include wheat grass, algae, and kimchi. Fresh wheat grass juice contains chlorophyll and live enzymes and destroys harmful bacteria in the digestive tract while ridding the body of waste matter and toxins. This juice is an excellent energizer, but the taste may take some getting used to. Algae, including spirulina, chlorella, and blue-green algae, are densely packed complete foods that contain proteins, carbohydrates, fats, amino acids, vitamins and minerals, and chlorophyll. They have cleansing properties that can reduce free radical activities.

Spirulina supplies nutrients that cleanse and heal the body, as well as provide proteins that are easily digested. Chlorella is rich in chlorophyll, acting as a detoxifier and providing vitamin B_{12}, essential to nerve health, red blood cell formation, and the production of energy in the body. Blue-green algae supply a high amount of concentrated nutrition, aid in digestion, assist in the detoxification of heavy metals, inhibit the growth of bacteria and yeast, and support the proliferation of antioxidant enzymes. Organic kimchi, a marinated cabbage, is mentioned because anecdotal reports by long-term survivors of AIDS include daily intake of this food. It is thought that its spiciness helps kill harmful bacteria, while supporting the growth of *Lactobacillus acidophillus*.

Sprouted Foods

Emphasizing fresh fruits and sprouted foods in your diet is important because these foods are enzyme-rich, contain oxygen, and are predigested. This means the proteins, fats, and carbohydrates are already broken down, which saves the body's digestive juices and enzymes. If you save this energy by consuming predigested foods, the body will have that much more energy to devote to the job of healing and repair.

Consuming sprouted foods is a simple way to increase the nutritional content of your diet, while saving energy devoted to the digestive process. All kinds of seeds can be sprouted, including alfalfa, aduki, barley, cabbage, lentil, millet, mungbean, pea, radish, sunflower, and many others. The process of sprouting is simple and includes soaking and rinsing seeds until they germinate.[15] Foods that are eaten raw and sprouted constitute the ultimate food. Not only are they easy to digest and the enzymes preserved, but they are loaded with life-giving nutrients.

The Hippocrates Health Institute in West Palm Beach, Florida, offers a life-giving nutritional program that emphasizes enzyme-rich foods and juices, as well as wheat grass therapy.[16] These foods help cleanse and detoxify the digestive tract and ingestion of fresh wheat grass juice helps rid the body of harmful toxins.

Brian Clement, the director of the Institute, says, "In a nutshell, I see environmental illness and chronic fatigue syndrome as slowly becoming a recurring condition in our overprocessed world. Through building and increasing healthy cells from a living diet, moderate exercise, and a positive attitude, one can remiss and hold off this modern plague."

Juicing

Juicing is the process of extracting the liquids found in fruits and vegetables and offers an efficient means of supplying you with a large quantity of enzymes and other nutrients while bypassing the immense physiological digestive effort needed to break down the fiber of the juice. Juicing is the easiest way for food to be absorbed and digested. Within minutes of consuming a freshly juiced drink, the nutrients enter your bloodstream and produce energy.

Ayurvedic and naturopathic physicians use juices therapeutically in treatment. Yet few traditional physicians understand the life-supporting benefits firsthand. One caution when drinking large amounts of juice is to monitor your pH. Since juicing tends to make the body alkaline, optimal urinary pH should be kept between 6.3 and 7.0.[17] It is suggested that people with yeast problems not take up juicing until these difficulties are under control. Juicing yields concentrated sugars from produce such as carrots and beets, which can exacerbate yeast growth.

What you select to juice depends on your physical needs and allergic sensitivities and you may wish to mix up to four juices in combination. Fruit juices act as cleansers and vegetable juices contain proteins that tone and build the body. Certain juices can tonify a particular organ: carrots, spinach, grapefruit, dandelion, parsley, beets, and mustard greens are good for the liver and gallbladder. Other juices like beet, wheat grass, apple, and cabbage are particularly cleansing, but need to be diluted or ingested in moderation. *Juicing for Life* (Garden City Park: Avery, 1992) by Cherie Calbom and Maureen Keane is an excellent book for the beginning juicer.

Judy, now well from CFS, reports that daily juicing of 1 to 4 glasses offers increased energy and mental clarity. For years Jamie had painful abscesses in her ears, nose, and mouth that would not resolve. Within 2 weeks of drinking fresh juices, the abscesses went away and have not returned. It may be that her body was finally able to absorb the enzymes it needed to heal.

Fasting

Fasting gives the digestive system a rest, allowing the body to pay greater attention to the mobilization of toxins that have been stored in fatty tissue, the liver, and other organs. Nutritionists report that 80% of the body's energy is devoted to digestion, so undertaking a fast diverts this energy, turning it inward to release and remove damaging chemicals from the body.

In fasting, the blood supply, relieved of its digestive responsibilities, can devote itself to the elimination of waste. During a fast the body must subsist on nutritional stores within the tissues and if the fast extends long enough the body burns glycogen, then fat, followed by protein stores in the body.

Fasting and Allergy

Fasting is not for everyone; those with diabetes or hypoglycemia should not fast without careful medical supervision. Fasting must be done safely and responsibly, as it can cause tissues to dump long-held waste into the bloodstream, taxing the liver and kidneys. Deciding to fast after an acute exposure to toxins can mobilize and release increased toxins, making you more ill than you already are.

Yet, a juice fast may be an excellent way to cleanse the body and allow it to rest, particularly in the face of ongoing allergic reactivity. Another option commonly used to alleviate chemical and food reactivity is a complete fast of only pure water taken for several days until allergic symptoms disappear. Undertaking the elimination diet, as previously outlined, gradually reexposes you to foods after a fast so you can discover which ones cause reactivity.

Some with CFS express concerns that fasting will further reduce already low energy levels. The fatigue and increased discomfort from fasting can be a positive sign that poisons are mobilizing out of the cells and ultimately out of the body. However, it's a good idea to anticipate a decrease in energy and thus consciously reduce stressors during this time.

If you undertake a fast, start by eating light meals a day or two before. Set your sights on a juice fast of 1 to 3 days. During this time your breath may emit a foul odor and your tongue may be coated with debris, as toxins are released. Some break out in pimples as a result of poisons leaving the body and intense headaches may be a part of detoxification.

Taking a baking soda and sea salt bath, coupled with dry brushing the skin, and deep breathing heightens detoxification. Massage and light exercise can help stimulate the lymphatic system in the cleansing process. Enemas or colonics are used during cleansing diets to support the removal of toxins and prevent the putrefaction of waste in the bowel.

Fasting 1 day a week for 24 hours provides an excellent opportunity to rest and repair with little discomfort. Should you choose to do this on a regular basis, the money you save could be used to treat yourself or to make a donation to an important cause. In this way, fasting can be a feast to share with someone else.

During the first few fasts, you may feel anxious about experiencing hunger. You may fear becoming confused, weak, or agitated. During the actual fast, compelling thoughts about your attachment to foods, or feeling the need to be in control may float to the surface. Permitting these thoughts to be recognized and appreciated can bring a meditative quality to the experience. The entire process of self-observation is made easier during a fast because there is more time to relax and pay attention instead of having to plan, shop, cook, and clean up after meals.

Termination of the fast is as important as the fast itself. Loading up with all foods you have been craving can flood your system with toxins and defeat the entire experience.

Healthy Food Ingestion and Digestion

Eating a balanced diet is an important tool for recovery, but it is only as valuable as the body's ability to digest the foods you eat. Proper food combinations—consuming digestively compatible foods in the same meal—facilitates digestion. Eating incompatible foods impairs your ability to digest them. Proteins require an acidic medium in order for the digestive enzyme pepsin to be effective. Salivary amylase, required for the digestion of starches and fats, is destroyed in an acidic environment. Likewise, lipase, an enzyme necessary to break down fats, functions poorly in an acidic medium. Attention to these facts will optimize digestion.

Keep in mind that different foods stay in the stomach for varying lengths of time. Fruits, when eaten alone, stay in the stomach an hour or less. Starches complete the digestive process in 2 to 3 hours. Proteins require about 4 to 6 hours. The digestive process is slowed if incompatible foods are eaten, causing impaired absorption.

Examples of incompatible food groups include: eating starches with fruits; proteins with starches; proteins in combination with other types of proteins such as nuts and meats; fruits with proteins; fats with proteins; sugars with proteins; and sugars with starch. This means that, contrary to Western eating habits, proteins and carbohydrates should not be eaten at the same time because they are poorly digested.

Fruits should be eaten alone, perhaps for breakfast, and acid fruits should not be combined with sweet fruits such as oranges and bananas. Melons should be eaten separate from all other fruits, as they are digested more rapidly. Vegetables combine with almost everything but fruits. Starches are the easiest to combine with each other; this means brown rice mixes well with cornbread and steamed carrots. Lunch should consist of a fruit or vegetable-starch meal. Dinner is considered the best time to eat foods that are more complex and difficult to break down.

For optimal digestion, stop eating when you have reached about three-fourths of your capacity. Stopping at this point will leave room for digestive enzymes to optimize their work. Don't eat again until the food from the previous meal in the stomach has been fully digested. Hunger is a signal that the food has been processed. If you are never hungry, you are never fully done with the job of digesting. When you eat right before going to bed, the food sits undigested in your stomach until the next morning.

Drinking fluids with your meal dilutes gastric secretions, making digestion more difficult. If you wish to drink, it's best to take fluids 15 to 30 minutes before or after a meal. Liquids are less disturbing to your body if taken at room temperature. Selima, who has severe digestive difficulties, takes Curing Pills, a Chinese medicine found in health food stores that helps resolve digestive discomfort, as well as acute and chronic gastrointestinal disorders.

Mealtime Digestive Tips

Here are simple steps that can enhance digestion:

1. Chewing food completely and slowly gives you a head start on the digestive process, as saliva produced by chewing begins the breakdown necessary for digestion.
2. Being fully "present" when eating allows you to relax and enjoy your meal. Focus totally on the act of eating rather than distracting yourself with stressful or peripheral activities. This means turning off the TV and closing your book.
3. Eating in a settled, quiet atmosphere makes it easier to digest your food.
4. Try to eat at the same time each day. Regularity helps improve digestion.
5. Eating too rapidly or too slowly disrupts the digestive process.
6. Sitting quietly at the end of the meal will permit the secretion of digestive enzymes.
7. Eat dinner at least 3 hours before going to bed. Your body cannot simultaneously rest and repair as well as digest foods while you sleep.

Cleaning Your Foods

Do you have any idea what's on your fruits and vegetables? For starters there is shellac, sodium orthophenyl phenate, polyethylene, germs, fungi, bacteria, metallics, and parasites. Fungicides and pesticides are also common. The foods purchased at supermarkets are also frequently coated with wax to protect and prolong their shelf life. This coating prevents moisture loss and inhibits mold, as well as decay and insect damage while foods are being shipped across the country to the grocery store.

It has been charged that these wax coatings are routinely mixed with pesticides, formaldehyde, and fungicides. Grocers are required to inform consumers as to the presence of this coating, yet few comply with this regulation. Often you cannot tell simply by looking if your apple has wax on it. So how do you know if your fruit is coated with wax? A fingernail scraping may tell you, but if you aren't certain, take a bit of the peel and dip it into boiling water. If it's wax-coated, water droplets will surface on the peel.

The message to the public is not to worry, that these coatings are safe. You are instructed to wash the foods in water and scrub them with a brush; yet poisonous materials bound in place by the wax are not water-soluble and the wax itself is indigestible. Most of us think a quick rinse in the sink removes poisonous residue left on fresh foods; however, this does little more than rearrange the poisons sealed onto the food's surface.

The unwitting ingestion of these foods is one of the ways that the body's toxic load is increased. For obvious reasons the chemically sensitive are in even greater danger, as allergic reactivity is coupled with the added weight of poisons that suffocate immune function. Ideally, you can avoid these wax-coated, pesticide-treated foods by eating organically grown foods. But, some organically grown foods are also chemically treated.

Once a food has been sprayed with pesticide, there is no known way to remove the residue. Even if you clean the outside, the pesticide becomes a part of the food itself.[18] If you cannot purchase unsprayed, organically grown produce, harmful substances can be partially removed through a cleansing soak, reducing the amount of toxins that might lodge in your body. Even if there is no spray on the food, vegetation can be polluted by irrigation or tap water that has been exposed to acid rain, chemicals in groundwater, and polluted air. In light of this you may prefer to do a routine cleansing soak on all foods you consume.

Procedure for Treating Foods

In order to remove residue from fruits, vegetables, and meats, it is advised that you soak them in a cleansing bath. In an effort to reduce chemical sensitivities, Judy uses The Fruit and Vegetable Safety Rinse, a natural product that helps remove pesticides, wax, and other chemical residues on the surface of produce. This is a blend of nontoxic, biodegradable food-grade wetting and chelation agents.[19] Several other options will be mentioned shortly.

The best way to treat food is to start by separating them into the following groups. Vegetables should be separated by placing leafy vegetables in one pile and root vegetables, heavy-skinned, or fibrous vegetables in another pile. This is because the timing of the bath is dependent on the thickness of the skin of the item to be soaked. Thin-skinned fruits such as berries, peaches, apricots, and plums go in one pile. Heavy-skinned fruits, all citrus, and bananas go in another.

Eggs tend to be allergy stimulating, in part because of the pesticide sprays used around the chickens. Salmonella bacteria can also be present in the egg. Eggs can be put in a cleansing soak for 15 to 20 minutes, which removes offending agents and gives them a better flavor. With this method, Elaine, who was formerly intolerant of eggs, can occasionally eat one. Meats are full of toxic matter, containing antibiotics and other medicines ingested or injected into the animal throughout its lifetime. Soaking fish and meats helps eliminate toxic residue, but it's inadvisable to soak ground meat.

Cleansing Formulas

Apple Cider Vinegar: As a natural disinfectant and cleanser, use 2–4 tablespoons per gallon of water, then soak 5–10 minutes, taking less time for thin-skinned and leafy foods. Next, rinse and dry thoroughly. Vinegar is natural, biodegradable, inexpensive, and removes most chemicals.

Hydrogen Peroxide 3% Strength: Food-grade hydrogen peroxide acts as an antiseptic. Using 2–4 tablespoons per gallon of water, soak for 10 minutes or less depending on skin thickness, then rinse and dry thoroughly. Peroxide helps remove bacteria, has no detergent properties, but is not as effective for the removal of chemicals.

Soap and Water (Neolife Green, or Shaklee's Basic H): These detergents are activated by squirting a small amount of liquid soap in water, mixing well, and scrubbing with a brush. When done, rinse well. This cleaning only removes some water-soluble and non-water-soluble chemicals found on the food's surface.

Sea Salt and Fresh Lemon Juice: Using cold water, add 4 tablespoons of sea salt and the juice of half a fresh lemon to make dilute hydrochloric acid, soak 5–10 minutes, rinse in cold water. This is a mild, nontoxic cleanser that works minimally on food surfaces.

Grapefruit Seed Extract (Paracan 144 and ParaMicrocidin are some brand names, and Nutribiotic is the liquid form): This biodegradable detergent calls for 1–2 teaspoons of extract to 2 gallons of water. Soak foods for 5 minutes, agitating the solution, then rinse and drain. Grapefruit seed extract has fungicidal, bactericidal, and antiparasitic properties, and is also an all-purpose household cleanser.

Preferably, purified or distilled water should be used for all soaks. When you remove foods from the cleansing bath, allow them to stand in purified water for 10 minutes before rinsing, then drain and dry completely before storing. Soaking foods for a prolonged interval will leach out water-soluble vitamins; consequently, don't leave them for more than a few minutes.

It can take time to become used to washing foods this way. After a day's work, a trip to the grocery store, and hauling the bags into the house, the last thing you may want is to add one more step. Elaine claims this step is well worth the reduction in her allergic sensitivities.

Vitamins, Herbs, and Supplements

The more you explore on your own, the more you may come to rely on nutritional supplements and herbs to enhance the process of healing and repair. Owing to the many options and conflicting pieces of information about supplements, it can be difficult to determine which ones will best aid your health. A supplement such as coenzyme Q10, an important energy-supplying enzyme, may benefit your friend but do absolutely nothing for you. You may also be so sensitive that you cannot tolerate the very supplements your body needs, as they can cause harmful reactions.

A major drawback to vitamins and supplements is their high cost. Wholesale suppliers of nutritional supplements offer vitamins and other remedies at a discount. On the other hand, local health food stores are a valuable source of practical health-related information, with pamphlets and individualized attention to your questions and concerns.

The efficacy of nutritional supplementation is dependent on whether the particular brand of supplement has been manufactured and tested to ensure that it will dissolve. Some nutrients block the absorption of other nutrients and some foods interfere with the absorption of certain kinds of supplements. In addition, your body may have trouble breaking down certain supplements in the intestinal tract so that they cannot be fully assimilated.

If you have difficulties with absorption of nutrients, you may need to test how well the capsule or pill dissolves. If the substance doesn't dissolve, you can waste hundreds of dollars taking supplements that are useless to your body. In order to be of benefit, the substance must dissolve within 30 minutes of ingestion. One way to clarify this is to ask your supplier about the standards of disintegration. You can also perform a home test by placing the tablet in a glass of lukewarm water and adding a little vinegar; without touching the tablet, stir the water for short intervals. The tablet should dissolve in 1 hour or less; if it doesn't, it won't be of much value to your body.

Another issue to note is the time of day that you ingest the supplement. Vitamin and mineral supplements are usually best absorbed when taken with food, rather than on an empty stomach, particularly if you have a sensitive digestive tract or get queasy when taking vitamins. Amino acids and acidophilus are most effective when taken without food so they won't compete with amino acids in foods, and so the food won't dilute their effect. Other fat-soluble supplements digest best in the presence of fat and fat-digesting enzymes, which means they should be taken after the meal.

Some report very positive changes when first taking a product and then in time fail to note any beneficial effects. If this occurs, it may be useful to experiment by putting yourself on an herbal holiday from time to time. This may mean taking a product for 2 to 4 weeks, going off it for 2 to 4 weeks, and then going back on.

Numerous supplements have been identified that heighten energy and specifically help those with EI and CFS feel better. Included here are some products that may be particularly beneficial in your recovery. This list is not exhaustive; many substances that are helpful for both EI and CFS are not described so you may wish to explore further. First, consult your physician in the use of any supplement.

Aloe Vera Juice

Whole-leaf, food-grade aloe vera juice helps combat the high incidence of maldigestion and digestive dysfunction common to EI and CFS. Undigested food remnants typically become irritants and cause inflammation of the mucosal wall of the intestines. Enzymes and chemicals are then released, injuring the intestinal wall, and causing increased intestinal mucosal permeability, which is known as having a "leaky gut." Undigested foods provide fuel for the overgrowth of fungal organisms such as candida and several types of parasites and their presence can result in increased food allergies, digestive disturbances, excessive mucus, and fatigue.

Acemannan, the active ingredient in cold-processed, whole-leaf aloe, acts as a powerful anti-inflammatory agent and neutralizes many of the enzymes responsible for damaging the mucosal wall. Aloe has viricidal, bactericidal, and fungicidal properties that can help control candida overgrowth. Acemannan also stimulates intestinal mobility helping move allergic proteins from the small intestine into the colon.

Beta-Carotene and Vitamin A

Foods and supplements rich in beta-carotene or vitamin A are effective at removing free radicals, the damaging substances found in cell membranes, and helping restore cellular fluidity, vital to energy production. Carotene is particularly medicinal for the liver, the organ that suffers the most from free radical damage. Carotene is converted to vitamin A, which, along with healing and strengthening mucous and cell membranes, improves the function of the thymus gland, the site where T cells are made.

Consuming two or more portions of orange-red-colored vegetables a day or drinking raw carrot juice will increase the number and activity of T-helper cells in the body and help heal the liver. Beta-carotene is commonly found in yellow and green vegetables and fruits such as yams, carrots, sweet potatoes, fish liver oils, beets, broccoli, apricots, cantaloupe, chard, dandelion greens, garlic, and spinach.

Coenzyme Q10

More commonly known as CoQ10, this enzyme catalyzes other enzymes into action. If the body has sufficient stores of CoQ10, it can supply the huge amount of energy necessary to perform the functions of the immune cells. Without the triggering force of CoQ10, there is no energy to sustain life, as it is needed in each cell to oxidize organic substances so that damaging oxidants can be neutralized. Besides providing energy for the cell, CoQ10 increases antibody levels necessary to fight invading pathogens.

CoQ10 is naturally produced by the liver and is found in all foods, but as a food source it's easily destroyed when cooked or processed. Primary supplies are animal tissue such as beef, pork, chicken, and fish. Plant sources include spinach, alfalfa, potatoes, sweet potatoes, and soybeans. It is also found in oils such as rice bran oil, soybean oil, corn, and wheat germ oils.

This enzyme is used by people with EI and CFS for its multiple benefits; most notably it energizes the cells and increases stamina and endurance. When Laura first started taking CoQ10, she was constantly exhausted; after 2 weeks she experienced a significant increase in energy and felt better. At one point she stopped taking the supplement, thinking it was no longer needed, and her energy took a nosedive so she began taking it again.

Echinacea

Echinacea is one of the most common natural remedies used to fight viral, fungal, and bacterial infections. It results in increased T-cell production, causing the destruction of bacteria or viruses, increasing natural killer cell activity, and increasing levels of circulating neutrophils. Its anti-inflammatory, antiviral, and antibacterial properties hold special benefits for CFS sufferers and many who are intolerant of antibiotics swear by it. Taken in tincture form, the tingling taste indicates a fresh batch of the extract. Generally it is best used for acute, short-term conditions such as colds, flu, and infections.

Gamma Globulin

This is not an herb, supplement, or vitamin but is listed because of its effectiveness in helping people with EI and CFS. Gamma globulin is a fraction of human blood that contains all of the antibodies. Intramuscular and intravenous gamma globulin given at 10 to 20 grams a week can intercept and destroy a variety of infectious agents, including viruses, bacteria, and candida. Intravenous gamma globulin is very expensive, about $1000 an infusion, and insurance companies are slow to pay because they consider treatments investigational. Despite the expense, David found that these regular infusions played an important part in his recovery from CFS.

Garlic

Garlic is a powerful herb that functions as a fungicide and a bactericide. It also destroys some parasites. Those who have trouble taking antibiotics prefer to take garlic when they have an infection. One drawback is that people around you may be offended by the odor; even odorless garlic can be detected by sensitive nostrils. If you can tolerate the smell, raw garlic is the most potent form, helpful in resolving yeast overgrowth and bacterial infections. Raw garlic can be irritating to the stomach or bladder, so it's best taken with food.

Germanium

Germanium is an element that acts as a strong antioxidant that helps to remove free radicals from the body. It carries oxygen directly to the tissues and cells where the oxygen then destroys cellular toxins. Germanium induces gamma-interferon production and increases NK cell activity. Since the body requires oxygen for fuel production, to maintain health, and to remove toxic matter, germanium can assist in performing these functions. Germanium is found in trace elements in garlic, ginseng, chlorella, comfrey, and other substances. There can be toxicity in using this substance, so it should be discontinued if diarrhea, nausea, and vomiting occur.

Ginseng

There are two main types of ginseng with slightly different effects: Siberian and Panax. Siberian ginseng is a rejuvenating herb taken to increase energy. Panax is taken to heighten alertness and concentration. Both are used for their adaptogen properties, helping increase the body's resistance to adverse influences, stimulating the immune system, and optimizing cellular fluidity. Studies show that endurance and recovery rates after physical exertion, as well as the ability to handle stressors, have increased with ingestion of ginseng. A word of caution: ginseng has been noted to exacerbate a cold, flu, or acute illness, making it worse and has side effects if not taken in moderation.

Goldenseal

This herb is an antibiotic with bactericidal properties that also aids in digestion and helps prevent gum disease. It helps increase the blood supply to the spleen and promotes the release of the spleen's immune-stimulating compounds. Used in conjunction with Echinacea it is a strong natural antibiotic. Goldenseal is particularly good for gastrointestinal and genitourinary infections, but it can cause an imbalance of the flora in the intestines, increasing the potential for yeast and fungal infections if taken for prolonged periods.

Grapefruit Seed Extracts

ParaMicrocidin, Citricidal, and Nutribiotic are brand names of grapefruit seed extracts. This extract is touted as the strongest antifungal, antibacterial agent found in nature. Although its mechanism of action is unknown, bacterial, fungal, and parasitic infestations can be resolved through its use.

There are multiple uses for this substance: it can be taken internally or used as a skin and household cleanser, produce wash, and dishwashing additive. It should not be used full strength, as it can be very irritating to sensitive tissue. Grapefruit seed extracts have no adverse side effects, which makes it preferable to parasite medications such as Flagel and Yodoxin which make many ill. Beware of the startlingly bitter taste of the liquid extract, which over time will bother you less.

Juice Plus

This is a whole food that offers five servings of many fruits and vegetables in capsule form. Manufactured through a unique process that preserves the enzymes, it is like juicing without the hassle. It contains antioxidants and is easier for some to absorb than ingesting the actual foods. Those who take it note increased energy, mental clarity, and stamina. Some report reduced pain and alleviation of depression.[20]

Lactobacillus acidophilus

In the healthy intestine there are hoards of bacteria and yeast that thrive and live happily in harmony with your body. When a person has *Candida albicans* or intestinal parasites, yeast and bacteria proliferate, consuming nutrients and producing toxins.

There are several forms of acidophilus and bifidus supplements that provide healthy flora for a bowel that has been overtaken by unhealthy microorganisms. Acidophilus is present in various foods, including yogurt, miso, and buttermilk. Reintroduction of healthy bacteria allows the bowel to heal and promotes a healthy environment that helps keep the yeast and bacteria in balance. Balanced intestinal flora can achieve dominance over candida overgrowth and heighten digestion and elimination.

Magnesium

Magnesium is essential for all energy-producing activities in cells. Its presence enables the cells to produce proteins that nourish and replicate themselves. These proteins are necessary when the body is attacked by invaders, as they act with other proteins in the blood to destroy invaders. Magnesium deficiency may be the cause of lethargy, pain, weakness, spasms, hyperirritability, and numbness commonly seen in CFS.

Magnesium supplements help replace lost body stores, but if you are unable to absorb magnesium your physician may choose to administer it intravenously, bypassing the digestive tract. Magnesium is found in nuts, seeds, sprouts, legumes, whole-grain cereals and breads, seafoods, dark green vegetables which are high in chlorophyll, pork, poultry, and eggs.

Max GLA, Flaxseed Oil, and Evening Primrose Oil

The polyunsaturated fatty acids gamma linoleic acid (GLA) and linoleic acid, oils essential for cellular metabolism, are contained in the above-named substances and are often recommended for immune disorders to help fight viruses. Essential fatty acids, which comprise part of the structure of all body tissues, are transformed into prostaglandins, which are crucial in regulating the function of every part of the body.

Fatty acids comprise most of the cell membranes and when you lack them in adequate amounts these membranes are unable to function adequately. In particular, they are important in nerve function and the maintenance of stable body temperature. GLA and linoleic acid are taken for chronic pain, inflammation, and premenstrual symptoms.

GLA helps flush fats and fat-soluble toxins out of the body, helps strengthen and balance the nervous system, and increases the immune response. Studies indicate that disordered metabolism of fatty acids may play a part in CFS. Those taking it report increased energy, reduced muscle weakness, fewer aches and pains, improved concentration, reduced depression, reduced palpations, and less dizziness. Food sources include flaxseeds and fish products.

Molybdenum

A nutritional deficiency of molybdenum can cause you to be sensitive to sulfite and rancid fat by-products. The liver enzyme aldehyde-dehydrogenase acts to break down aldehydes and those with EI have difficulty producing it in sufficient amounts needed to metabolize these toxins. Wines, some seafood (especially shrimp), lettuce, and many processed foods contain sulfites which are used to preserve foods. Many people have allergic sensitivities to these foods because of the inability to neutralize sulfites and rancid fats. Molybdenum taken intravenously or by injection neutralizes the effect of sulfites and can increase your ability to tolerate other antigens. Sources of molybdenum include organ meats, whole grains, legumes, leafy vegetables, and hard water.

Pau d'Arco

Pau d'arco tea has important fungicidal properties. Available in capsules, tea bags, powder, or bark form, it is also known as taheebo, ipes, ipe roxa, and trumpet bush. It is beneficial for those with candida as well as immune dysregulation and helps stimulate the immune system.

Reishi Mushroom

Ganoderm lucidum, also known as the King of Fu Zheng herbs, is used to strengthen the innate defenses of the body and increase overall enduring strength. Reishi, like CoQ10, is used for a variety of purposes, but with CFS it is used to treat chronic weakness, helps restore vital energy, and helps stimulate the immune system.

Reliv Now

This is a balanced nutritional supplement that offers easily absorbed vitamins, minerals, proteins, herbs, and enzymes mixed in a powerful combination. Available in powder form that can be mixed with juice or water, individuals taking it report increased energy and greater mental clarity. It should not be taken to the neglect of normal dietary habits and it is advised to consult your physician first.[21]

Royal Jelly

This jelly produced by bees is the substance used to feed their queen. A regular dose of this jelly can alleviate discomfort by cleansing the body, increasing circulation, and aiding in the disposal of body waste. It has disinfectant, antifungal, and antimicrobial properties as well as being a strong diuretic. Royal jelly affects people differently, by bringing abnormal bodily functions back to balance as needed. With CFS, it is suggested to take this substance for at least 3 months to experience the cumulative effect of increased energy and mental alertness. It is advised to start cautiously; because of its detoxification properties, you may feel worse for a time.

Saint-John's-Wort

Also known as *Hypericum perforatum*, this medicinal herb has antibacterial, antiviral, anti-inflammatory, antidepressant, and mood-stabilizing properties. It is also used to alleviate a wide variety or premenstrual and menstrual discomforts. Octacosinol present in the herb may increase oxygenation of tissue. It can be ingested in powder, tincture, or tea form and provides excellent protection when you feel a virus coming on. Though there is no known level of human toxicity, it can cause photosensitivity in fair-skinned individuals.

Shiitake Mushroom

This mushroom is useful in increasing the body's resistance to infection. Lentinan, a polysaccharide found in the mushroom, has immune-stimulating and antitumor capabilities. It stimulates macrophage activity, increases interferon production, increases T-cell production, and enhances helper T-cell activity.

Lentinus edodes mycelium (LEM), the extract of the immature mushroom, inhibits viral infections and stimulates the immune system, acting in a manner similar to the Reishi mushroom. LEM is particularly useful for CFS sufferers who are often deficient in T cells. LEM is also effective in prompting the production of antibodies and improving liver function.

Interferon is produced by lentinan and also activates NK cells, increasing their activity and number. You may recall that NK cells are white blood cells that are responsible for fighting virus-infected cells and many with EI and CFS are deficient in NK cell activity. LEM is extremely expensive and, since it must be taken for several months before noting an effect, you may spend a great deal of money to discover whether it helps. The whole shiitake mushroom is sold in grocery stores and can be added to meals, producing the same beneficial effects.

Soil-Based Microorganisms

These stimulate the immune response by helping cleanse and heal the digestive tract. Their presence in the GI tract helps boost nutritional assimilation by implanting beneficial bacteria into the bowel wall, thereby stimulating the body's ability to absorb and use important nutrients and rid the intestines of pathogenic materials. This supplement contains an array of micronutrients and phytoplankton that purportedly enhance digestion, increase energy, improve mental clarity, and increase resistance to infection. It is aggressive against mold, yeast, fungi, and viruses and stimulates cellular self-repair as well as providing antioxidants.[22]

Supplemental Cellular Oxygen

Oxygen is vital to the body's metabolism of food and to help fight disease. It acts to keep cells alive, increases immune function, produces energy, and aids in the detoxification and nutritional process. You may think it's enough to breathe fresh air, eat well, and engage in exercise in order to oxygenate the body, but stress from illness, toxic pollution, and runaway emotions can increase oxygen needs.

Cancer, viruses, candida, and parasites are anaerobic and cannot proliferate in an oxygen-saturated environment. One way people become oxygen deficient is through improper breathing. When you breathe improperly, the body does not receive adequate oxygen and carbon monoxide is formed, eventually rendering the body incapable of resisting the toxic effects of bacteria, viruses, and environmental toxins. Oxygen-saturated supplements help increase energy and help fight diseases. Magozone, Oxy-Max, Genesis 1000, and Homozone are the brand names of a few oxygen-based supplements that help boost health, increase energy, aid recovery, and increase the absorption of nutrients vital to the return of health.

Vitamin C

Vitamin C, also called ascorbic acid, is essential in production of collagen, which is a protein needed to form connective tissue in ligaments, skin, and bones. Vitamin C is particularly useful for people with EI and CFS because of its ability to increase immune function and, in turn, help fight bacterial and viral infection. Vitamin C also allows the adrenal glands to work more efficiently. As with vitamins A and E, it functions as an antioxidant, helping the liver to detoxify and remove free radicals from the body.

Vitamin C can have an immediate effect on the reduction of acute allergic reactivity because it stimulates certain T-cell activities and inhibits suppressor T-cell action following exposure to toxins. For several years Jamie has received intravenous vitamin C on a routine basis, which has significantly reduced allergic symptoms by detoxifying chemicals and removing free radicals. Given intravenously it is easier to absorb because it bypasses the digestive system. Vitamin C food sources include cantaloupe, citrus fruits, bell peppers, strawberries, green leafy vegetables, potatoes, sweet potatoes, and cauliflower.

Zinc

Sherry Rogers, MD, from the Center for Environmental Medicine discovered that zinc deficiency is common among the chemically sensitive.[23] Zinc, an important mineral that fortifies the thymus, is required by other nutrients for the detoxification processes of the body. Zinc doesn't last long in the body and must be replaced daily.

Summary

What you eat has a great influence on your health, and eating healthy foods may be the single most important thing you can do to influence your body states. This chapter has just touched the tip of the iceberg regarding healthy dietary practices. Hopefully, it will provoke you to think about the kinds of things you put in your body and lead you to make sensible dietary choices. Acid–alkaline balance as well as healthy food combination is as important as cleaning up your diet. The supplements, herbs, and vitamins mentioned are substances that have assisted others in their recovery.

Endnotes

[1]Lynn Lawson, *Staying Well in a Toxic World* (Chicago: The Noble Press, 1993) 245.

[2]John Robbins, *Diet for a New America* (Walpole: Stillpoint, 1989) 343.

[3]John McDougall and Mary McDougall, *The McDougall Plan* (Clinton: New Win, 1983) 151.

[4]John Stauber, interview KUSP, Santa Cruz, CA, 27 Nov. 1995.

[5]Gregory Pouls, address, "Environmental Solutions," Pacific Cultural Center, Santa Cruz, 17 Jan. 1996.

[6]McDougall, 17.

[7]McDougall, 114–115.

[8]McDougall, 146.

[9]Humbart Santillo, *Intuitive Eating* (Prescott: Hohm, 1993) 36.

[10]Lawson, 246.

[11]Theron Randolph and Ralph Moss, *An Alternative Approach to Allergies* (New York: Harper & Row, 1989) 70.

[12]Randolph, 88.

[13]Santillo, 85.

[14]For information about the Zone-favorable diet, call (800) 346-2703.

[15]For information on sprouting, contact The Sprout House, 40 Railroad Street, Great Barrington, MA 01230.

[16]Contact the Hippocrates Health Institute, 1443 Palmdale Court, West Palm Beach, FL 33411, (800) 842-2125.

[17]Santillo, 227.

[18]Randolph, 72.

[19]The Fruit and Vegetable Safety Rinse can be ordered through Safe Horizons, (800) 800-1200 for product information.

[20]Juice Plus is available through local distributors or by calling (415) 885-5200.

[21]Reliv Now is available by calling (800) 735-4887.

[22]Sources for SBO's include Natur-Earth, available from Healing Within Products at (415) 454-6655, Flora Source from Golden Health Products at (800) 780-1198, and Earth Manna purchased from a general distributor at (800) 735-4887.

[23]Sherry Rogers, *The EI Syndrome* (Syracuse: Prestige, 1986).

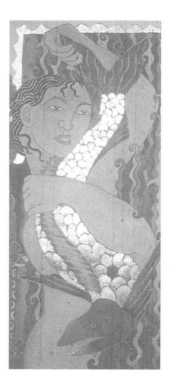

Chapter Ten

General Hazards

*t*his chapter examines some hazardous substances in detail so that you will know how to mitigate against their harmful effects. Like cofactors that contribute to illness, these substances may only have subtle influences, but taken in toto they can make the difference between ongoing illness and health. Many of these hazards are accepted as a normal part of our existence, yet they pose an insidious health threat. Once you recognize their impact on your body, you can be proactive in making conscious choices to avoid them.

Air

The EPA set a goal to reduce the nation's waste by 25% by 1992, yet total emissions in the United States continue to increase by 1% each year. Our country is responsible for the largest portion of man-made contributions to the greenhouse effect, at 21%. Second is the former USSR, with emissions at 14%. Carbon dioxide emissions will more than double by 2025 from 5.24 to 12.8 billion tons a year.[1]

In 1970 Congress passed the Clean Air Act, aimed at controlling emissions of major chemical pollutants as well as particulates. In some respects our air is cleaner, but the death rate from nonsmoking lung disease is on the rise. Studies have revealed that cities reporting the highest levels of ultrafine particulates, those smaller than 2.5 microns, had the highest death rates from lung and heart disease, at 15% higher than cities reporting the cleanest air.[2] Small particles are more hazardous because they lodge deeper in the lungs, interfering with the ability to take in oxygen and release carbon dioxide.

This is just one hazard. The air you breathe is composed of all kinds of substances: air is no longer just air. Toxic chemicals are found in the air in your home and in public places. Outdoor pollution comes from factories, automobile exhaust, and the runoff from pesticides that drain from farmlands and vaporize into the atmosphere. Indoor air pollutants are more prevalent in buildings as they become more energy efficient, while becoming more concentrated with pollutants which magnifies health hazards. Air toxins kill trees, crops, animals, and pollute the skies, lakes, and rivers. On a human level, polluted air damages the respiratory system, poisons the blood, and alters cellular DNA.

Air Interventions

The best you can do to reduce the effect of indoor air pollution on your health is to keep your environment well ventilated, or better yet, spend as much time outdoors as possible. Make certain your heat source is properly vented to the outside. If you have the money, an air purifier can be a big help. The street you live on should be as traffic free as possible. When outside, stay away from freeways and industrial areas. If you ride a bicycle, choose routes with less auto traffic in order to avoid exhaust fumes.

Health experts are pushing for the tightening of clean air standards. To this end the American Lung Association successfully sued the EPA, forcing them to complete its overdue air-quality report by 1997, paying specific attention to air particulate standards. It may be time to give your congressional representatives a call to voice your concerns.

Carbon Monoxide

Carbon monoxide is a dangerous colorless, odorless gas that is produced by incomplete combustion. It comes from automotive exhaust, gas flames, and wood smoke and is an insidious killer that is absorbed into the bloodstream by way of the lungs, attaching to red blood cells to combine with hemoglobin and thus reducing the body's ability to absorb oxygen. Over time, if enough carbon monoxide accumulates in the blood, oxygenation cannot occur, leading to asphyxiation and death.

The buildup of carbon monoxide in the blood taxes the cardiovascular system and hinders reflexes. Low-level exposures can cause headaches, fatigue, and flulike symptoms. Mental fogginess, dizziness, weakness, nausea, and vomiting may also occur. Chronic exposures can create a long-lasting general malaise which is the result of compromised oxygenation to the tissues. Besides automobiles, carbon monoxide is emitted from wood stoves and is a by-product of natural gas heating and other appliances.

Carbon Monoxide Interventions

The way to reduce exposure is to eliminate all sources of exhaust into your living area. Proper ventilation of your home, maintaining your appliances and heating systems, as well as cleaning the chimney will keep carbon monoxide from building up in your body. Routinely check your car for exhaust leaks, as a leak may allow poisonous fumes into the passenger compartment. Older cars are more apt to have this problem.

Garages that are attached to the home allow hazardous fumes to seep into the living space from parked cars or from stored materials. To prevent this, your car should be parked in a shelter that is not connected to your home. When idling in your auto at an intersection, allow a greater distance from the vehicle in front of you to avoid a face full of exhaust fumes. As a passenger, sit in the front seat rather than in back, where there is more exhaust.

Clothing

Clothes might seem to be safe, but they can be a source of extreme reactivity. People with EI must wear cotton clothing that is undyed, contains no flame retardant, and is pesticide- and formaldehyde-free. Acrylic may be found on cotton thread and plastic buttons can cause problems. Formaldehyde is used not just in permanent-press clothing, but in nearly all garments. Clothing and furniture fabrics commonly contain formaldehyde, which increases their ease of care but may make you sick. Fabrics also contain synthetic dyes made from polluting petrochemicals and heavy metals.

It is difficult to identify clothes that have been processed in this way, because there is no such information on the label. The odor of the fabric, particularly after it is removed from the dryer, can provide a clue as to the presence of formaldehyde. Selima became acutely ill shortly after wearing a new nightgown that she had forgotten to wash before wearing. If you cannot sleep at night, the reason may be the treated cotton sheets or your sleepwear. It has been found that bleached cotton fabrics release the toxin dioxin. A good rule would be: the fewer processes and chemicals involved in manufacture, the more natural and safe the garment.

Suffering the illnesses of EI and CFS lends new meaning to the expression, "Fashion victim no more." Stylish clothes are traded in favor of comfort, warmth, and utilitarian function. You may not always look sharp in terms of sophistication, coordination, and taste, but healthy clothing choices can enable you to feel alive and energized.

James Swan, author of the book *Sacred Places* (Santa Fe: Bear & Co., 1990), performed muscle testing on healthy individuals using different fabrics and found that muscle strength significantly weakened when in contact with synthetic fibers. For those with EI, the prevalence of toxic material in fabric makes it important to select cotton clothing and materials that are safe.

Clothing Interventions

Gradually replace old clothes with natural fibers of untreated cotton, linen, or wool. Natural fabrics tend to have a more balanced energizing feeling. Wearing loose-fitting as well as cotton fiber clothes enables the body to breathe and thus eliminate toxins through the skin. Fabrics of mixed composition can be okay for some, whereas others may be sensitive to natural wool products; therefore, just because an item is natural, don't rule it out as a source of reactivity.

If you can find them, choose organically grown, unbleached, undyed, formaldehyde-free cottons without pesticides, herbicides, or defoliants. If not, new clothes and linens should be washed repeatedly to remove formaldehyde and pesticide residue. To make these clothes completely safe, they must be washed repeatedly in nontoxic detergent. Washing in borax or baking soda will remove odors caused by chemicals as well as help remove permanent-press treatments.

Since new clothes are often treated with harmful substances, purchasing used clothes can be an effective means of avoiding toxins. Theresa's friend buys used clothing for her at flea market and rummage sales.

One way to test a garment is to place the palm of your hand on a fabric for a minute or two. If you suddenly note that your nerves are on edge, or you feel tingly, or sense a drop in energy, you may be experiencing allergic reactivity. Such reactivity may not occur in all people with chemical sensitivities; for some it is more subtle or may take longer to surface.

Ongoing care of your clothes is important. They should be washed with biodegradable products, avoiding spot removers and bleach. Chemical residues can be left on clothing by using traditional detergents, producing respiratory and skin irritation, in addition to the negative impact they have on the environment. Avoid dry cleaning, as the process relies heavily on chemicals. If there is no other alternative to dry cleaning, you may want to air out garments in order to disperse the fumes.

Electromagnetic Radiation

We are living in an electromagnetic soup, surrounded by unseen fields that vibrate within our bodies. Electromagnetic frequencies (EMFs) are a normal part of the earth, and consequently impact our bodies. Every shift in environmental EMFs directly affects how your body functions.

All electrical devices produce electrical and magnetic energy that travels as waves, moving through anything in its path. These fields have been found to interfere with the body's biological cycles and cause imbalance. Power lines are the most obvious source of EMFs, yet one-third to one-half of EMF radiation comes from household appliances and improper grounding of household wiring.

All forms of radiation interfere with cellular activity and are immunosuppressive. Radiation acts to destroy B cells, which produce antibodies. Radiation can come from gamma rays, microwaves, X rays, and radioactive materials. Radio frequencies are also generated by radio, TV, as well as microwave transmitters. Other things that emit EMFs and cause neurological damage include fluorescent lights, heating pads, electric blankets, microwave ovens, and video terminals. While the impact of an electric blanket may be very low, the dose is cumulative, over time adding to the total body burden and enhancing illness.

It is nearly impossible to avoid contact with these forces. Try driving your car without passing by any power or telephone lines. Repeated exposures to EMFs have been documented to cause health problems: electricians, phone and power linemen, and electrical engineers develop brain tumors, leukemia, and cancers at a much higher rate than those who are not as closely exposed.[3]

In 1990 the EPA reported that the 60-hertz magnetic fields from power lines can cause cancer.[3] Research reported in *The American Journal of Epidemiology* by Nancy Wertheimer, Ph.D., and Edward Leeper, Ph.D., notes that children living close to high-voltage power lines died of cancer at twice the rate of children living near low-current wires.[4]

Sherry, who struggles with EI, points out, "Electrical wiring is so all-pervasive in our society that few of us consider its damaging effects. But I'm concerned about the cumulative electromagnetic effects of my home because we've converted to electrical wiring and heating." Her intolerance of natural gas has forced her to rely exclusively on electricity in her home.

Electromagnetic radiation is of particular concern for those with EI because so many of their homes have been converted to electric heat and power in order to avoid the hazards of allergic reactivity to gas and other substances. For unknown reasons, people with EI tend to be more sensitive to EMFs to the extent that some hear and feel the vibrational noise and sensations resultant from these energies. This radiation can cause irritability, light sensitivity, and fatigue.

In the past, the hazards of EMFs were downplayed or ridiculed. There is an understandable reluctance to heed these risks, as the financial consequences would force our society to revamp its emphasis on electromagnetic support.

EMF Protection

Gauss meters are hand-held devices that measure the strength of magnetic fields. Rather than purchasing a meter, you may contact your local electrical utility, who will send someone to measure these levels free of charge.

The best way to protect yourself from these frequencies is to increase your physical distance from the relevant devices, or limit exposures. It has been suggested that you not live in a community that has a nearby power plant and, if possible, not live near any power lines.

Reduce the number and use of EMF-producing appliances and machines in your home. When you are near such an appliance, emissions are high; by stepping back a few feet, the strength of the field diminishes. EMF-emitting appliances near your bed are a particular concern. Situate electrical devices such as digital clocks away from the bed and remove electrical blankets. Elaine wears a protective polarizer pendant that absorbs harmful EMFs.[5]

Formaldehyde

Formaldehyde, a colorless gas, is the most common indoor air contaminant. At one time it was primarily used as an embalming fluid, but it has proven to be a versatile chemical and is now found in hundreds of products, including cosmetics, plastics, carpeting, paints, insulation, wood, paper, particleboard, permanent-press fabrics, plywood, toothpaste, and even tea bags.[6]

Other products that contain formaldehyde are: antiperspirants, antiseptics, mouthwash, fertilizers, soap, shampoo, air fresheners, clothing, dyes, insecticides, dry cleaning, rug cleaning, vitamins, paper products, milk, ice cream, furniture fabric, eggs, glue, furniture stuffing, dishes, and prescription medications. Other uses of formaldehyde are as a fungicide or preservative in foods. Formaldehyde is used to treat permanent-press fabrics and on fireproof materials. Traces of formaldehyde are even carried in our food, air, and water. You probably never realized how all-pervasive it is, but its presence slowly, quietly erodes the health of everyone who comes in contact with it.

Checking labels will not tell you if minute amounts of the substance are contained in a product. Formaldehyde is found in so many things it's difficult to avoid contact. Formaldehyde production in the United States has gone from 987 million pounds in 1951 to 6730 million pounds in 1988.[7] In 1983, after years of minimizing its harmful effects, the EPA declared formaldehyde to be "a potential carcinogen in humans."[8] Immunologists Jack Thrasher, PhD, and Alan Broughton, MD, have studied the effects of chemicals such as formaldehyde on the immune system and suggest that there are measurable immunological changes associated with chemical exposures and that formaldehyde can cause a subtle but chronic activation of the immune system.[9] This means toxic chemicals such as formaldehyde can cause immune dysfunction.

Once in contact with the body, formaldehyde is absorbed into the organs where toxic aggravation occurs. As an irritant, it affects the eyes, nose, throat, and lungs. In addition to making other illnesses worse, it can cause dizziness, depression, and neurological difficulties, and brief exposures can render those with EI incoherent. The insidious effects may account for respiratory difficulties and headaches which are, at times, dismissed as psychosomatic.

Hospitals can be the worst place for people who are sensitive to formaldehyde. Linens and floors are lathered with materials containing this substance. It wasn't until much later that Josh, a hospital oncology nurse who developed CFS, realized how debilitating the sparkling clean floors, walls, and surfaces coated with formaldehyde had been. Josh now knows that years of toxic exposures eroded his health.

After Josh transferred out of oncology, he worked in the nursing administration office until shortly after new particleboard desks were installed. Brief exposures rendered him senseless with fatigue and his brain seemed to short-circuit. Symptoms were not alleviated until the culprit was identified and removed; the desks had been treated with formaldehyde.

Formaldehyde Interventions

Formaldehyde has an unmistakable pungent odor, but even if you cannot smell it, it may be causing harm. Those who are chemically sensitive can often smell the fumes, while the average person cannot. When you are having a reaction and cannot identify the source, you may be reacting to substances that have been treated with it. The only way to control its effect in the environment is to avoid contact with materials that contain it.

Removing all formaldehyde-treated articles in your environment requires reading labels. Cosmetics may list formaldehyde as quaternium-15 or quaternium 8-14. Also avoid the substance listed as DMDM hydantoin, which is a preservative that can release formaldehyde. Since food products may not identify the presence of formaldehyde, it is best to avoid packaged or canned products and to eat foods that are as whole and untreated as possible.

Aside from identifying culprits and isolating them from contact, there are other things that can be done. Airing out a room, or an object treated with formaldehyde may alleviate acute discomfort, but data show that it takes approximately 5 years to release 80% of the fumes. Increased heat and light heighten outgassing. The use of an air purifier will also remove some of the formaldehyde and chemical fumes from an environment.

Sensitive people with EI often move to new homes in the hope that their health will improve. Instead, they may become more ill as a result of the outgassing of formaldehyde commonly used in new construction. Some nontoxic paints and sealants, when applied to cabinets, walls, and furniture, can seal in outgassing fumes, but it is better to live in an older home that has fully outgassed. It is also advised that you avoid stores that sell clothing and rubber products.

Heavy Metals

When heavy metals such as cadmium, aluminum, lead, and mercury are absorbed by the body, they reduce immune function by suppressing the phagocyte response, interfering with the formation and function of antibodies, and increasing susceptibility to infection. When heavy metals overload the system, the capability of organs such as the liver and spleen is compromised, which interferes with their ability to act to reduce the toxic load. In addition, other toxins, such as radioactive isotopes, latch onto heavy metals, binding each other into the body.[10] And radionics experts contend that parasites and candida are bound in place in the presence of the heavy metal mercury.

For example, lead toxicity can cause acute and long-term deficits. It's estimated that 38 million people in the United States have significant levels of lead in their bodies.[11] Lead inhibits the synthesis of blood, and can cause serious neurological deficits in children. It can be airborne or ingested as a result of lead dust flaking off lead-painted walls or from foods grown in soil high in lead content. Airborne lead outdoors often originates from gasoline additives, but this has been controlled since the 1980s.

Food, water, and air are increasingly contaminated with lead, cadmium, and mercury. Car exhaust and industrial residues release heavy metals into the atmosphere. Arsenic and lead can damage the central nervous system and increase debilitating symptoms, and the damaging effects of mercury are discussed in the next section. The clinical picture created by the presence of excessive amounts of heavy metals include allergies, fatigue, hair loss, excessive fluid retention, and susceptibility to viral infections.

Heavy Metal Interventions

Remove lead-based paint from your environment with the help of a professional well-versed in protective measures. Do not burn painted or treated wood, which will release toxins into the atmosphere and possibly into your lungs.

The good news is that a cleansing diet and supplements can help eliminate heavy metals from your body. By restricting your intake of organic foods and drinking fresh water, you can help reduce the accumulation of heavy metals in your body. General detoxification measures mentioned throughout this book can keep heavy metal accumulation to a minimum and the interventions of The Environmental Health Center in Dallas, Texas, can help detoxification from extreme exposures.

Mercury

Mercury is a toxic heavy metal with mutagenic properties, capable of causing physical defects in those who come in contact with it.[12] When dental fillings, which contain approximately 50% mercury, are exposed to air, vaporization of mercury occurs. These fumes can then be inhaled or swallowed and enter tissues of the body.

Mercury is not just found in dental work, but also in water and air. It is present in automobile exhaust, cosmetics, and various foods, seafood and freshwater fish in particular. It is used in foods and medications as a preservative. Polyester clothing, deodorants, wood preservatives, hair dye and makeup, pesticides, and fungicides can all contain mercury. It is present in flashlight batteries. When you dispose of batteries, mercury leaks into landfill disposal sites and enters groundwater.

Dental Mercury

All silver dental fillings are composed of mercury because it is easy to use and is less expensive. There is increasing evidence to support the damaging and toxic effects that mercury can have on the immune system. Mercury's effects include DNA damage,[13] structural changes in proteins and disruption of cellular communication,[14] and introduction of free radicals.[15] Damage has been known to occur even with low levels of exposure. Despite this knowledge, there are continued assurances of mercury safety from the dental and medical community.

Mercury is considered highly poisonous when found outside the mouth. The EPA actually prohibits dentists from disposing of mercury particles down the sewer, but doesn't prohibit mercury from being placed in the human mouth. How can this be so? Politics and economics seem to hold the answer.

The Amalgam Wars began in the United States in the 1830s when the side effects of mercurial ointments used against syphilis were commonly known. Opponents claimed that mercury content would harm teeth, the oral cavity, and general health. Proponents argued that it was safe and cheap, offering the working class another option to the extraction of decaying teeth. The Amalgam Wars reemerged in the late 1970s, emphasizing concerns about the galvanic currents in the mouth caused by different metals.[16]

The American Dental Association urges dentists to follow careful protocols regarding the handling and storage of mercury amalgams, and they conduct annual screenings to determine if dentists have absorbed high levels of mercury. Despite its toxicity outside of the body, the public is told that mercury, when set in the mouth, does not leave the amalgam. What is difficult to understand is how mercury can be safe in your mouth when it is considered a deadly toxin anywhere else.

When mercury does vaporize or break off in small amounts, dentists assert that it is not enough to cause harm. How about for those who are extremely sensitive? In the case of people with EI, it is possible to be allergic to small amounts of mercury. Hal Huggins, Colorado Springs dentist and founder of the Toxic Element Research Foundation, says research shows that 20% or more of the population is allergic to mercury.[17] While tests can ascertain the presence of abnormally high levels of mercury, difficulty occurs when reactivity to mercury cannot be clinically measured but still constitutes an allergic or toxic presence. This means it's possible to be reactive to mercury without being exposed to toxic levels.

Where It Goes—Clinical Findings

Over time the mercury content of your fillings decreases, leaving the filling site as it is released by the process of consuming hot liquids or foods, polishing and brushing teeth, and chewing during eating. Placement, polishing, and grinding of amalgam fillings causes an increase in mercury exposure, lasting for days or months after treatment.[18] Where does this mercury go? Mercury is then vaporized and swallowed, inhaled, or absorbed through the lungs into the bloodstream. It accumulates in the vital organs and body tissues, causing damage. The most common sites for the storage of mercury are the brain, kidney, thyroid, pituitary, liver, heart, and blood.

Why should you be disturbed by the presence of mercury in tissue? If your health is good, you probably are not being harmed by its presence because your immune system is able to counteract the damaging effects. If your health is compromised, toxicity from amalgam can pull your immune capability down. One study found that amalgam fillings placed in the mouths of monkeys caused significant increases in antibiotic-resistant bacteria.[19]

Studies have also linked the mercury poisoning from amalgams to renal failure. Animal research studies show that the presence of amalgam fillings in sheep reduced their kidney function by half while the control group that received glass ionomer fillings retained normal renal function.[20] The greater the amount of mercury fillings in the mouth, the higher were the levels of mercury deposits found in the brain and kidneys.[21] Autopsy studies indicate that people with silver fillings show a two- to threefold greater mercury level than those with porcelain or gold fillings.[22]

Mercury is known to be toxic to living cells. Harmful effects most frequently noted involve immune system as well as nervous system damage. Mercury inhibits the absorption and utilization of nutrients, leading to a variety of pathophysiological disturbances. Amalgam fillings can also cause electrical currents to be generated, interfering with the electrical conduction of the nervous system.

Symptoms of Mercury Toxicity

The following is a list of signs and symptoms of mercury toxicity:

1. Immune deficiency—fatigue, allergies, chronic infections
2. Neurological effects—depression, difficulty concentrating, headaches, loss of memory
3. Psychological disturbances—depression, irritability
4. Glandular—cold hands and feet, low body temperature, swollen glands
5. Cardiovascular—chest pain, irregular heartbeat
6. Miscellaneous—joint pain, fatigue, digestive problems, facial pain, pyorrhea

It bears note that these symptoms overlap with the CDC criteria for CFS. Multiple sclerosis is believed by some to be triggered by undiagnosed mercury toxicity. Sherry, who has EI, has a chronically low body temperature, a typical response to mercury contamination. Symptomatic similarities make mercury toxicity difficult to distinguish from EI and CFS.

Diagnosis

Mercury poisoning from low dose chronic exposure is difficult to diagnose because mercury absorbed by the body is excreted at a slow rate. Over a period of years the body reaches its capacity and clinical signs of illness become apparent. Several tests can help uncover evidence of mercury toxicity. Urinalysis for mercury includes assessing urine mercury levels to determine if the body is able to excrete it. Hair analysis involves measuring levels of mercury in the hair to assess if there has been a heavy exposure. Blood studies may show abnormal immune activity, which helps round out the diagnostic picture.

Relief on an Empty Wallet

Some, but not all, chronic fatigue and allergically sensitive people have been known to get better after removal of their dental amalgams. Sherry, mentioned previously, had trouble eradicating her candidiasis, but got well once her dental amalgams were removed. Others report that seemingly unrelated problems, such as extreme joint pain, foul breath, persistent tremors, and metallic taste, improved after their mercury fillings were removed.

Studies show that amalgam removal allows the T-lymphocyte ratio to increase. T lymphocytes are important in mediating cellular immunity, as well as secreting factors that trigger various other sequences necessary to immune regulation. Replacing old fillings can be extremely expensive: dental insurance seldom covers replacement of amalgams without measurable evidence of medical necessity. Gold fillings are very expensive but they are a replacement substance that doesn't cause toxic reactivity. Some dentists are using a composite resin material that seems to be tolerated by people with chemical sensitivities.

Removeal of amalgams is not a decision that should be made lightly. Removal of fillings can release mercury into the body in greater amounts, further compromising your immune system. The stress of having them removed has been known to make some more ill, particularly if the fillings are not removed properly. A San Francisco Bay Area chiropractor became temporarily paralyzed after improper amalgam removal. If not done with extreme care, removal of mercury can cause dangerous exacerbation of acute symptoms as the poison is released into circulation. There are safe protocols that manage and control this release. Dentists administer oxygen, which reduces the chances of breathing mercury vapor. Intravenous vitamin C used during the procedure helps bind and excrete the mercury as it is released during extraction.

Even if you don't experience an exacerbation of symptoms, each time a filling is replaced a greater portion of the tooth is lost, increasing general body trauma and stress. In addition, for those with sensitivities, root canals are known to be packed with substances that contain phenol and formaldehyde. Traditional dentists, failing to grasp the nature of chemical sensitivities, don't understand that it's possible to have an allergic sensitivity to these substances. One healthy woman underwent a root canal procedure and subsequently experienced multiple viral infections and colds which persisted until she had the procedure redone, eliminating the amalgam packing.

Sherry's health, which had been bad following exposure to fumigants, became acutely worse immediately after a root canal procedure and several fillings. Rather than subsiding, the pain grew worse with each filling. It wasn't until subsequent dental amalgam testing for sensitivities that the problem of allergic reactivity was uncovered. Once the root canal procedure was redone with nonreactive materials, the pain subsided.

Mercury Interventions

Under the supervision of a health practitioner, Jamie, the therapist, was able to reduce the load of mercury in her body by using noninvasive measures. During that time she was too ill to safely tolerate the removal of her amalgams. Mercury detoxification protocols should be undertaken under the supervision of a practitioner who understands the process. While detoxification doesn't permanently solve the ongoing problem of mercury leeching out of your fillings, it can reduce the accumulated body burden.

In this process, supplements can be taken that bind with mercury to remove it from tissues, enabling it to be excreted. Important antitoxicity nutrients include zinc, selenium, pectin, and algin, a substance in sea vegetables. These supplements bind with mercury and escort it out of the body. Using detoxification measures can enhance your health and avoid the excessive expense of replacing fillings. Undertaking a detoxification program causes considerably less physical discomfort than if you have the fillings extracted. When old fillings finally wear out, you may want to have your dentist replace them with nonallergic substances.

One of the quickest ways to protect yourself from mercury vapors is to stop chewing gum. The chewing process causes friction, which continually stimulates the release of mercury vapor from the fillings into surrounding tissue. Another intervention includes reducing the mercury content of your diet. A primary source of ingested mercury is from fish, especially shellfish and tuna. Consuming farm-raised fish will help avoid mercury.

The health of the intestine is important to the excretion of mercury. If bowel flora is abnormal, mercury that could be excreted via the feces becomes reabsorbed, making its way back to the liver. Acidophilus supplements, yogurt, and buttermilk will help to maintain proper intestinal balance. A high-fiber diet hastens the exit of toxic mercury residue from the bowel.

Toxins that remain in a sluggish bowel become reabsorbed and recirculated, returning to tissue. Routinely drinking 6–8 glasses of nonfluoridated water daily will also help eliminate toxic matter. Reducing stress in your life will prevent the body from becoming depleted of necessary nutrients. Engaging in exercise that works up a sweat at least three times a week will also enable you to eliminate toxins. In addition, steam baths and saunas can be of value.

While it doesn't appear that dental practice in the United States will change in the near future, there is hope on the horizon. Responding to the health concerns, Sweden and Germany have banned mercury in dental fillings. Perhaps one day other countries will see the light as well.

Mold

There are over 100,000 types of molds and fungi, which are ubiquitous organisms that are able to grow on anything. Mold spores are living organisms that are difficult to eradicate and once they take hold, they grow and spread, contaminating adjacent materials. High ambient moisture levels make mold contamination a significant problem; and sensitivity to the spores is difficult to control because they are so prevalent, making them difficult to contain and destroy. Despite efforts to eradicate them, they can hide dormant for long intervals, and then after a wet spell they can emerge everywhere.

Exposure to molds and fungi has toxic effects ranging from brief irritation to immunosuppression and cancer.[23] Molds are Laura's worst source of allergic reactivity; brief exposure to spores can cause serious respiratory distress and make it difficult for her to think clearly for weeks. Exposure can come from ingesting mold-laden food, inhalation of fungus spores, and through the skin.

Favorable breeding grounds for mold include humid, moist locations with the right temperature, condensation, and food source for them to thrive. Mold and mildew grow on organic material as well as paint, fabrics, wood, and synthetic surfaces covered with grease and dirt. Mulch piles and dirt, as well as musty damp places are favorite mold locations. Household dust contains mold spores. Foods high in mold include: bread, vinegar, ferments, cheeses, dried foods, alcohol, and chocolate. Humidifiers found in ventilation systems can be a source of mold proliferation, the spores then being vented to all regions of a building.

Mold Interventions

Avoiding mold-infested environments can help keep exposures to a minimum. By identifying sources of mold as well as removing them or making structural changes in your home, you can isolate or clean up the problem. Keeping your home as warm and moisture-free as possible will greatly reduce mold growth. Shower curtains and bathrooms are typical sites of infestation, and trash containers and house plant dirt can be other sources. Stuffed furniture, including mattresses, are other places that hold spores.

Newspapers should be recycled or thrown out because mold accumulates in the pages. Directing outdoor drain spouts away from the house can reduce the opportunity for mold to grow up in the walls and under the house. Living areas that are clean, dry, and full of light will inhibit mold growth. Furniture should be placed away from walls so that air can circulate around all sides to prevent mold from proliferating on the walls and in the fabric. Dehumidifiers placed in damp areas such as basements can help remove moisture from the air, reducing the proliferation of spores. Since a dehumidifier extracts moisture from the air by collecting it in the machine, it may also become a breeding ground for mold.

Frequent cleaning of your home prevents the accumulation of mold and dust. Since vacuum cleaners blow mold particles through the filter into the air, surfaces should be wiped or mopped with a damp sponge or cloth instead. Feather dusters only loosen dust and disperse spores into the air and brooms do the same thing.

You may wish to wear a mask to protect from inhaling spores when cleaning or working in the yard. Placing charcoal in strategic damp locations, such as book-cases, will help absorb moisture. If you can tolerate them, products such as borax, Bon Ami, Zephiran, baking soda, and vinegar can be used to destroy or clean mold. You may have to clean periodically, as mold tends to reoccur.

Natural Gas

Sherry cannot go into buildings that have gas heat; she can have seizures even if the heat is off. Likewise, Theresa must avoid the public library because the building is heated with gas. Natural gas is one of the most insidious culprits causing sensitivities. The word *natural* can be cause for confusion; though natural, this gas is toxic to the body and synthetic chemicals have been added. Gas water heaters, heating systems, kitchen stoves, and clothes dryers are major contributors to household air contamination.

Since natural gas fumes have no odor, mercaptans are added to alert you when there is a leak. Mercaptans give off a characteristic pungent odor, making it easier to detect small quantities of escaping gas. When gas burns completely, it consumes oxygen, producing carbon dioxide, nitrogen oxides, and sulfur oxides. When combustion is incomplete, the result is carbon monoxide, a deadly gas that interferes with the blood's ability to transport oxygen. When appliances leak imperceptibly, there can be an increase in the buildup of carbon monoxide in the body over time.

It is not uncommon for fittings to leak undetectable amounts of gas, which can be a central reason for the persistence of your symptoms. When you have a gas stove in a vented kitchen, the carbon monoxide and nitrogen dioxide levels can be as high as those in Los Angeles during a smog alert.[24] Pilot lights produce less total pollution than ignited stove burners, but in poorly ventilated spaces a buildup of airborne pollutants inevitably occurs. Even in a well-ventilated building with a gas system in good repair, emissions are a significant source of indoor pollution.

Though a leaking gas line is a life-threatening matter, an insidious threat is the day-to-day inhalation of small amounts of this same poison. Skillful advertising attempts to convince you that natural gas is safe, yet studies at the University of California show that carbon monoxide and nitrogen dioxide can become danger-ously high when a gas oven is heated to 350 degrees for 1 hour.[25] Gas is generally the worst heat source for sensitive people. Many seemingly healthy people are also harmed, but don't see this as the source of their low energy and general malaise.

Natural Gas Interventions

Those with EI who don't get better after adhering to all of the other recommended physical and environmental detoxification approaches should consider their household gas systems a possible source of their ongoing difficulties. Gas heat can be a frequent cause of hidden allergies, making your ideal heat source an electrical system. Theresa even becomes ill eating foods that have been cooked over gas heat.

Your local gas utility company can be contacted to test for leaks, but they lack the ability to detect microscopic quantities of gas that escape from improperly sealed fittings and tend to minimize the risk. To the average person, this leakage may mean nothing; yet to someone as sensitive as Sherry, a minute leak can be fatal.

The problem may not be resolved by simply turning off the gas: to make a difference the system must be removed from the environment. Proper venting of gas appliances to the outside can help reduce fumes, but it does not entirely solve the problem. Removing the gas system is the solution, but it can pose a major expense, and there is no guarantee that removal will enhance health. The removal of Laura's gas range resulted in a significant improvement in her health.

Ideally, there should be no gas pipes in your home. Electrical heating is more expensive, but is the lesser of the two evils with regard to causing harm to your health. Electric appliances—space heaters, dryers, stoves, ovens, and water heaters—work well for persons with EI. In particular, radiant ceramic heaters have worked well for Theresa and Laura, because they don't emit fumes.[26]

Ozone

High in the earth's stratosphere is a natural thin layer of ozone that absorbs ultraviolet rays, which can damage human skin and eyes. This layer is being depleted because of the release of chlorofluorocarbons by refrigerators, air conditioners, industry, aerosol cans, and auto exhaust. The human race is just now waking up to the significance of the destruction of this protective layer.

Ozone, down below on earth, is major agent in the formation of smog. Ozone builds up on earth because of the interaction of sunlight and the pollution of hydrocarbons, mostly produced by automobiles. Its presence or absence upsets the balance of the earth's temperature, atmosphere, weather patterns, and life itself. Today there is too much ozone filling our lungs and too little up above filtering out damaging rays.

It is confusing to understand that ozone is both damaging and beneficial. As a form of electrically energized oxygen, ozone is created by nature and purifies the air through electrical discharges that cause oxidation. The benefits of ozone are also touted in air purification systems in the form of ion and ozone generators specifically designed to disperse pure ozone into the air.

Despite highly positive claims, there are no standards regulating the safety of these machines; the only guideline for their use is to turn down the volume control if you notice an acrid odor. Employees of one ozone machine manufacturer have sued their employer for respiratory damage believed to have been the result of ongoing contact with high levels of ozone emitted by these machines. Healthy people are being harmed by ozone levels far less than the EPA standard of 120 parts per billion.

Symptoms of overexposure include respiratory ailments, nausea, premature aging of skin, and headaches. Excessive ozone exposure causes a slow burn, scarring of your lungs. Copiers and laser printers expose office workers to many times the safe level of ozone. Workers in close proximity with these pieces of equipment are advised to contact the manufacturer to find out how frequently the internal filter should be changed, as they often become clogged, which results in higher ozone emissions.

Ozone Interventions

Until there is more information as to the long-term effects of ozone exposure, you can best protect yourself from ozone exposure by avoiding contact with machines and objects that emit the substance. Regarding protection from ultraviolet rays, strike a balance between too much and too little exposure to sunlight. If you are concerned about the larger picture, collect information from sources including the EPA Right to Know Hot Line (see The United States Environmental Protection Agency in Appendix II) and lobby elected officials for tougher clean air standards.

Perfume as Nerve Gas

"Not wearing perfume is better for those you come in contact with. It is also a political statement. Saying no to the cosmetics industry includes saying no to the concept of women as sex objects," notes an ex-advertising executive who became ill with CFS. Perfume is a multi-billion-dollar industry that sells what some might call poison to women.

Did you know that perfumes and cosmetics contain dyes and preservatives, including heavy metals and formaldehyde, that are absorbed into the skin when applied? It is also true that certain musk fragrances have neurotoxic effects and cause the breakdown of nerve cells and the myelin sheath of the nervous system.[27] These neurotoxic reactions range from sneezing to life-threatening seizures.

In addition, about 95% of all ingredients in most fragrances and cosmetics are synthetic compounds that have not been tested by the FDA for safety.[27] It is believed that many substances used in perfumes, after shaves, detergents, and soaps may cause cancer, birth defects, central nervous system disorders, allergic reactions, and toxic effects.

When the perfume smell wears off, you are still not safe; the body has merely adjusted to the fumes. You absorb chemical fumes not only through the nose, but also through the skin. Fumes can cause damage even when you cannot detect them. Some fail to realize they are allergic to cosmetics and lotions, until they stop using them and then resume application which evokes allergic reactivity.

Perfume Interventions

Fortunately there are growing numbers of natural cosmetic products made without synthetic ingredients or natural scents that can be found in vitamin, herbal, and health stores. In the face of chemical sensitivities, it is best not to wear any perfume or after shave, but it is not possible to control the decisions made by those with whom you come in contact. A passing whiff of perfume can send Laura to bed for days.

"Our society is accustomed to using stronger smells to cover up other smells. Telling someone that you are being harmed by their perfume or deodorant becomes very personal. When you explain this it's hard for them to grasp that their perfume can make you nauseated and dizzy for days after exposure. People become personally insulted by my efforts to avoid a reaction, but they are invading my sensory space," comments Laura.

She advocates in favor of speaking up. "It's important to tell people that it isn't personal; it's just that my body cannot tolerate their odor. It doesn't stop there, because if they invite you into their house you have to say, 'It's also your cleaning, your furniture, and your food.' This is not an Emily Post disease; you're hitting the basics; but I find it impossible to cover up and make nice when I'm wilting inside."

Speaking up in meetings and advocating against perfume and after shave use can be important. Most people don't have any idea that they're causing harm. One woman with chemical sensitivities decided to sue a major clothing retailer for mailing her aromatic advertisements.[28] The presence of their perfumed supplement caused violent allergic reactivity.

Current U.S. Postal Service regulations allow fragrance strips to be mailed only if they are activated by opening a glued flap or by removing overlying paper. California law prohibits scented mailings unless they are sufficiently sealed to block out inadvertent inhalation. Despite these laws, magazines and catalogs continue to be scented. Scented mail wafts onto bills and important letters, making it difficult to isolate the offending piece without bringing the odor in your home.

Pesticides

According to the World Health Organization, from 1 million to 25 million people suffer from pesticide poisoning a year.[29] In 1995, *The Crop Duster*, published by Pesticide Watch, noted, "A new study is being reviewed by the EPA which shows that the pesticide malathion causes liver tumors in mice."[30] It has been estimated that as many as 20,000 people in the United States each year will develop cancer from pesticide residues on their foods.[31] These pesticides, insecticides, herbicides, and fungicides are all substances used to kill living things.

Mostly, pesticides are used on crops, but they are also found in nearly every public place you can think of. Pesticides are encountered in the home, workplace, and businesses, as well as in the food and water you consume, the clothes you wear, and the air you breathe. Hospitals and movie theaters are known to spray for ants. Pesticides are used in fumigating homes, mosquito-abatement, and pest-strips.

Over half of all pesticides used are sprayed on corn and soybean crops that are used to feed livestock. Animals consume these crops and you eat the animal, which is thus a major source of pesticide residue. Unexplained chronic illnesses can result from unsuspected daily contact and minute quantities of residue can be problematic for the chemically sensitive. This is a growing concern because pesticide use has tripled between 1965 and 1985.[32]

Researchers from the University of Newcastle in Australia published a study that found CFS patients to have 45% higher levels of certain pesticides than found in normal controls.[33] Exposure to pesticides and herbicides can cause varied psychological and neurological symptoms such as mental confusion, depression, headaches, and abnormal nerve function. These substances are difficult to excrete through the already overburdened liver and become stored in the fat cells of the body where they remain indefinitely.

Sherry's last healthy day in over 12 years came when the apartment she lived in was fumigated for termites. The primary site of infestation, receiving the heaviest treatment, was right under her bedroom and she was not informed until after the work was done. Abruptly after that she lost control of her muscles and had difficulty breathing, and was on continuous oxygen.

Consider methyl bromide, which is classified by the EPA as a Category 1 acute toxin, the most deadly classification of substances. Methyl bromide is a colorless, odorless gas that is used primarily in agricultural fumigants. California strawberry farmers are one of the largest users of methyl bromide and this fruit has the highest combined score for pesticide contamination and toxicity of all fruits and vegetables. During strawberry fumigation, this substance is injected into the soil and covered with plastic tarpaulins. It is estimated that 50% of the gas escapes, posing an immediate health hazard to those nearby.[34] Eventually it dissipates and reaches the stratosphere where it destroys the ozone layer.

The acute effects of this poison include headaches, nausea, vomiting, dizziness, and blurred vision, and can be fatal. The impact is cumulative and considered to be dangerous in low-level exposures. Long-term effects can damage the central nervous system, heart, kidneys, lungs, and reproductive system, and it is a suspected carcinogen. In 1984 the Birth Defect Prevention Act required that manufacturers of over 200 high-priority pesticides submit toxicity studies within 5 years or face cancellation of the registration and subsequent use of their product. In 1991 a one-time, 5-year extension to March of 1996 was granted for many chemicals, including methyl bromide. To date no study has been done. Congress has now okayed another extension.

Pesticide Interventions

If pesticides are so pervasive, how do you avoid exposures? Avoiding places known to use pesticides is the first step. Other interventions include purchasing a water filter that removes pesticides. Eating organically grown foods and using the procedure for cleaning your foods will reduce the burden to your body. Ingestion of fresh juices can help, as the juicing process separates the fibers that hold the pesticides. Some homeopathic remedies can also help remove the damaging substances from your cells.

Minimize the use of insecticides around your home, and if you must, use less toxic forms such as boric acid. Keep your environment clean so that pests will not be attracted to your home. Avoid travel on airlines, which routinely spray insecticides in the plane cabin. Try to educate your neighbors as to alternatives to spraying their yards and lawns with these poisons. Most insects are beneficial and learning to live in harmony with them may hold part of the answer.

Researchers at Florida's Institute of Food and Agricultural Sciences are moving in the direction of sustainable agriculture, that is, farming done at the lowest cost to natural resources. To this end, friendly insects, water-based soap sprays, and natural repellants such as garlic extracts are replacing the use of toxic chemicals on many farms. Pest-resistant plants and physical barriers that control the pests but do not harm the environment are also being used. These efforts at "integrated pest management" allow growers to rely less on chemicals and are cutting production costs as well.

Phenol and Petroleum-Based Products

Phenol is an organic compound made from coal tar commonly used in epoxy, drugs, gasoline additives, perfume, and as a preservative in medications and foods. Phenol is used in molded articles such as telephone parts, children's toys, dishes, and laminated boards. Reportedly phenol is present in mouthwash as well as disinfectants. It is frequently used in household cleaning products, as well as in dyes. It is even used in the manufacture of nylon. It should be noted that phenol is one of the unstable substances that outgas from plastics.

Petroleum is used not just in your car, but also in engine and gas oils, paint, kerosene, floor waxes, and plastics. It's in nearly every synthetic object man has invented. Synthetic fabrics, crayons, rubber boots, contact lenses, appliances, food wrappers and containers, pens, and electric blankets are a few more products containing plastics that can emit harmful fumes.

Plastics pose a problem because they are so widespread and are hidden in other products that seem to be safe. Small molecules break off from the larger plastic polymers, causing the emission of fumes. When agents are added to keep plastics soft and flexible, outgassing is more intense. It has become common to wrap foods in plastic wrap or to place foodstuffs in plastic containers and plastic wrap, but fumes outgas, being absorbed into the foods. Theresa becomes quite sick when she eats foods stored in this manner. Plastic becomes more harmful and offensive when it is heated, which intensifies the release of the molecules.

Contact with plastics and phenol products can cause nausea, arrhythmias, emotional lability, and respiratory difficulties. Theresa's small child is attracted to plastic toys and Theresa is reactive to the fumes emitted by these toys. It has been no small feat to gradually introduce old, fully outgassed plastic toys into her home for her daughter's enjoyment while balancing her own health needs.

Newsprint

The print in newspapers and most books contains petroleum products. The simple act of reading can become an impossible task if you have EI, as the fumes can make you ill. The less sensitive read by holding printed material at arm's length to put as much distance between their nose and the print as possible. Reading boxes, purchased commercially or made by adapting a glass picture frame to cover reading material, can help isolate newsprint fumes. Gloves can also be worn to avoid contact with the ink. Theresa is so intolerant of newsprint fumes that she can only listen to talking books on tape and Laura has friends read the newspaper to her. If you are not as sensitive, try to air the newspaper or book in the sun for a week or two. Placing reading materials in the oven at 180 degrees for 20 minutes can accelerate the outgassing of fumes. There has been an increased demand for soy-based ink books which, if printed on dioxin-free paper, can make reading materials more accessible for those who are chemically sensitive.

Petroleum and Phenol Interventions

Once again, it's best to avoid contact with substances that outgas fumes. Hard plastics are less likely to be problematic. The process of receiving antigen injections to control allergic reactivity may unwittingly introduce the preservative phenol into your body. Phenol injections can make you feel worse, and consequently it is important to request phenol-free solutions. Although they are more difficult to prepare and cannot be stored for long periods, phenol-free solutions are available. Before taking any substance, check the label; phenol should be listed in the medication contents, and if it is not listed, ask.

Positive Ions

Have you ever noticed that around the time of a full moon, or when it's windy, or just before a storm, you feel irritable, uncomfortable, and tense? Does driving on the freeway or contact with synthetic substances prompt tension and irritability? You may be experiencing the impact of positive ions created by synthetic substances. These synthetic substances, prevalent in certain environments, take away your life force, depleting and draining you because of the adverse impact of positive ions.

Positive ions are abundant in closed-ventilation buildings where the air is recirculated and the windows are sealed, and where there are mostly synthetic materials. Central heating and air conditioning systems destroy negative ions. When you spend all day inside this artificial environment, you are affected by this critically disturbed ion balance, which may account for your headaches and lethargy. Excessive positive ions are also more dense in auto traffic. A ride in an elevator can cause you to feel poorly when you get off. A stuffy room can cause you to feel tense and edgy or groggy, and inattentive.

Ions are electrically charged particles, either positive or negative, that are generated by the natural radiation from the earth and sun, water and light. Ions are short lived and require constant replenishing from nature. A negative ion, formed when an electron becomes attached to an oxygen molecule, can vitalize and refresh you in much the same way that purifiers clean air. Positive ions have been noted to depress the movement of cilia in the body, whereas negative ions stimulate the movement of cilia. Ions effect the release of serotonin which regulates blood pressure, inflammation, mood states, and the impulses of the nervous system.[35]

Positive Ion Interventions

Many with EI opt to create negative ion-saturated living environments in order to relieve symptoms. People with allergic sensitivities prefer to live near the ocean or in the mountains where the air is most pure and there are higher concentrations of negative ions. Negative ions are those that heal and restore you, but they cannot be replenished in places where cement and synthetic environments are pervasive.

It is the subtle, intangible healing effect of negative ions that causes you to be drawn to bodies of water or the mountains. In these environments people experience increased energy and generally feel more optimistic and robust. If you cannot get to these places, you may wish to install a negative ion generator or air purifier in your home or work space. Using a purifier can cause an increased sense of well-being, heightened energy, and increased relaxation.

Water

Half of our drinking water comes from lakes and streams and we are drinking the same water from places that are subject to industrial waste and pesticide runoff. Groundwater can also be damaged by leaking gas tanks and toxic waste. The EPA estimates that 42 million people drink water that exceeds the safety level for lead.[36] There are increasing amounts of toxic chemicals present in drinking water. Fluoride, chloroform, and other chlorine-containing compounds are found in the water you drink. There is particular concern about studies linking cancer and heart disease to chlorine, the chemical commonly used to disinfect drinking water. In fact, it is such a matter of concern that Greenpeace is calling for the global phaseout of chlorine.[37]

Fluoride is often found in water and may be useful in preventing tooth decay, but it also enters the stomach, bones, heart, brain, kidneys, and tissues. And, according to the National Cancer Institute, fluoride can cause cancer faster than any other chemical. Since fluoride is a known insecticide and causes genetic mutations and birth defects, what is it doing in the water supply?

Waterborne illnesses are on the rise. An outbreak of illness afflicting 400,000 people occurred in 1993 in Milwaukee caused by *Cryptosporidium.* In this outbreak, over 100 people died. An outbreak of the bacterium *E. coli* was reported in July of the same year in New York City.[38] Chlorine is useless against *Cryptosporidium* and *Giardia,* two protozoan cysts found in water supplies.

The hygiene of our water supply is vital to health and the sustaining of all life. Drinking impure damaged water creates an impure damaged body, making it disturbing that so much of our drinking water contains contaminants and chemicals.

Theresa and Laura are "allergic" to the tap water in their homes. They become sick from the chlorinated fumes and cannot turn on the spigot without the use of purification systems. Not only is drinking water a concern, but reports show that showering is a major source of human toxicity, as it exposes people to chlorine and its fumes.[39]

As water supplies become more polluted, standards protecting us from unsafe drinking water continue to be inadequate. Until recently, the public had the notion that whatever came through the tap was safe to drink. Yet, healthy skepticism is necessary if you are to find out what contaminants and purifying agents are present in your tap water.

Your local water utility is required to inform you of the results of its water testing. Once you access information regarding water quality, you can search for appropriate water purification equipment to remedy the problem. This should be done keeping in mind that water pipes contain deposits and materials unique to your household, and old pipes contain greater amounts of rust and residue that break off into the water. Even if you don't drink directly from the tap, your skin absorbs chemicals when you bathe or shower.

Water Interventions

There is a growing market for water filtration and purification systems that can be installed in the home. Different systems remove different substances: filtration systems prevent the breathing of chlorine fumes and remove other contaminants and water purifiers remove pollutants. Treating the entire water system with reverse osmosis and charcoal filtration helps remove plasticizers and chlorine fumes. It should be noted that purchasing a water filtration system does not mean you are safe from contaminants; the filter often acts as a breeding ground for bacteria and mold.

So what is safe to drink? Spring water, touted as safe, is free of chemicals but may have pesticide residue or excessive amounts of minerals. Boiled tap water is better for you than water taken straight from the faucet, but this procedure can be a time-consuming nuisance.

So far, distilled is the purest water available, which means it has been boiled, turned into steam, and condensed. In the condensation process impurities are left behind when the liquid returns back into the container as precipitation. When water precipitates, heavy metals and sediments stay at the bottom of the container, separating out because they are too heavy to rise with the steam. The process of boiling destroys bacteria and mold, making it more pure and chemical-free.

Private water purification companies have begun to cash in on the growing public concern and awareness that groundwater has become more contaminated. The quality of the drinking water at any particular distributor should always be subject to question. These water distributors say they "distill" their water, but this does not necessarily mean they boil the water, the step essential to the removal of certain impurities. You may want to have this water tested or ask to see the company's water quality standard report.

Make sure you get the real thing. The purity of steam distilled water is an important factor in promoting health. Theresa distills her family's water using a large home-distiller so that she is certain of the water's quality. Distilled water has the property of pulling inorganic minerals out, while allowing organic minerals to remain in the tissue. Other types of water carry inert minerals into the body while distilled water transports the minerals out, thereby cleansing the arteries, lungs, liver, and kidneys.[40] Despite the good news about distilled water, it doesn't contain the minerals that are present in most drinking water so you must seek them elsewhere. This means you may want to replace the minerals found in ordinary water through diet and supplements.

Despite evidence that supports the use of distilled water, the issue of water safety is a complex and controversial subject. There is much evidence linking drinking water without minerals, also known as soft water, to significant increases in the risk of heart disease. Also, in an energetic sense, distilled water is considered to be dead or lifeless. Because of these concerns some feel that filtered water is a healthier option.

Storing water in plastic bottles can pose a hazard, as these containers are contaminated with chemicals such as formaldehyde that can leach into the water. Outgassing is intensified if the container sits in the sun. You may be able to taste the plastic in the water when it has been stored in these containers. It's best to store drinking water in glass or stainless steel containers because there is no outgassing. This is complicated by the fact that several years ago companies stopped making glass five-gallon water bottles, so they may be difficult to find.

Carbon filters, straining devices mounted onto the cold water line leading to your kitchen sink, work to purify water automatically. The problem is that these cannot be trusted to remove all bacteria and viruses and some brands work better than others. Laura uses a Multi-Pure filter that removes lead, asbestos, pesticides, chemicals, bacteria, and microscopic impurities, yet retains natural minerals.[41] Equinox brand filters have performed even better in laboratory tests. The Doulton water filter is reported to be the only system capable of filtering bacteria the size of cryptosporidium, and some believe it to be one of the best systems available.[42]

Large amounts of chlorine are absorbed through the skin and lungs from breathing vapors while bathing or showering. It is important to have a shower or bathtub filter in order to prevent the absorption of chlorine through the skin and lungs.

Summary

Various types of environmental hazards from petrochemicals to EMFs to heavy metals are becoming more common worldwide. As a rule, traditional medicine has not been aware that these substances are harmful, but they are waking up to concerns regarding these health hazards. The best you can do is educate yourself and seek to minimize the impact these substances have on your health.

Endnotes

[1]U.S. Environmental Protection Agency, Office of Community and Public Affairs, "Environmentally Induced Diseases," *EPA Journal* Mar.–Apr. 1990.

[2]Michael Castleman, "Tiny Particles, Big Problems," *Sierra* Nov.–Dec. 1995: 26–27.

[3]Paul Brodeur, "Danger in the Schoolyard," *Family Circle* Sept. 1990: 64.

[4]N. Wertheimer and E. Leeper, *Am J Epidemiol* 109 (1979): 273–284.

[5]For information regarding polarizer pendant and other related products, contact William Bennett, Springlife Polarity Products, P.O. Box 2181, Aptos, CA 95001, (800) 987-9425.

[6]Theron Randolph and Ralph Moss, *An Alternative Approach to Allergies* (New York: Harper & Row, 1989) 62.

[7]Lynn Lawson, *Staying Well in a Toxic World* (Chicago: The Noble Press, 1995) 187.

[8]Lawson, 188.

[9]Lawson, 191.

[10]Richard Gerber, Vibrational Medicine (Santa Fe: Bear & Co., 1988) 263.

[11]Sara Shannon, *Good Health in a Toxic World* (New York: Warner, 1994) 232.

[12]Sam Ziff *et al.*, "The Hazards of Silver/Mercury Dental Fillings; Mercury Detoxification," *Bio Probe 1990*.

[13]O. Canto *et al.*, "Mechanisms of $HgCl^2$ Cytoxicity in Cultured Mammalian Cells," *Mol Pharmacol* 26 (1984): 60–68.

[14]A. Rossi *et al.*, "Modifications of Cell Signaling in the Cytoxicity of Metals," *Pharmacol Toxicol* 68 (1993): 424–429.

[15]A. Bansal *et al.*, "Lipid Peroxidation and Activities of Antioxygenic Enzymes In-Vitro in Mercuric Chloride Treated Human Erythrocytes," *Bull Environ Contam Toxicol* 48 (1992): 89–94.

[16]Harald Hamre, study by E. Lain and G. Caughron, "Electrogalvanic Phenomenon of the Oral Cavity Caused by Dissimilar Metallic Restorations," *J Am Dent* 23 (1936): 1641–1652, "Mercury Exposure from Dental Amalgam and Chronic Fatigue Syndrome—A Possible Connection?" *The CFIDS Journal* Fall 1994: 44–47.

[17]Carrie Topliffe, "Silver Fillings: Poison in Your Mouth?" *Candida Research and Dysbiosis Foundation.*

[18]J. Richards and P. Warren, "Mercury Vapor Released During the Removal of Old Amalgam Restorations," *Br Dent* 159 (1985): 231–232.

[19]A. Summers *et al.*, "Mercury Released from Dental "Silver" Fillings Provokes an Increase in Mercury and Antibiotic Resistant Bacteria in Oral and Intestinal Floras of Primates," *Antimicrob Agents Chemother* 37.4 (1993): 825–834.

[20]*The Human Ecologist*, quote from newsletter, *Rocky Mountain Environmental Health Association* Nov.–Dec. 1990: 28.

[21]R. Schiele *et al.*, "Studies of the Mercury Content in the Brain and Kidney Related to Number and Condition of Amalgam Fillings," *Med Dent Med* (12 Mar. 1984).

[22]Frank Green, "Is Your Mouth Full of Toxic Teeth?" *The San Diego Union* 29 Dec. 1990: E1, E5.

[23]U.S. Environmental Protection Agency, "Indoor Air Pollution" (Washington, DC: EPA) 12.

[24]Lawson, 142.

[25]Theron Randolph and Ralph Moss, study by Marshall Mandell and Lynn Scanlonn, *Dr. Mandell's 5-Day Allergy Relief System* (New York: Thomas Crowell, 1979) 188, *An Alternative Approach to Allergies* (New York: Harper & Row, 1989) 239.

[26]For information regarding ceramic heaters, contact Radiant Heater Corporation, P.O. Box 60, Greenport, NY 11914, (516) 924-0444 or (800) 331-6408.

[27]U.S. Congress, office of Ron Wyden, "Is Perfume Getting You Down? Now is the Opportunity to Speak Up," *Cosmetic Safety* (Washington, DC: U.S. Congress, 1989).

[28]"Retailer Sued for an Olfactory Offense," *Santa Cruz Sentinel* 6 Feb. 1992: A-9.

[29]Lawson, 206.

[30]Janet Dauble, "Pesticide Update," *Share Care and Prayer* Jan.–May 1995: 35–36.

[31]Lawson, 210.

[32]Theron Randolph and Ralph Moss, notes from Samuel Epstein's book, *The Politics of Cancer* (San Francisco: Sierra Club, 1978); *An Alternative Approach to Allergies* (New York: Harper & Row, 1989) 66.

[33]Molly Holzschlag, "Pesticides May be Part of CFIDS Etiology," *HEALTHwatch* 6.1 Jan. 1996: 1–2.

[34]Joyce Vandevere and Karen Light, "Methyl Bromide:Huge Profits for a Few or Public Health?" *The Ventana* Feb. 1996: 6–7, 25.

[35]Phyllis Saifer and Marla Zellerbach, *Detox* (Los Angeles: J.P. Tarcher, 1984) 73–74.

[36]Anita Slomski, "Is Your Home Poisoning You?" *Consumer Digest* Sept.–Oct. 1989: 65.

[37]Joe Thornton, "Chlorine, Human Health and the Environment" (Washington, DC: Greenpeace, 1993).

[38]"Water Borne Illnesses are on the Rise," *The New York Times* 29 July 1993.

[39]Gregory Pouls, address, "Environmental Solutions," Pacific Cultural Center, Santa Cruz, 17 Jan. 1996.

[40]Jack Soltanoff, *Natural Healing* (New York: Warner Books, 1988) 226.

[41]For information regarding Multi-Pure products, call (800) 622-9205.

[42]For more information about the Doulton water filter, call (800) 888-4353.

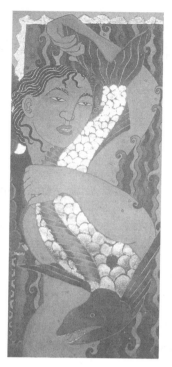

*Chapter
Eleven*

*Practical
Matters*

*f*inancial worries pose a major concern. It is impossible to measure the overall financial impact of these illnesses on your own life, let alone the economy at large. Not only do you suffer from the personal financial burden caused by these illnesses, but the contribution and productivity of those who are ill is lost to the larger society as well. By multiplying the not so hidden cost of this illness by the two to five million people reported to be sick and adding the social and economic damage done to families, there is a profound socioeconomic impact.

These illnesses are expensive. As previously noted, Dr. Byron Hyde, physician in Ottawa, Canada, estimates a loss of $100 billion in salaries in the United States and Canada.[1] One support group compared notes and the 12 participants with EI and CFS found that nonreimbursable medical care and alternative treatments cost them from $2000 to $25,000 a year. Ongoing medical care can deplete a family's financial reserves, even causing bankruptcy.

Gloria and her husband will probably have to sell their beautiful home, as they cannot make the payments on one income. With all of Gloria's old medical bills still to be paid, they cannot borrow more money in order to meet their mortgage payments. Understandably, she is reluctant to return to teaching because the stress of the job had everything to do with the onset of her illness. "Going back to teaching means choosing between health and money and this isn't a choice I'm willing to make."

"People who start out with savings before this disease hits are broke before it's over," notes Laura, who has Crohn's, severe EI, and is in recovery from CFS. "I have had to become very creative, flexible, and frugal in keeping financially solvent."

There are several forms of assistance available for those with disabilities. Mortgage payments can be restructured, pharmaceutical companies have plans offering free or discounted medication, and student loans can be forgiven. Utility companies have reduced bill plans for people with low incomes and state and federal agencies have services not widely known. There are also community resources such as the Lions Clubs, United Way, local social and health services departments, as well as self-help publications available in the library.

This chapter explores not only the financial impact of these illnesses on your life, but also the practicalities of survival. How to get medical insurance companies to pay is as important as figuring out how to create a less toxic home. You will need to consider whether its worth risking toxic exposures and taxing your body by continuing to work. Electing to gear down career expectations can enable you to work in a less stressful, perhaps less chemically loaded environment. But in doing this, you must consider that you are opting to reduce your income and thus your ability to meet health care expenses.

Medical Insurance

Many people who suffer from EI or CFS cannot work full-time and others are completely bedridden and cannot work at all. Many cannot get insurance coverage, or cannot afford to pay the premiums. Even when there is coverage, carriers often decline to pay for nontraditional interventions, despite the fact that they alleviate symptoms. Even when insurance does pay, compensation is erratic and rules for honoring claims change, making it difficult to count on reimbursement over time.

Elaine and her husband budget $300 a month for nonreimbursed medical expenses above their insurance premiums. This is so she can have access to acupuncture, supplements, intravenous vitamins, replacing air purifier filters, and occasional hands-on healing sessions. Even then this is not enough, and occasionally they have to dip into savings. At one time, Judy, who has had CFS and still struggles with EI, had no medical insurance and was also not eligible to collect disability payments. At that time she borrowed money from her credit cards. When she could no longer play this shell game, she came close to being homeless and was still unable to convince Medi-Cal and social security of her need, and her applications were repeatedly turned down. All that time she had to go without medical care.

County-funded medical care is available for those who have no medical insurance or who are awaiting Medi-Cal or Medicaid eligibility. Medi-Cal and Medicaid are state-funded insurance policies for low income individuals. This coverage takes care of the basics, but is often insufficient to meet your unusual healthcare needs or if you need the attention of a nonprovider physician who understands the quirks of EI and CFS. Still, this coverage is better than having no coverage at all. Then there are people like Elaine, who receives weekly intravenous vitamin C infusions needed to reduce allergic reactivity, but even her private medical insurance refuses to pay for this.

Some insurance carriers such as Blue Shield have an annual open enrollment drive that enables those with preexisting conditions to seek medical coverage. Premiums are usually expensive, but worth securing. Avoid allowing current insurance to lapse, as it is difficult to acquire coverage once this occurs.

Getting Insurance Companies to Pay

Most people who are ill will not fight if their medical claims are denied. When you receive a letter of denial, it is easy to take the company's word for it, accepting that you are not entitled to reimbursement. Many people with EI and CFS opt to suffer without treatment rather than confront and disagree with their insurance carrier.

There are no penalties for decisions made by insurance companies that err in their own favor by declining to honor valid claims. Insurance companies are immune from prosecution for damages incurred when they refuse to pay you, even if they are later found to be wrong. However, you may not realize you have the right to appeal denied claims. In order to summon the energy to fight a denial, it may be necessary to establish firmly in your mind that you deserve compensation. You are paying for coverage so if the claim is within the terms of the contract the company is required to pay.

The documentation required to submit an appeal can be daunting, thereby discouraging you from even trying. Initiating an appeal takes time and effort. You may have the time but this added stressor can make it impossible to cope with other parts of your life. At this point you must weigh whether an appeal is worth the effort; only you will know the answer. When the bills are complex and numerous, there is a lot more money at stake, a compelling reason to appeal.

Going to battle can be exhausting and discouraging, but it can also be an empowering and hopeful experience to successfully win an appeal. By looking at the process as an interesting challenge, you may be able to turn a potentially stressful experience into an informative adventure.

It can be quite a feat to get insurance to pay for some of the more extraordinary services for EI and CFS that are regarded to be experimental, nontraditional, or include vitamin or herbal supplements. Consider intravenous vitamin C treatments which have proven to be helpful in relieving allergic reactions, as well as improving overall immune function. Insurance companies often turn down these claims, citing that they come under the heading of vitamins, or experimental treatment.

For years Josh received intravenous infusions of vitamin C, on a weekly basis at a cost of $85 a treatment. That's $4420 a year out of his own pocket just for intravenous fluids. Despite insurance's refusal to pay, the treatments have made such a difference in his health that he has continued them. On the other hand, Elaine's insurance carrier pays for these beneficial treatments because her physician bills each treatment as an office visit.

So that you don't waste unnecessary energy and time on futile efforts to be reimbursed, try to recognize which appeals are likely to be successful and which are not. After years of Jamie receiving routine chiropractic adjustments to help alleviate spinal and joint pain, her insurance carrier abruptly decided these treatments did not meet medical necessity. Certain of her right to service, she appealed and was turned down three times. Many months and many letters later, the insurance company hired an independent specialist to examine her at their expense. "All along I was certain that I was right, but it was like felling Goliath to finally succeed. What a confirmation of my right to care," gloated Jamie when the specialist examined all the documentation, performed a physical exam, and decided in her favor.

The first step in challenging a denial is to review all of the reasons why you should be covered. This can be done by examining your insurance policy to determine what services are excluded and what items are allowed. Learn all you can about your particular policy, noting what time limits you must adhere to in order to submit a written appeal. Most submissions and appeals must take place within a year of the date of service, although some require a letter within 30 days. In preparing your letter, include all pertinent factual information, then state your arguments, citing why the insurance company should pay.

Persuasive arguments are critical. If you are being denied coverage for interventions that are considered experimental, gather information as to how many physicians use this particular treatment. Specify what positive results have been achieved and note how safe and effective the treatment has been. You can get this information from your physician, reference librarian, newspapers, medical journals, and organizations dealing with EI and CFS.

Let the insurance company know what impact the treatment has had on improving your health. Explain how this intervention will ultimately reduce your overall medical claims and that denial of this treatment will interfere with your ability to maintain wellness. The humanity of their decision should also be emphasized. If going without reimbursement means you will not be able to function at your job, or will suffer increased discomfort, state this clearly in your letter.

At times, carriers pay for initial treatments, only to deny later claims for the same service. You can argue, since they paid for the initial treatments and later denied coverage for the same treatment, they are in violation of what is known as an "implied contract." If a company initially pays and the client depends on this implied agreement, incurring further debts as a result of treatment, there is an "implied contract." The insurance company is breaking that contract when it reverses its initial decision and refuses to pay for subsequent services.

Even if you cannot formulate a clear argument for coverage, you should write an appeal, simply requesting that they reconsider their denial. Writing the appeal in angry harsh words is like shooting yourself in the foot: while it may make you feel better to vent your hostility, it can interfere with achieving desired results. You will be most successful if you sound as appreciative and positive as possible, conveying a certain faith in the adjuster's good intentions. Sometimes it helps to write two letters, one that takes care of all the frustration and anger you may feel, and one that is positive and hopeful. Then send the one that best supports your success.

Insurance companies are known to decline to pay because the diagnosis of the illness has not been substantiated by clinical tests. You may have to ask your physician for copies of tests that support the presence of your illness or ask that confirmatory tests be performed if they have not previously been done. Requesting that your physician routinely write a prescription for all nontraditional interventions that might be questioned will help support an appeal. Send a copy of this prescription with the insurance claim to help substantiate medical necessity.

If the claim is denied, you still must reimburse the physician for his services. Try to avoid resenting or blaming him for ordering unreimbursable tests and supplements by understanding what you are getting into before you agree to tests and added expenses. Even if a treatment has been helpful, there is a tendency to direct frustration over nonreimbursement toward the physician who certainly deserves to be paid.

It can be an onerous task to keep track of claims and to hound the companies. It's understandably common for insurance carriers to lose track of claims, so you should keep track of all bills. This can be accomplished by maintaining a ledger that includes all healthcare expenses and the dates of claim submissions. Be sure to keep copies of all letters and prescriptions you send and receive in the process of an appeal.

When speaking by phone to the claims office, make sure you get the name of the person you are dealing with so he or she can be recontacted for follow-up queries. Another reason to get a name is to later send a letter of appreciation if the person has been helpful in handling a complex matter. Your thoughtfulness can fuel the person's incentive to fulfill what seems to be thankless, impersonal work.

If the matter is small, yet you don't want to let it drop, take it to small-claims court. Their fee includes only the filing costs and the process is oriented toward the layperson. Check with your county courthouse as to the particulars of this process. The maximum amount awarded may vary according to state.

The state insurance commissioner provides free investigation and review of formal complaints against state-certified insurance providers or you may wish to contact your local congressperson's office for help. Both of these numbers, listed in the government section of the phone book, may get results when you have not been successful on your own.

Social Security Disability

There are two mind-sets with regard to accessing disability. The concept of being disabled carries with it a certain self-fulfilling prophecy which emphasizes the need to prove dysfunction. Having to prove that you are disabled can heighten attachment to the illness. If you think of yourself as being disabled, you may become more disabled. In this way, accepting the label can hamper your recovery.

While on short-term disability leave, unable to work because of EI and CFS, Jamie worried that she might appear to be too healthy on occasions when her boss or co-workers visited. She exaggerated symptoms so she wouldn't look or act too energetic. Despite feeling terrible, she looked the picture of health and she was afraid they'd think she was well enough to return to work. Meanwhile, the more she tried to act ill, the worse she felt and the stronger she found herself holding onto the image of herself as a sick person.

The other school of thought is that if you need financial assistance you are certainly deserving, but may have to steel yourself and summon the courage to request help. Many with EI and CFS are too disabled to work; it's not a matter of choice, they simply cannot. It's scary to see the bills roll in and the money roll out, and not be able to work.

In some instances, continuing to work causes greater incapacity. Time away from work offers the opportunity to rest in order to enhance the healing process, yet this decision is often reached with great resistance and anxiety. Selima became so ill that the choice was no longer her own. When she finally took time off and went on disability, in a subtle way she too noticed a certain attachment to the image of herself as being ill. "It was like trying to do two contradictory things at once. Supporting my recovery, while also trying to prove I was too ill to work. My body was totally confused." Then there is also the stigma attached to being on disability that may include a loss of self-esteem and self-image.

Initiating the disability application process means you have, to some extent, come to accept the illness. Filing is a tangible admission of the reality of the illness that calls a halt to any sort of denial. This can open the floodgates for you to grieve the loss of function, the loss of life-style, and the loss of self-definition.

Once you move through denial, your resistance may continue to come from a sense that you are not entitled. You have probably already paid into social security disability through years of employment, making it your right to seek this help. If you are unable to work and feel that you are eligible for disability, apply and keep at it.

When Josh, the oncology nurse with CFS, became too sick to work, he repeatedly tried over the course of 3 years to get on disability. "I was turned down the second time because they said I still had the use of my arms and legs. What finally qualified me was giving my car to a friend. Ironic, isn't it? My lack of transportation now makes it impossible for me to secure employment, but it did the trick. Because the system was so backed up, a judge just signed my papers without the usual hearing." A successful veteran of the experience, he has several tips for those applying for disability:

1. Take a look at your fear of applying for disability. By taking this step you are no longer defined by what you do, but who you are. Examine what this means to your self-image and loss of identity. This can also mean accepting powerlessness over your illness in a deep way.

2. Accept the fact that the process will take a long time and that meanwhile you will be poor.

3. You must have no taxable income and must spend down your savings. You may have to sell your car and then apply for general assistance in order to get by while you await a hearing.

4. In order to qualify, you must be able to prove in a court that you can no longer work at all and that your disability will last a year or more.

5. Get an attorney to help. No attorney can charge for her services before the case is settled, which means anyone can get legal counsel. The attorney's fees are deducted from your settlement. It can make a big difference to get legal support in this mind-boggling process.

6. Don't be discouraged if you receive denials, which are common. Be prepared to take the appeal through numerous stages, even up to the administrative judge level. The system is designed to weed out people who are not truly in need. Fortunately, the settlement is retroactive from the date you file.

It has been easier for people with CFS to get on disability based on documented treatment for depression than for CFS. "I know three people who got on disability faster than I did because they opted to go that route. Sure this illness causes depression, but that isn't what makes me unable to work," notes Josh. The lack of support that legitimizes these illnesses makes it difficult to access disability. And, make no mistake about it—it is difficult to get on disability. For some, this prospect alone is a deterrent, particularly when feeling utterly depleted.

It helps to reframe your mind-set, seeing this task as your current job. Tenacity is a quality that will be required of you when dealing with insurance claims and disability benefits, and most of all, in finding the patience to return to health. There is a close relationship between tenacity and feeling that you are deserving. Don't get the word *deserving* confused with *entitlement*, which is what happens when you think someone owes you something. Deserving means you are comfortable asking for something out of a sense of respect for yourself.

When you believe you are deserving, it's easier to find the energy to stand up for yourself, not giving up when your request is turned down. Instead of taking "no" for an answer, when you are deserving it means establishing a plan to find another way to get what's fair. In this process, don't waste precious energy on efforts that are bound to fail, unless you are just looking for a way to vent irritation. When you vent your irritation, aside from leaving you more frustrated, you'll lose the incentive to stand up for yourself the next time around even though you are deserving. Harnessing tenacity is a part of harnessing your power. Tenacity is necessary to help your entire being heal.

Income Tax Information

This section is offered to help open your eyes to the possibility that you can write off some of your illness-related medical expenses. The process of becoming well and maintaining your health can require that you make significant changes in your home, diet, and personal care habits. Your physician may inform you of the need to convert your home from gas to an electric heating system and household appliances may need to be replaced. You may need to remove a formaldehyde-treated carpet, or all of the particleboard in the walls. Or you may be told you would benefit from routine massage, a special diet, or a certain kind of shampoo.

These directions from your physician may require large financial expenditures, some of which can be considerably mitigated if you understand and use the medical deduction portion of your income tax form. If these changes are needed because of medical necessity, they can be treated as a partial or full medical deduction.

"You may include in medical expenses amounts you pay for special equipment installed in your home or for improvements, if the main reason is for medical care. Permanent improvements that increase the value of the property may be partly deductible as medical expenses. The amount paid for the improvement is reduced by the increase in the value of the property. The rest is the medical expense," according to the Internal Revenue Service, which offers a publication specifying what medical deductions you can write off.[2]

Save all receipts for any items you are deducting; if you don't have proper documentation, the deduction can be disallowed. You may prefer to keep track of all of your expenses by keeping a ledger. If you are on a medically prescribed diet, you can take an itemized medical deduction for the extra cost of the foods.

Those who must eat less chemically contaminated foods are seldom questioned about the deduction; but when other household members who are not ill claim this same deduction, there can be problems. To resolve this, your physician can list on the prescription the fact that all household members need to be on the diet, citing their names. This is acceptable because the act of cooking standard foods in the same household can cause reactivity for the ill person.

Every time you deduct an item that is of medical necessity, you must have a written statement from your physician that will support the deduction. This is handled by having the physician write a prescription or letter specifying the changes that are needed to sustain your health. Keep a copy of this information with your income tax forms. If necessary, obtain any other supporting documentation from your building contractor, hospital, realtor, pharmacist, landlord, or anyone else as necessary. Retain all of these records for at least 7 years after filing your taxes. What you are legally allowed to deduct can be subject to interpretation and may change from one year to the next, so you may wish to contact your accountant to clarify what items are acceptable.

Work and Identity

Gloria, in recovery from CFS, says her illness forced her to reevaluate how she defines success. "When I became ill I was teaching full time and caring for my mother who eventually passed away. I took responsibility for her life and feelings, as well as my own, all my students, my husband's, and my children's. I took responsibility for all sorts of people and less responsibility for my own emotions to the extent that my own feelings were deeply hidden. Then I hit the wall."

She went on to comment, "I grew up with the idea that who I was was very much associated with how successful I was and how much I helped other people and never learned to take care of me." One notable, consistent quality that links EI and CFS sufferers is that they often are superresponsible, hard-working people. Many who have been ill note that their sense of self-definition has been largely derived from the work they perform.

Are you driven, achievement-oriented, and a workaholic? Undoubtedly, you have always been very good at your work and have a terrific need to be successful. Despite your gifts, your body may not be in balance with the way you live. Running faster, pushing harder makes it difficult to stop and listen to the messages your body is sending you.

Dr. Randy Baker, who specializes in EI and CFS, notes, "A high percentage of those who are ill come from dysfunctional families. In these families of origin there may have been physical, emotional, or sexual abuse which eventually stressed the immune system and can result in EI and/or CFS." People from dysfunctional families are typically known to be unusually conscientious and overinvest in their work, which makes it easier to avoid painful relationships. In this way, it's more comfortable to place an inappropriate emphasis on the impersonal world of work because work causes fewer interpersonal conflicts for you to have to control. Since there may have been many interpersonal conflicts in childhood, it's easy to see why you might try to keep these experiences at arm's length as an adult.

For years Josh worked as a supervising nurse in an acute medical hospital. On the job he was exposed to X rays, cleaning solvents, electronic equipment, and pathogens. He was also subtly exposed to the psychic disturbance of the physically ill. Gradually, he experienced increased headaches, not suspecting that toxic exposures were causing damage. Over time, the stress of his job broke down the weak link of his genetic predisposition. And his personal life was in a shambles. Refusing to think of himself as a quitter, he kept pushing harder, "It was impossible to imagine giving up the identity I'd worked so hard to create."

Working in an unfulfilling job is as destructive as forcing yourself to perform in a work environment that has toxic chemicals. By tradition, much of your self-identity and esteem has been bound up in the material contributions you make in the world. Many find self-worth in their job to the extent that who they are is inextricably bound up in what they do. Like Gloria, the ex-teacher with CFS; you may have had to completely burn out before being forced to reexamine compensatory patterns. When Gloria could no longer work, she had no idea who she was and her illness forced her to define herself by new standards.

EI and CFS can completely chew up and spit out your identity. Unable to work and without an income, it becomes necessary to formulate a self image based on your true deeper strengths, rather than on what you do. When you meet someone for the first time, what do you want to know first? If you are like everyone else, you ask, "What do you do?" The response causes you to form an opinion of that person, regarding them with varying degrees of respect depending on their title.

Then how do you describe yourself when you are only able to stay awake a few hours a day or cannot leave home? There are no identifying characteristics that allow you to create a positive picture of yourself. You will need to decide to consciously reshape this externally imposed vision.

Finding a way to support yourself when you cannot work also poses a serious problem. The prospect of being indigent is both humiliating and frightening, adding yet another burden to an already overburdened existence. At one point, Judy, now recovered from CFS, had no idea how she would pay next month's rent; with only $100 in the bank, she was too sick to work. The fear surrounding this issue only made her health worse.

Having a chronic illness holds no special place of consideration at home or on the job. This is especially true at work; since you are being paid to do your share, there is no relief when you feel poorly. If you are often out sick or unable to work to maximum ability, it's easy to feel guilty. As Audrey, who had CFS, became more ill, she felt compelled to find ways to work more efficiently; coming in at 7 A.M. before the phones began to ring, she hoped to get ahead. Some force themselves to do extra work when they feel better to make up for downtime.

Many try hard to keep up, passing as healthy individuals by day, but out prostrate by night. "All my nonwork hours were devoted to resting in order to recover from my job," notes Jamie. "On weekends I would start to relax and feel better; by Sunday I'd feel almost human. But by the end of Monday, returning to all that toxic stress, the cycle would begin again."

Of course, you could find another job, or just quit. But the stress of finding new employment seems overwhelming and more stressful. How could you summon the energy to find another job when you can barely keep going at the one you have?

You could start by examining your options in your current work situation. Give yourself permission to request a desk near an open window, or ask someone else to do your photocopying for you. If necessary, explain to co-workers that toxic fumes impair your ability to function in a normal manner. The average person has no understanding of how difficult it is to do the job in the face of overwhelming fatigue and outgassed fumes. No one will look out for you so it's up to you to look out for yourself. It may be possible to assert yourself in small ways that make the workplace more tolerable.

Unless there is another reliable income source or you are on disability, quitting work can create more difficulties than it resolves. Those who are single often have no safety net; there is no one to support them. Part-time employment may be ideal for those who can work, allowing sufficient flexibility for time off to devote to healing.

If you've taken a leave, you may want to engage your employer prior to your return to figure out how to make the job work, given your limitations. A gradual return to work offers a great opportunity to figure out if you are able to keep pace and manage job stress. This may mean starting out with a minimum number of hours, gradually adding more over a period of weeks. Some elect to work for a period of time in a less demanding position in order to reduce stress.

Perhaps flexible work hours that permit you to be there when you are well and leave when the job is done will work for you. A change in spending habits that reduces your financial needs, a job change within the system, or a new job in a less toxic or stressful environment can support you into recovery.

Gloria originally decided to take a leave of absence from her teaching job, but this ultimately jeopardized her job standing. In a job search, it may detract from your desirability as a prospective new employee to mention a previous extended leave. Let's face it: who would you hire as a new employee? One who is known to take an excessive number of sick days and has multiple health complaints? Or one who has no problem working up to speed?

For the security conscious, there is also the issue of job benefits. Quitting a job that provides sick leave pay and medical coverage is risky. Medical insurance is a lifeline many cannot afford to be without. Seeking coverage from a new carrier runs the risk of their refusal to pay for your preexisting condition.

Gearing Down

Struggling to hold onto the image of yourself as upwardly mobile may mean you have to hit bottom before you are ready to let go. That stubborn resistance may include attachment to the idea that letting go of career goals signifies failure; meanwhile your health and sanity continue to tumble downward.

All of the money and esteem in the world cannot make up for the fact that you are too miserable to enjoy the fruits of your labors. Having to earn a certain amount of money becomes insignificant if you cannot enjoy your life. A fast track career is fluff when the life underneath is empty and full of suffering. Once you free yourself, the notions of who you are and what you are worth are no longer bound up with external striving. What becomes important is to have a full and happy life.

Once you accept that it is impossible to keep holding on, you may decide to move a rung or two down the career ladder to a less stressful job. Though the work may be less financially rewarding, you may be able to choose something more congruent with your heart's desire. Moving down the career ladder may mean freeing up your ideas of who you are or who you were meant to be in order to give yourself permission to settle for something better. Instead of continuing to strive for an elusive, external dream, your aspirations can now be realized on an inner level.

Illness can force you to clarify values, leading to the realization that it is more important to invest energy in yourself. In time, even when you recover, you may find the old way no longer fits and opt for a less complicated, less stressful life. When you undertake to simplify your life, the "shoulds" that are often not your own, but echoes of parental and societal expectations, fall away as you become more congruent with your real needs.

Like it or not, illness has forced you to pay attention to what matters most. When this happens, life becomes pretty basic. Rather than worrying about collecting accolades, financial success, and material objects, it becomes easier to see and honor the truth within. Discarding old values that no longer serve means you must toss aside your old definition of "success"; it is just an illusion you have agreed to create. Making this choice requires that you find the courage to buy out of a system that says who you are and what you are worth is bound up with what you do.

Living with greater honesty and congruence, there is more energy to attend to what really matters. A natural by-product of increased congruence is to begin to entertain concerns as to what kind of contribution you wish to make to the greater world. As your inner process becomes more harmonious, you are inevitably moved to reconnect in a harmonious manner with the rest of the planet. When you feel full and well loved, it is inevitable that your attention and compassion will be drawn toward others. Service flows outward as a natural progression of the completion you experience within.

The Work Environment

Hazards in the physical environment affect everyone. Just because you have the overt symptoms of EI doesn't mean you are the only one whose immune system is being harmed by the environment. Most people are not aware that their headaches, visual difficulties, and lethargy may be the result of environmental contamination.

In the interest of energy efficiency, offices and homes are built airtight, but there is growing concern that trapped air, contaminated by household chemicals, finishes, synthetic materials, plastics, and construction materials, is damaging to the body. In 1987 the Environmental Protection Agency (EPA) issued a report stating that pollution in homes and buildings is 2 to 5 times higher indoors than outside and may cause serious acute and chronic illnesses.[3]

If you are suffering from a weakened immune system, you are particularly vulnerable to the toxins found in unhealthy buildings. Common symptoms of an allergic, toxic response include: irritation and dryness of mucous membranes of the eyes, nose, and throat, dry skin, mental clouding, fatigue, difficulty concentrating, headaches, nausea, dizziness, and persistent colds.

Most concerns emphasize air quality, but there are other hazards as well. Formaldehyde molecules are released from particleboard, plastics, furniture, and carpets. Conductive magnetic and static effects created by electric phenomena can supply minute charges to the body, as well as result in an abundance of positive ions. Radon is emitted from cement and chemical fumes are emitted from paints, sealant, foam padding, building materials, and caulking.

Air stagnation can result in the buildup of carbon dioxide and a reduction of oxygen. Newsprint, air fresheners, chemicals from copy machines and cleaning products can also increase the toxic load. Cleaning fluids can linger in the air for hours and tests show that toilet bowl cleaner can cause a reduction in animal respiratory rate.[4] Anderson Laboratories in Massachusetts performed tests on 350 carpets and found adverse health effects on test animals, including death.[4] Ironically, in 1993, several EPA employees were awarded $950,000 for respiratory and neurological disorders caused by the installation of carpets and renovations in their Washington, DC headquarters.[5]

Older buildings can also be hazardous with their lead-based paint, poor ventilation, and the presence of mold growing in the walls and ventilation system. Environmental emissions can vary with temperature changes and air stagnation. Buildings located near major roadways are a magnet for toxic fumes. When a building is erected in a damp, shady location, mold and fungus can grow in the walls and carpets. And proximity to diesel generators can cause contact with fumes that nauseate even the healthiest.

An employer can be understandably reluctant to try to remedy an environmental problem because it often means added expense. This action may also indirectly acknowledge culpability, setting a precedent for the expectation of future upgrades. However, The Americans with Disabilities Act requires that employers provide reasonable work accommodations for individuals who have documented work-related health problems. To this end, Jamie's employers purchased an air purifier for her when they moved into a new, closed-ventilation building.

A 1984 World Health Organization report suggests that as many as 30% of new and remodeled buildings worldwide may generate excessive complaints related to poor indoor air quality.[6] Since this is a pervasive problem, you may need to join forces with co-workers and, if you have one, your union, as well as consult with public health officials for support to develop solutions. In the short term, what can you do to protect yourself? The following suggestions for yourself and your employers can help reduce indoor health hazards:

1. Identify and remove toxic materials from your surrounding area
2. Use nontoxic cleaning supplies
3. Have windows that open, increase ventilation, and improve the supply of fresh air
4. Maintain and properly clean ventilation systems
5. Restrict or prohibit smoking in work sites
6. Properly vent photocopy and fax fumes
7. Discourage wearing perfume and cologne
8. If possible, change gas heating sources to a less toxic system

Home Environments

Eliminating or reducing chemicals and hazardous materials in the home is the best way to reduce your toxic load. Reducing the toxic burden to your body will support your immune system to do its job protecting you. To this end, you may have to make radical changes in household furnishings.

For example, Theresa, who has severe EI, has a sparingly furnished home: all of the odds and ends that create the personality of a home must be kept in tin containers, stored high on shelves. In this way, she cannot be harmed by the marking pens, plastic objects, and papers that emit fumes and gather dust.

Household furniture is made of inert substances. In the dining area, canvas director's chairs surround a metal-and-glass dining table and an unusual-looking electric heater resembling a solar panel lines one wall.

Theresa cannot handle books because the odor from the print makes her sick; instead she listens to books on tape. Even after 10 years the old worn carpet in the living room still causes her to react; as a result she seldom enters this room. Fortunately, she is detached from material possessions, having the capacity to live simply and fully with great acceptance, despite the severe restrictions of her illness.

What a surprise to note that homes are more polluted indoors than the outside environment. As homes become more energy efficient, this enclosed environment can become a health hazard. Making your home airtight cuts off the fresh air supply needed to cleanse the environment. As more airtight, energy-efficient homes are built, gasses are more thoroughly trapped inside, increasing the toxic effects. The populace has yet to grasp the long-range effects of surrounding themselves with these substances that are unwittingly making them sick.

These indoor health hazards are insidious but extremely damaging to your well-being. Electric currents can change your mood and alter cellular activity. Common household products can cause allergic reactivity and natural gas has been known to produce cardiac arrhythmias and seizures. Advertising fails to note that many cleaning products have damaging effects on the body.

Older homes covered with lead-based paint can cause lead poisoning, impairing neurological function. Painting over a lead-based paint does not solve the problem because the lead eventually leaches through. Lead is used in the solder of food cans, as well as in some forms of regular gasoline. Some homes have been insulated with asbestos and roof and floor tiles can be made of this substance. Asbestos, known for its insulating ability, causes problems when it deteriorates, becoming a powder that can be inhaled. Once asbestos enters the body, it remains in the lungs and can result in lung and digestive tract cancers.

Radon emissions pose another concern as the second leading cause of lung cancer after cigarette smoking. Radon is an odorless, colorless, tasteless gas that results from the decay of radium. The EPA estimates that as many as six million homes throughout the United States have elevated levels of radon.[7]

Cleaning up and removing toxins from your home is the main thing you can do to reduce your body's total burden of toxins. Unfortunately, people often blame the wrong things for their problems, in part because it can be difficult to identify sources of reactivity. You may not know that a substance is causing you harm until it is removed and you feel better.

A good rule of thumb is that the more natural and fewer synthetics a product contains, the safer it is to use. Start by removing all standard brand detergents, replacing them with less toxic cleaning materials. Employing water-based floor finishes and using nontoxic paints can make a difference. When purchasing furniture, select stable materials such as untreated woods, aluminum, glass, and metal, which don't give off damaging fumes. Gradually replace linens, furniture, and cleaning supplies with more natural products.

advantageous as well as detrimental. A NASA study concluded
1 remove up to 80% of toxic indoor air within 24 hours.[8] Spider
drons help remove formaldehyde fumes and the presence of
e carbon monoxide from the air, converting it to oxygen. Yet,
clay pots which hold moisture can also be a source of mold. To
...us problem, replace clay pots with hard plastic or ceramic ones.

A continuous supply of fresh air is necessary to remove and dilute accumulated household toxins. In addition to keeping windows open, you may want to purchase an air purifier, an excellent way to remove dust and mold. With all of the different kinds that are on the market, it can be a daunting task to select the right one. Theresa, who has used different types of air purifiers over 13 years, recommends contacting Jim Nigra of Nigra Enterprises before making a purchase.[9]

There will still be other things you can do to change your environment that will improve your health. Your gas appliances can be a hidden source of continued allergic reactions, yet it can be expensive to convert to other systems. Periodic inspection and maintenance of your furnace, water heater, clothes dryer, and stove could prevent leaks and such equipment should be vented directly outside. Fireplace and wood stove flues should also be regularly inspected and cleaned.

Waking up tired is a clue that a nearby substance is causing reactivity. You may be reacting to animal dander, mold, or dust mites, which are arthropods that thrive on the dust and moisture in your bed linen. Keeping living areas dry will inhibit their proliferation. Creating an allergy-free oasis in your bedroom is probably the best thing you can do, since nearly a third of your life is spent there. Tips on how to create such an oasis were discussed in a previous section.

Less Toxic Furnishings and Products

Furnishings

Furniture should be outgassed, using untreated hardwood, metal, aluminum, or glass materials, or old objects. Most cushioned furniture has been treated with flame retardant and waterproofing substances. Polished or waxed furniture or anything that outgasses should be removed from your home.

Removing household carpets reduces the outgassing of formaldehyde and the accumulation of dust, mold, and dust mites. Electrostatic activity caused by walking on the carpet generates harmful positive ions. Use cotton throw rugs that can be placed in the wash.

Frequent cleaning of your home will reduce environmental contaminants and removal of carpets will reduce the accumulation of dust and dust mites. Though frequent cleaning of your home reduces environmental contaminants, vacuum cleaners raise dust. So the built-in, wall socket vacuum system, or a vacuum that filters small particles, such as the Nilfisk GS 90, can be helpful.[10]

Construction Materials

There is a growing number of wall paints that don't outgas; including casein, a milk product, and alkyd paints, which are best for reactive people. Commercial paints, latex in particular, can cause ongoing sensitivities. Once paint is applied to a surface, it can take years to fully outgas; then it's time to paint again.

It is best to paint and refinish floors, as well as perform household repairs, during warm seasons so that the house can be open to allow fresh air to circulate. In addition, warmer temperatures help speed up the neutralization process. Hiring a handyman to perform these tasks while you stay elsewhere reduces exposure to toxins.

Floors should be made of nontreated hardwood or glazed ceramic tile, which does not outgas or emit an electric charge. Wax floor finish should be avoided, using water-based finish instead. Even water-based finish carries an odor that can be irritating, so you may want to experiment by testing it on a small area at first.

Seemingly inoffensive construction materials release toxic chemicals. Some building materials contain arsenic, which can be fatal in small amounts. Wood, considered a natural substance, has often been treated to protect from insects, fungus, mold, and weather. Consequently, pesticides, fungicides, and formaldehyde are a normal part of wood materials used to build your home, giving off fumes for years to come. Careful selection of construction materials can avoid this problem: redwood and cedar are naturally insect resistant and don't need to be treated.

Household Cleaning Products

Many household products on the market today have long-range harmful effects on the body and advertising fails to inform you that damage can occur. Despite this lack of disclosure, public awareness has gradually begun to direct the consumer to accept products that don't damage health or the environment. Fortunately, there are increasing numbers of biodegradable and natural household products on the market. Seventh Generation is one such company that sells cleaning supplies developed with your health in mind along with the health of the planet.[11] A rule of thumb in making such a purchase is that the more natural the product, the less likely it will harm you or the environment.

Avoid scented or perfume-containing products, as well as those containing petroleum by-products. Natural or organic products clean just as well as heavy-duty detergents. Products such as Dr. Bronner's peppermint soap and New Age Biodegradable Cleanser can be used to wash dishes, hands, or vegetables.

It's possible to make your own cleansers and disinfectants. White vinegar, effective against mold, is an excellent all-purpose cleaner. Baking soda removes odors, and can be used for scouring. Borax is a disinfectant that acts as a nontoxic cleaning agent and can replace bleach and commercial detergent. Zephiran chloride, 17% aqueous solution, when mixed with water is effective against mold and bacteria.

You should bear in mind that a product considered to be safe for one person may not be safe for you. When you first use a cleanser, disinfectant, soap, or lotion, start by applying a small amount of it, and don't put it on your body until you are certain you are not reactive. Even when employing natural substances, it is best to open windows and wear gloves.

Careful consideration of what you put on or around your body will reduce reactivity and make you a conscious consumer. Before you make a purchase, evaluate its impact both on the environment as well as on your body. Take into consideration the ethics of the manufacturer and assess the product's recycling potential before making a purchase. Since there is much more for you to know that is not found on these pages, consult any of the books by Debra Lynn Dadd, including *Nontoxic, Natural, and Earthwise* (Los Angeles: J. P. Tarcher, 1990), for more details regarding safe products.

When removing toxic materials from your home, it's not possible to do so all at once; you'll be overwhelmed if you try. Make a list of the most bothersome toxins, starting in the bedroom and removing these first. Once they are gone, take time to notice if you feel better. This can be subtle, so don't dismiss an object's impact.

Simple Things to Protect from Toxic Exposures

1. Request visitors refrain from wearing perfume or after shave, and that they smoke outside.
2. Keep your home as dust free as possible.
3. Grow house plants: 20 plants will help remove impurities in the air in a 2000 square foot house. Make sure the pots are not ceramic, as this is a source of mold.
4. Close bedroom closet doors when you go to bed at night.
5. Purchase domestic, organically grown fruits and vegetables; imported foods contain chemicals often banned in the United States.
6. Avoid scented, tinted toilet paper, paper towels, and facial tissue. Use only biodegradable, undyed, unscented products.
7. Avoid making your home airtight; open windows daily and sleep with a window open.
8. When using household cleansers and cleaning products, including non-toxic products, open windows and doors to allow fumes to escape.
9. Cut down on chemicals used in your home; dispose of unnecessary or unusual household products, or store them away from your living space.
10. Only use carpet shampoo, as well as flea and insect bombs when absolutely necessary.
11. Have your household and drinking water checked for impurities and change your water source if necessary.
12. Use steel, copper, glass, or cast iron for cooking as aluminum and Teflon can leach into foods and be absorbed by the body.
13. Leave the garage door open after pulling the car in to disperse exhaust fumes.
14. Sleep in a low EMF field area to avoid unnecessary exposures. Keep electrical devices such as digital clocks away from the bed and remove electrical blankets.

15. Install an air filtration or air purification system.
16. Maintain and properly clean ventilation systems.
17. Use water-heated radiators or electric heaters; they are safer than gas heat.
18. Sit a safe distance from the computer monitor and TV.
19. Unplug appliances when not in use.

Public Exposures

When Theresa takes her daughter to story hour at the library, she must stand outside because of her sensitivity to gas heat. In good weather, she can stand outside her church to listen to the service; inside, the incense, perfume, and the like would be toxic to her. In order to stay well, it is often easier for Theresa to remain isolated.

There are so many variables for the chemically sensitive to consider when leaving home. You may need to scope out new environments ahead of time to ensure your safety. You may need to question friends about your intended destination to determine if it is safe. You may need to know beforehand if a building has been newly painted or renovated and have to ask about the building's heat source. Gas heat, even when it's turned off, may prohibit you from entering. Movie theaters often spray insecticides and the public library may have just installed new carpeting. Your destination, while it seems benign to friends, can harm you if you don't take proper precautions.

How you get to your destination poses another series of difficulties. Laura drives an old vehicle, with outgassed fabric, rather than leather or plastic seats. In addition, she has blocked off the outside air flow to prevent outside fumes from entering the car. She travels with a portable air purifier and carries an oxygen tank for emergencies.

Cars pour out exhaust fumes that can render you senseless as you drive or walk. Some resolve this problem by wearing a mask or holding a cotton handkerchief to their nose. Although you may feel awkward, such protective devices can enable you to remain mobile.

One way to avoid public exposure is to shop by phone or by catalogue. In order to shop this way, you must have a credit card or be willing to mail a check. Be sure that purchases are returnable without hassle when shopping by mail as well as when making direct purchases. Laura prearranges to meet sales clerks outside shops that contain toxic fumes and enters some stores at early hours when she is not competing with other customers for service.

Summary

This chapter has explored ways to advocate for yourself in terms of medical insurance, income tax deductions, and securing disability. We have also examined ways to reduce or eliminate toxic exposures in the home, in public places, and at work. Self-advocacy is the key: the more you speak up to protect yourself, the more you will have the opportunity to heal. You will be most effective if you advocate on your behalf giving reasonable consideration to the feelings and needs of others.

Endnotes

[1]Kimberly Kenney, ed., "CFIDS Historical Perspective and World View," *The CFIDS Chronicle* Spring 1991: 64.

[2]Contact the IRS, whose number is found in the front of your phone book, for their free publication, "Medical and Dental Expenses Publication 520."

[3]Lance Wallace, "Total Exposure Assessment Methodology Study," U.S. Environmental Protection Agency, Sept. 1987.

[4]Janet Dauble, ed., American Academy Environmental Meeting comments on Anderson Laboratory's studies, 9–12 Oct. 1993, *Share Care and Prayer* Mar.–Sept. 1994: 13–16.

[5]Prosecuting attorney, Mark Proctor, (904) 435-7000.

[6]U.S. Environmental Protection Agency, Office of Air and Radiation, "Indoor Air Facts No 4: Sick Building Syndrome" (Washington, DC: EPA, 1991).

[7]U.S. Environmental Protection Agency, Office of Air and Radiation, "Indoor Air Pollution: An Introduction for Health Professionals" (Washington, DC: EPA).

[8]*50 Simple Things You can do to Save the Earth* (Berkeley: Earthworks, 1989).

[9]For information on air purifiers, call Jim Nigra at Nigra Enterprises, 5699 Kanan Road, Agoura, CA 91301-3328, (818) 889-6877.

[10]Nontoxic Environments sells Nilfisk GS 90 vacuums, as well as building and household products for the chemically sensitive. Contact them at P.O. Box 384, Newmarket, NH 03857, (800) 789-4348.

[11]For information regarding Seventh Generation products, contact them at 49 Hercules Drive, Colchester, VT 05446-1672, (800) 456-1177.

Part Four

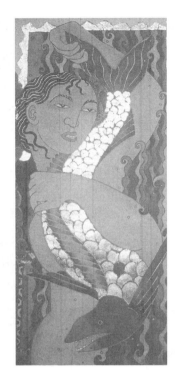

*Examining
and Changing
Your Beliefs*

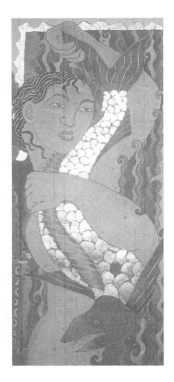

*Chapter
Twelve*

*Mental and
Emotional
Factors*

*t*he role of the mind is of great importance in the healing process. Psychoneuroimmunology is the scientific field that studies the influence of the mind and emotions on immune function. Throughout Part IV of this book you will be encouraged to examine some of the mental and emotional factors that may be interfering with your recovery. Harboring so called "negative emotions" such as anger, fear, despair, depression, and grief has an adverse impact on the body. Positive emotions such as joy and love have healing effects on health.[1] Learning to fully feel and appropriately express a full spectrum of feelings is important to your return to health.

Instead of seeing yourself as a victim of uncontrollable emotions and circumstances, you may discover tools that will help you take charge of how you perceive this very difficult experience. Changing your relationship to pain and suffering will have an enormous impact on your progress. You are no longer a victim when you assume responsibility for the choices you make.

Stress

"It wasn't until I recognized and took responsibility for how stressed out I was that I could see that it was largely a matter of choice. . . . I no longer needed to prove that

I was okay by putting myself into such difficult situations." Jamie worked for years in an acute psychiatric hospital where she was constantly vigilant and afraid, but failed to recognize the harm. In the morning she would leave for work feeling okay, only to crawl home into bed at the end of the day. Work and recovery from work became her entire life.

Consider Audrey, who went from one disaster to another prior to becoming ill: shortly after her father died, her marriage ended, then her business failed, and her health took a tailspin. Stress was the byword of her existence. "I was running faster and pushing harder to the extent that I never stopped to grieve all my losses."

Stress causes increased secretions of adrenal hormones, adrenaline and corticosteroids. These hormones inhibit white blood cells and can cause the thymus gland to shrink, increasing susceptibility to infections and the suppression of immune function. When stress is long-lasting or excessive, the control mechanisms that counteract everyday stress go awry. Pushing yourself too hard over an extended period can drain your body of cortisol reserves.

In 1991 Mark Demitrack, MD, of the University of Michigan, reported a study indicating that people with CFS have low levels of cortisol secretion.[2] Cortisol inhibits the activity of the immune system, and low levels may cause immune activation. This means that when you encounter stressful circumstances, including viral and bacterial agents, or overexert yourself, your body will have difficulty coping with the stress. Unlike with healthy people, there is no reserve of cortisol available to cushion the impact.

Studies show that overstimulation of the adrenal cortex occurs when there is a prolonged expanse of time in which people have no sense of control over their circumstances. Examples of this include Holocaust survivors where the fight-or-flight mechanism goes into overdrive for a prolonged interval, depleting the immune system. Prolonged stress weakens organs, depletes adrenal glucocorticoid stores, alters gastrointestinal physiology, and diminishes the capability to digest foods. Stress triggers the release of chemical messages from the brain that act to suppress the immune system. Emotional stress causes changes in physiological chemistry that affect all bodily functions.

Ongoing stress does not cause EI and CFS but it does exacerbate symptoms. Illness may become worse at times when life is fraught with worries, concerns, and physical endeavors that tax the body. In the face of prolonged, multiple stressors, your body may expend energy faster than it can regenerate it. No longer able to fight off even a mild threat, it breaks down.

You may have become abruptly ill after undergoing a prolonged or acute episode of emotional or physical stress. Stress of any kind helps to set the stage for illness: Sherry became ill with EI after her home was fumigated; Gloria was incapacitated with CFS after caring for her mother and being exposed to new carpet fumes.

Dr. Hans Selye pioneered our understanding of stress in the 1930s, determining that certain amounts of stress are necessary for optimal health. When this level is exceeded, dysfunction results. Stress in the form of tension and strain is a normal, inevitable aspect of existence, and there are many types of stress that can have an influence on your health. These threats may be real or may be unconsciously perceived as potentially harmful.

Undergoing a constant state of stress can make it difficult to fulfill your needs. Stress can also impair your ability to integrate what's happening to you in a useful manner. When you are not able to respond directly to sources of stress, you may become susceptible to illness. Over time, unresolved stressors accumulate and become driven into the body, manifesting as allergic reactions, extreme fatigue, and depression.

One of the first symptoms of stress is fatigue. Fatigue is a message to stop and attend to what is harming you. You may not realize you are being harmed; the eroding effects of stress can be both subtle and cumulative. It may not be possible to isolate a single stressor as being causative, but multiple and varied stressors play a large role in the onset and persistence of EI and CFS, reactivating viral illness and intensifying allergic reactions.

Yet, stress can also be a catalyst for growth and health. Time and again, those with EI and CFS report, though they would never have voluntarily chosen it, these illnesses have forced them to make choices toward greater peace and joy. "Since I became ill I've found my best self; more so than if I'd continued nursing. Illness has forced me to examine my priorities. Immersion in my writing has made this one of the most blessed and richest times of my life," notes Josh, now a freelance writer and poet.

The important part of psychological stress is to recognize that to a large extent it is in the mind of the beholder. Your unique perception of a difficult experience is based on your sense of the level of threat to your well-being and depends on the effectiveness of your coping strategies. People who are able to cope with stress tend to have fewer stress-related physical symptoms and higher levels of immune function.[3]

How you respond to everyday situations determines the amount of stress you accumulate. For unknown reasons, those with EI and CFS tend to internalize stress into their bodies. An emotional upset for Laura immediately shows up as heightened allergic reactivity. Learning to externalize stressors in an appropriate manner can reduce the potential for illness. Without denying your feelings, consider the possibility that your negative thinking is simply a habit. When you recognize the destructive nature of this habit, you may then elect to interrupt the cycle.

Your life can be considerably less burdened when you change your perspective about the things that disturb you. How you choose to react to stress is more important than the stress itself. When something is bothering you that cannot be changed or directly controlled, it is possible to alter your attitude and how you respond. This means accepting the things you cannot change, and making positive choices as to how you wish to respond to uncontrollable experiences.

Understanding the role of conscious control over your response to stress can make you more capable of returning to health. The external world is no longer able to make you ill when you identify and reduce external stressors, releasing their power over you. Recognition of stressors in your life will help interrupt the process.

Stress may include excessive attachment to drama that offers excitement, but erodes physical health. The thrill and self-importance that come from being privy to every office scandal or family drama have a downside that exhausts and eventually depletes you. Being involved in drama prevents you from facing deeper, uncomfortable matters and from getting on with your life. It can agitate, depress, and divert energies that could better be used by focusing attention on your true needs. Extracting yourself from these dramas will give you more energy to attend to life.

A frequent source of stress is an overly busy, tightly scheduled life-style, a common thread for those with CFS. If this is true for you, simplification is the key. A more simplified life means fewer dramas and a resultant lack of stress. Illness may have already forced simplification. Within a simplified life-style you have the opportunity to make ongoing choices that emphasize balance.

In order to achieve this, you must build an internal regulatory mechanism, a voice that continually whispers in your ear, giving cues as to what is important and what is not, about where to let go and where to hold fast. The net result is that your body will no longer be the passive recipient of the dictates of your old habits or of externally imposed obligations and expectations.

The next time you feel anxious and overwhelmed, stop and notice what's going on and what tasks are nonessential, and what obligations can be set aside. Very little is essential, while much of doing and rushing is the result of self-imposed expectations and illusion. These self-created values are usually the small, silly, inconsequential trappings you think you can't live without. You will free up an enormous amount of energy by reducing your attachment to trivia. When you do this, subverted life energy is freed up to focus on what is really consequential to your life.

Fine tuning your awareness will alert you to the impact of particular stressors on your health. Recognition of activities that deplete you offers the opportunity to remove them. For example, Judy notes that talking on the phone when she's tired further depletes her and that she does better sending notes and talking on the phone only when rested.

Learning to manage stress will reduce its damaging effects on your immune system. Removing stressors and adding activities that fuel and sustain you is key to health maintenance. Pacing yourself, avoiding too many life changes at once, strengthening your personal boundaries, and enjoying yourself will go a long way toward reducing stress in your life.

Good Grief

"Once I accepted that I had lost everything, things started to get better. I wasn't frightened anymore. The process of mourning all of my losses was an essential part of getting well. Until you mourn you are still denying reality, hoping things will be different. Until you mourn fully and deeply you can't accept what's going on," says Audrey, recovered from cancer and CFS and now a cancer support counselor.

Grief is a natural, healing reaction to the multiple losses incurred through illness. With CFS and EI, loss can include almost anything: a loss of body image; a loss of autonomy; for some, the loss of fingerprints; the loss of hopes and dreams; and the threat of further, ongoing multiple losses. Your loss of health may precipitate the loss of employment, money, spouse, relationships, a role within the family, or self-esteem.

Many people with EI and CFS have had to completely let go of their old way of life. It's common to mourn the loss of the many years you have had to attend to your illness. You may lose a sense of who you are in the world and of the accomplishments that once defined you.

However, grieving can impair your life in the same way as depression. Audrey found it important to allow herself to go through this experience but to avoid becoming stuck in it. Yet, she could not begin the process of getting well until she mourned fully and deeply. Grieving is a process that permits healing to take place and mourning is the way grief and loss can be resolved. Choosing to enter into this experience, rather than resisting, enables you to move through and out the other side into healing. Holding grief at bay causes pain and suffering to be held in place and can lead to pathological disturbance.

There will be cause for grieving as long as you have breath. Much of life is learning to cope with loss. It is how you deal with grief and loss that holds the key to whether you rage against what is, or move forward and embrace all that life has to offer. Moving into those dark, painful spaces will make it possible to move on. Finding the greater meaning of your experience is the cornerstone to acceptance leading to resolution. Usually grieving cannot be rushed; like composting, it's an organic process.

Depression

"Depression is a common cause of the symptoms I had, so my family assumed all that was wrong was that I was depressed. I thought that if I talked enough about what was bothering me it would lift. Nothing I did helped," says Gloria, ex-teacher in recovery from CFS. Depression as stuck sadness is what happens when you know something is wrong but you cannot find the way out. When you are depressed, EI and CFS symptoms worsen because of a sense of disempowerment. Lacking the ability to mobilize so as to change your circumstances creates a pervasive sense of hopelessness.

Many people with EI and CFS have difficulty making a shift toward the affirmative or in finding meaning. Lacking energy and undergoing constant allergic reactivity can make it difficult to mobilize enthusiasm for anything. Every event and task looks insurmountable and is glazed over with negativity when you are depressed. Once it catches hold, it spirals into itself, setting all other areas of life aflame, leaving no area untouched.

Depression can arise as a result of chemical changes caused by the disease process or as a result of your assessment of your situation. Other CFS- and EI-related causes of depression include: a deep sense of loss, or multiple losses, repressed emotions, individual biological changes, early life experiences that set the stage for future patterns, environmental stressors, changes in personal identity, social isolation, response to medications, and allergic reactions. Depression also plays a major role in causing fatigue.

With CFS there has been a bitter debate which led some physicians to conclude that CFS is simply a manifestation of mental illness. True, studies have documented the presence of depression, anxiety, and panic attacks in CFS patients,[4] but this does not substantiate the presence of mental illness.

It has been suggested that people with CFS and possibly EI may be physiologically predisposed to depression. This brings up the chicken-and-the-egg dilemma: did the depression make you ill or did the illness make you depressed? Increasingly, information suggests that biochemical brain involvement is the root cause of depression in persons with EI and CFS. It is also clear biochemically that immune system dysregulation and depression can go together.

For those with EI and CFS, depression markedly differs from the clinical depression profile in which depressed people typically lack any interest or motivation. On the contrary, EI and CFS sufferers possess an abundance of will and desire, and are interested in life, despite illness. In contrast to other forms of clinical depression, your mind says "go" but your body rebels.

It's difficult to sort out which symptoms are caused by the illness and which are strictly related to depression. For instance, someone with pain typically regards this symptom as just the physical experience of pain. Yet, pain can also be related to depression, because discomfort intensifies in the face of depression.

In the case of EI and CFS, depression and its attendant symptoms are a pervasive aspect of the illness. The interplay between viral symptoms and stressors links depression to organic impairment caused by the virus. Depression can also arise from allergic reactivity or it can be the result of isolation, common with those who are ill. It may also result from the fact that environmental or interpersonal supports are not available or adequate.

For some, depression is anger turned unconsciously inward onto the self. Feelings of anger can be so unacceptable that they become distorted and not even recognized as such. Anger may also result from being overwhelmed by the challenges that the illness has caused.

Identity and Depression

One young support group member reported that it was impossible to find any sense of self-worth since she had become ill with CFS. Not able to work, and sleeping 20 hours a day, all sense of who she was vanished. These illnesses can rob you of your identity and sense of self-value. One of humankind's deepest needs is for self-worth. Most people find self-worth and definition through work, or in relationships, or through the contributions they make. When you cannot contribute, it is difficult to define yourself.

Depression occurs when you lose self-esteem and perspective and a sense of who you are. Perhaps the most devastating aspect of depression for those with a chronic illness is that it is easy to cave into the notion that the depression is here to stay. If you remember one thing about depression, try to hold onto the thought that it's not a permanent state. It is always reversible.

Having survived the ups and downs of these long illnesses, it is important to remind yourself of the transitory nature of depression, that you've survived rough times in the past and good times can come again. This knowledge will make it is easier to tolerate discomfort and depression.

Interventions for Depression

The good news about depression is that it is treatable and can be helped with therapy, medications, support, and other alternatives. And more importantly, the thoughts you choose to emphasize will impact your overall health. If you constantly bemoan your fatigue, like a self-fulfilling prophecy, your body chemistry and your mind will align into a configuration that supports this state. This means you can also tune your mind to the possibility that you can have more energy and a willingness to move through stuck places that resist this concept.

Past coping mechanisms offer a good indicator of how you can best deal with your illness. Examining old habits and patterns will tell you about your coping patterns. This can be explored by asking yourself several questions and answering them with unflinching courage, giving you a greater understanding of the choices you've made regarding your illness. Are you motivated to change? Is this depression a part of a larger life pattern? Is it possible that this depression serves you in some way? What internal strengths do you have that can be useful to mobilize at this time? What do you know about yourself that will help you to change? This process of identifying and naming your thoughts and feelings may enable you reclaim a sense of perspective, personal value, and an ability to impact the illness.

Further assessment and mobilization of your internal and external resource network is central to change. Are people there for you? How can you use their talents to serve as effective helpers? How can you use your own talents, despite physical limitations, to work toward change? Are you willing to take risks to make these changes?

Look at yourself as dispassionately as possible. Examine your current losses and how you have historically handled difficulties. Take a look at your support system and at your self-esteem. Who is out there for you? How do you feel about yourself? Chances are good you don't feel too great about yourself, but don't stop there. When that is done, examine your strengths and consider what motivates you. If you cannot find any strengths or motivators in the present, reach into the past to locate some.

The next step is to establish a treatment plan, incorporating your strengths and motivators, a plan that includes your support network. Make sure your treatment plan includes measurable, realistic goals so you can see tangible results in a short period of time. Be careful to keep the plan simple so you don't set yourself up to fail, identifying one simple thing you might be able to do for yourself. It may be that dangling your legs over the side of the bed for a few minutes or combing your hair is enough. What's important is that the results be tangible and that you don't have to work too hard to achieve them. Without the evidence of results, you may be inclined to give up.

David, who had CFS and was deeply depressed for months, shares his success: "I saw a therapist who put me on an antidepressant. When that failed, I went to my friends who tried to jolly me out of my state. And when that didn't work, I joined a support group, which didn't do any good. What finally helped was writing down and appreciating all my accomplishments, no matter how small." Acknowledging and appreciating what was working, rather than obsessing about all the things that were not, he was able to break the cycle of depression. You may make your own list of personal gains as a supportive witness to your achievements.

In order to work through depression, you must honor your feelings by noticing or expressing them appropriately. This may require you to be true to yourself and to cease creating a logjam of "shoulds" and adhering to the expectations of others. Initially, when you allow yourself to examine and express these feelings, you may feel more overwhelmed and depressed. Repressed feelings intensify because you are allowing them to surface. Sticking with this agenda can be difficult; but once the logjam is broken, it will become easier.

Part of what shifts in the process of moving out of depression is learning how to appreciate and honor yourself, regardless of what is going on around you or what you may feel physically. It is common to fear that permitting unacceptable feelings to emerge will damage you. Actually, the opposite is true; the actions you take to avoid those feelings can be more harmful than the feelings themselves. When feelings are disowned, depression can intensify.

Your job is not to try to cheer up and sweep feelings away, but to pay attention to them. As you notice and express yourself, each success will build on the next, giving you greater energy and confidence. Allow yourself to feel the glow of your accomplishments, requesting feedback from those around you as well.

Depression can be alleviated by structuring your day so there are events you can look forward to. This allows you to have fun, offers new hope, a sense of reward and accomplishment, and increases your energy. The events you choose can be very simple; one woman with CFS felt exceptionally good after simply sitting in her garden. Try daily to find some small thing that takes you outside your regular routine.

Illness will make you a master at letting go; this is one of its great lessons. It's impossible to hold the expectation of a smooth recovery too tightly. You have to be prepared to let go every time you have a setback. Inevitably the course of your healing will change many times before you are through. Many of us are years off schedule. Be open to surprises and changes, as healing is seldom a linear process.

When you become discouraged about your lack of progress, look back and recognize the small, incremental gains. Laura used to feel awful every day, then it was every other day, and now there will be one day a month when she feels terrible; that's progress! Look for subtle shifts in your energy and improvements that were not there a while back. Examining the overall trend can give you a lift even when you feel awful at the moment.

The Pleasure Principle

Making time on a regular basis to treat yourself to things you enjoy and engaging in events that energize you can help break the cycle of depression. Set aside a few minutes every day to attend to nurturing yourself, regardless of fatigue and depression. To do this you must stop putting work, chores, and the business of your life first and take time out.

Putting yourself first may run contrary to all of your training that says if you want to be lovable, you must place the needs of others first. These acts of self-kindness do not mean you are selfish or neglectful of others. Inevitably, by treating yourself with loving-kindness you will notice a greater depth to loving others.

Take yourself out on dates, even though you may in reality have to stay in. Plan something special on a regular basis—fix your favorite meal, rent a video or go to a movie, take a long hot bath, dress up in fancy clothes, or snuggle up in front of the fire and read. You can spend this time in prayer, or using affirmations, or in reflective appreciation, walking, listening to music, or just checking in with yourself.

What this is all about is learning to value your own company and treasuring your own self-worth. It is possible to use this time to send loving affirmative thoughts into parts of your body that are struggling. Celebrating yourself will lighten your life, giving you much to draw on during lean times. Carving a space for pleasure will relieve stress and give you something to look forward to.

You may wonder how you'll find the ability to have fun since you scarcely have the energy to perform many of the things necessary to stay afloat. All that is necessary is to give yourself permission to create time for those things that feed and renew you. Even the practical time you spend soaking in the bathtub can be used for relaxation and solitude. These soaks can give you the opportunity to read, meditate, or, if you are a bit daring, chant and sing.

Examine your life, considering what makes you feel good. Once you find a way to insert pleasurable activity into your everyday existence, you will notice increased energy and optimism. It will then be possible to tackle more mundane, unappealing tasks with greater ease.

Take an Energy Inventory

By examining your patterns of self-nurturing, you may gain insight as to the ways you lose energy. You may be exhausting precious energy reserves on pursuits that drain rather than feed you, for example, by engaging in activities that you don't want to do or that are mundane. Energy can be lost as a result of negative thinking or by holding a vision of yourself as a victim of illness.

Start by taking an energy inventory, noticing all of the things that energize or drain you. At times you may be going along at a pretty good clip when suddenly you are utterly exhausted and need to rest. What happened to all of that abundant energy? How did you become drained? Tracking back through events that occurred before and after your loss of steam can offer valuable insights.

Exhaustion can come when you are doing something you resent or resist. You may lose energy when you are fearful or when you fail to verbalize what needs to be said, disowning your feelings. If you don't eat balanced meals, you may feel drained. Perhaps you are surrounded by people who feed on the energy of others, leaving you depleted. You may be exhausted from continually giving the "shoulds" in your life first priority. These "shoulds" may cause the buildup of toxic rigidity that stresses the immune system. Losing energy may be a way of letting you know that you need to attend to certain matters you've been avoiding.

Recognition of the places and events that cause you to lose energy can alert you to stay on track with your true needs. Don't continue to stay on the phone past the time when you want to be off. Stop saying "yes" when you mean "no." Pleasing yourself will give greater vitality, honesty, and congruence to your relationships. Feeding yourself by selecting life-giving and energizing activities is an excellent way to feel better about life.

The Idealized Self

As a child, you probably came to the conclusion that you had to behave in certain ways in order to receive love. In this process a false, idealized, self was created in an effort to be worthy of love and to avoid unhappiness. As an adult, this may have translated into pretending to be what you are not, keeping your true self under wraps so as to be lovable. The ongoing strain to maintain this false front is much like building a house without a foundation and leaves who you really are out of the picture.

What is this idealized self? Often disguised as aggression, pride, hostility, or overambitiousness, it is the external expression of your efforts to cover up for a sense of unworthiness. You will not be able to release the idealized self until you recognize the subtle, seductive, often unconscious ways that it is woven into the fabric of your being. You may not even be aware of the pressure of the idealized self, the fear, shame, tension, and confusion that it causes.

Much of life is spent thinking we need this false self in order to be happy and safe and we exert tremendous efforts to preserve it. Yet, as you begin to tune in to all of the damage this false self has done, you will be more capable of dissolving it. Your personal crisis of health may play a big part in helping to uncover and release it. As you struggle with your changed self-image, trying to match the inner with the outer, you will become familiar with the false self-esteem you have tried to create through all of your efforts at doing. Illness offers the opportunity to evaporate the self-definition that comes from doing, allowing you just to be.

Illness forces you to redefine yourself. By examining and answering the essential question, "Who am I?" you will awaken and tune in to your core. When you awaken this aspect, what you once held in esteem will now be seen as prideful pretense. The very center of your being is the part of you that is truly whole, and is the only part of you that functions with all of your abilities intact. The more you live from this center, the more superfluous the false self becomes. Giving up your mask will change your perspective about many things; much of life will shift and there will be startling effects. When you live from your center, you will no longer have to hide your true self from yourself and others. Finding who you are is what the journey of healing is all about. As you find the courage to be your real self, you will no longer be plagued with depression and doubts. Instead, you will find peace and will function as a whole being.

Psychiatric Therapy

When you are grieving or depressed, you don't want someone telling you to cheer up, you want to be heard. The act of articulating your feelings and being heard creates a shift in perspective, making it possible to mobilize toward change. An even stronger benefit that results when you find a safe place to express yourself is the physiological relaxation and release that occurs when you liberate energies that you had been using to suppress feelings.

Being heard includes finding a safe setting in which to express yourself. This means finding a therapist who understands and acknowledges the reality and unique stressors of your illness. "The biggest challenge in doing therapy with someone with EI is that a lot of symptoms manifest as emotional states. So in choosing a therapist you would need to select one who is familiar with how the central nervous system response [to an excitant] can mimic emotional states," notes Annette Hulett, MFCC, therapist in private practice who is chemically sensitive herself.

She further states, "In working with a therapist you need to realize that emotional states can be physiologically triggered. Then engage the therapist as a consultant—someone who can help you learn to discriminate between what's truly an emotional issue and what is a physical issue that activates an emotional state." Annette's advice to therapists is that they must be prepared to deal with a lot of irrational rage as well as the client's judgment and blame of themselves and others. The work of the therapist is to interrupt this pattern.

Select a therapist who validates the reality of these illnesses; but also one who expects you to take charge of your healing rather than supporting you to lose yourself into illness. A good therapeutic relationship should not lead to dependency but toward greater autonomy. Be a cautious consumer when seeking counseling, as you can waste precious time and deplete already low funds trying to find a compatible match. Jamie, a therapist herself, notes, "I wasted an enormous amount of time and money trying to convince my therapist that I was all right." The best way to find a good therapist is to get referrals from people whose opinions you respect and those who have had needs similar to yours.

Much may be required of you as you engage in this process, for it is never easy to examine painful parts of your life. You will do a disservice to the experience if your try to minimize or cut corners. It's important to stay open and receptive to feedback, as this will make it easier to find solutions to your difficulties.

It's difficult to ask for help, particularly in a world that rewards and reveres autonomy so highly. Asking takes courage and humility; by asking you're placing yourself in a vulnerable, receiving role. There is also the implication that you have to be "crazy" to seek psychiatric counseling. Further, some physicians believe that these problems are all in the mind. So the act of succumbing to therapeutic assistance implies that those physicians were right in the first place. Despite the stigma of psychotherapy, it can be invaluable in helping you resolve difficulties and in sorting out and changing personal beliefs that you are not able to handle on your own.

Professional counseling can help you understand feelings and sort out what to do about them. Self-defeating behaviors can be examined and stuck relationships can be given permission to change. Life-style changes can be implemented and you can receive help in changing behaviors that no longer serve your life. Counseling can assist you to see what you need to do to get your life back on track. The experience also allows for greater perspective and acceptance of the truth about self-deluding behavior patterns.

Like getting a crash course in self-parenting, therapy can help improve your judgment as to what is okay to disclose and what needs only to be internally acknowledged. The ravages of these illnesses may find you breaking rules of acceptable behavior as you give in to mercurial mood swings and therapy can assist you to keep your emotions appropriately in check.

Medications

Small doses of antidepressant drugs are used with CFS, to break the cycle of depression, relieve pain, and help with sleep. Many with EI are not able to tolerate the synthetic materials used in medications for them to be of benefit. Medications are not to be seen as ends in themselves, as they do not cure the underlying cause of the depression. However, a medication can help alter the body chemistry back to a more normal state. It is advised to take an antidepressant in conjunction with professional counseling to achieve greater benefit.

Dr. John Gillette, Chief of Psychiatry for Santa Cruz County Mental Health, notes, "It's difficult to be sure in the case of CFS if the depression is secondary to the illness or secondary to life-style adaptations required by the illness. When serious depression is present, many people will be helped significantly by the use of antidepressants. Generally the medications that work best are Prozac, Zoloft, Paxil, Effexor, and Serzone because of the low level of side effects."

Another favorite antidepressant in treating CFS is low-dose Sinequan, taken to facilitate sleep, improve sleep quality, and decrease fatigue during the day. It is a tricyclic antidepressant that also has powerful antihistamine and anti-inflammatory effects.

Each person has a unique response to a given drug and tolerance will vary. In addition, for some antidepressants, 2 to 6 weeks is required before a blood level is built up so that an effect can be noted. Thus, you must exercise patience in trying to find the correct medication at the correct dose.

Low doses of the hypnotics Halcion or Restoril have offered some remarkable symptomatic relief, but can be habituating. Xanax, Klonopin, and even magnesium can help minimize the production of cytokines, which are thought to produce many of the symptoms of EI and CFS. The herb Saint John's-wort can be used to improve mood and relieve depression. Its effectiveness in alleviating depression has been noted to be greater than that produced by some standard prescription drugs such as Elavil.[5] In addition, it does not have the disturbing side effects of these prescription drugs.

Peer Support

Despite the isolation imposed by illness, your world expands when you pick up the phone and reach out for support. The phone is an important self-help avenue widely used by EI and CFS sufferers. Informal phone networks can actually become the backbone of your social contact, linking you to others who share your circumstances. It is a lifeline for those who can rarely leave home, normalizing what is an abnormal existence. Much of Theresa's social life occurs over the phone, keeping her connected to a world she cannot participate in.

One thing to watch out for is that you not take on the suffering of fellow callers. Laura has to work hard not to take on the distress of others; this is done by learning to just listen, rather than trying to fix. Sometimes this phone contact has been the only thing that has prevented her from giving up. Discussing coping strategies and shared experiences with people who know exactly what you're talking about can be a great relief. All you have to do is pick up the phone and reach out.

Support groups are also a vital resource for those who can tolerate direct contact. There can be empowerment in coming together which reduces feelings of isolation and energizes the body. Finding compassion for someone else can also propel you from a self-involved, depressed state.

Other Helps

It is possible to change the chemical balance of the brain by directing thoughts in a positive manner. In this way, affirmations and positive thoughts can help lift you out of a depressed state. The chemical serotonin, which helps to regulate moods, is transmitted when positive feelings are experienced. Similar to endorphins, it can also relieve pain. Cultivating positive thoughts can increase endurance and stimulate physiological energy, which can help alleviate depression. Physical exercise can promote an increased sense of control that offers an attendant increase in energy, and it's difficult to be depressed when your body is suffused with energy. *The Depression Book* (Murphys: Zen Monastery and Interfaith Retreat Center, 1991) is a wonderful resource for those willing to examine how they might be the cause of their own suffering and offers help to move past those stuck places into acceptance and compassion.

Light Therapy

Light from the sun has powerful energizing and healing effects. It is an electromagnetic radiation in the wavelength range including infrared, visible, ultraviolet, and X rays. Infrared is the heat that you feel in sunlight. Visible light is of various wavelengths that produce different biochemical effects that are dependent on the absorption of particular wavelengths of light. Ultraviolet light is part of the light spectrum that has the most impact on the body; depending on the wavelength, it can nourish or harm the immune system.

Your body absorbs light through the eyes and the optic nerve, sending messages to the pineal gland, the hypothalamus, the pituitary, and the rest of the endocrine system depending on the wavelength of light. Skin receptors respond to light, affecting nearly all physiological activities. Red blood cells at the surface of the skin are also light sensitive.

Light is essential to your well-being, and it acts as a nutrient. When you spend time in the sun, you may notice feeling better for days. When you are deprived of the sun, as in the winter months, you may notice an adverse influence on your mood and energy level. People, plants, and animals that are deprived of light die. Most of us spend our daylight hours indoors under white fluorescent light, which filters out other wavelengths of light. This lighting is harmful to your health—causing eye strain, fatigue, headaches, and decreased productivity—and emits a steady stream of radiation. To make matters worse, red blood cells become depleted of oxygen after exposure to video display terminals.

There has been exciting news that light therapy has a positive impact on people with immune illnesses such as CFS, AIDS, Gulf War syndrome, cancer, and leukemia. Studies show that full-spectrum light contributes to the healing process on both mental and physical levels. Light is important in refreshing and nourishing the nervous system and energizing the cells. Light acts as an antibacterial agent, increases oxygen transport to the blood, reduces cholesterol levels and blood pressure, feeds the pineal gland, and thereby enhances immune capability, increases white and red blood cell counts, and stimulates the activity of enzymes as well as the thyroid.

Seasonal affective disorder (SAD) is a physical illness caused by lack of sunlight. During the winter, i.e., when there is less light, the body produces more melatonin, resulting in SAD, characterized by decreased energy, irritability, anxiety, sleepiness, and depression. To offset SAD as well as other forms of depression, light therapy is now becoming more accepted in the mainstream as an adjunctive form of psychiatric treatment.

The use of full-spectrum lighting suppresses melatonin production by the pineal gland. Supplemental melatonin has been of increased interest in assisting people with sleep disorders, as it has a sedative effect and supports sleep. Melatonin also has immune stimulating qualities which slow down the aging process and reduce stress. Yet, when it is produced in excessive amounts, it can cause a depressed physiological state.

Dr. Jordan Goetz, former department chair of internal medicine at Vandenburg Air Force Base, prescribes the full-spectrum light box to be used several hours a day in cases of depression.[6] In addition, light treatment can potentiate antidepressant medications. Elaine, who has EI and CFS, was pleased to find that her depression lifted within 2 weeks of starting light therapy and that medical insurance covered the cost of the light system. Another woman, a support group member, noted that the full-spectrum light box gave her increased energy and enabled her to normalize her sleeping cycle. Using a radiation-shielded, full-spectrum light box will heighten the health-enhancing properties of light without being at risk of damaging effects.

Help for Pain and Suffering

Many with EI and CFS experience muscle and joint pain, as well as long-term and transient pain throughout the body. When pain is present, you may elect to tighten into despair, anger, and frustration, but there is much you can do to draw the experience into yourself that will afford some relief. For example, breathing into your pain allows you to relax, transforming the discomfort merely into energy and information. Conscious breathing will bring your attention into this moment and the next, preventing you from becoming engulfed and despairing of projections into the future. Following the breath allows greater clarity which will enable you to alter your body state from one of tension to one of relaxation.

Relaxing into pain can initially intensify distress, but relaxation also transforms it. Feelings of sorrow can be noted as they travel from the jaws to the throat. Knots of tension can be recognized as unshed tears or deep unresolved anger and grief. That place of holding in your neck or shoulders or anywhere else may cover a deeper feeling of utter loneliness or disconnection. In the process of connecting with and allowing yourself to become aware, pain may be recognized as a misguided attempt to divert attention from unexpressed true feelings of sadness, rage, or emptiness.

By softening into any sort of discomfort through the breath, discomfort may be recognized as blocked energy, which then begins to flow and move to other parts of the body. Being present with your pain frees it, transforming it into energy which can change in subtle ways until it eventually evaporates. Once you recognize the tremendous power of your awareness, you are no longer a victim and can mobilize and change your relationship to your discomfort.

Closing down by tightening the body in an effort to ward off discomfort intensifies it. The more you close down, the more firmly defined the pain becomes. Each time you breathe into the pain, it softens a little more and there is less terror. Fear as resistance tightens the body into a quivering mass of tension, which is the exact opposite of what should be done to achieve relief.

Pain is anchored in place and intensified by fear. Notice the energy you expend to avoid pain and discomfort. Undoubtedly those places where you've tried to avoid feeling pain are places where you feel fearful, stuck, and powerless. Examine what your worst fear about the pain might be. Are you afraid that the pain will steadily worsen and do irreparable damage?

Changing your relationship to your fear enables it to be revealed for what it is: suppressed feelings, places of disempowerment, or withholding that anchor discomfort in place. Much of life is spent working desperately to avoid the experience of those stuck spaces and now you're choosing to stop running. Instinct had told you to harden against it, to disown it, thinking this would make it go away; instead you can elect to turn around and face it.

Making this shift gives you a certain degree of control. Rather than being frightened by discomfort, you can surrender to the sensations. Just notice the energy and feel the movement. When you surrender, you reframe the experience to one of curiosity and attention. As you watch it shift and move, pain becomes less threatening; just offering friendly information.

Learning to own and speak to the pain can enable you to alter your perception of what it is. Ask the pain what it's doing in your face, or your joints. Be prepared to permit it to tell you fully what it is doing and what it wants. This pain may persist until you listen to what it tells you. Once you notice what stimulates it, you can work to resolve those causative factors.

The source of your suffering is often the result of denying your heart. Permitting yourself to experience the pain by moving into your heart, into those hardened, stuck spaces can be a source of comfort and greater expansiveness. Breathing into your heart, into your pain helps evaporate the boundaries that separate you from yourself.

As you inhale, imagine your body filling with golden light that enters every cell of your entire being. When you open to an area, the discomfort may temporarily intensify; but rather than cut off the unpleasant sensations, move your attention to the heart of your suffering, pouring love and light into the area. Being present with your suffering allows you to experience the moment fully and completely. It may seem paradoxical to enter into the pain and focus on it in order to achieve release. But, the more you can be present in your experience of the moment, the more you will be simply allowing the flow.

Like everything in life, pain is constantly changing: it comes and goes, changing shape and size from one moment to the next. For the next week keep a diary, noting the times when the pain is at its worst and the times when it is less intense. Keep track of what you are doing both when the pain is at its worst and when it's less intense.

By keeping a log, you may see a pattern. Perhaps it worsens when you are performing acts that are not congruent with your true desires. Notice if you are suppressing feelings or not maintaining healthy boundaries. What you are doing with your thoughts and actions has a tremendous impact on how you feel physically. By noting patterns that increase discomfort, you can then make decisions to reduce triggering factors and increase influences and events that enable you to feel better.

Despite overt efforts at avoidance, when the experience of pain and suffering is past it may be difficult to let the memory of it go. As uncomfortable as it is to acknowledge, you may be holding onto your suffering with pride and reverence as if it is a treasured wound. Undergoing years of discomfort has come to define who and what you are, and it is hard not to be attached. Pain is a familiar experience. The treasured memories of the pain are carried into the present because you may have made a pact never to forget. Mostly, holding onto the memory of past suffering carries with it old residue of fear and separation that prevents you from living fully.

Much of the experience of suffering is a matter of choice and habit. When you understand this, you can also choose to change. You may even be in the habit of taking on the suffering of others to elevate yourself, or alleviate others, or to lose yourself in the process. Allowing yourself to explore how your attachment serves you will enable you to make choices that move beyond this need.

Acceptance has a lot to do with the size and shape of pain and suffering in your life. Acceptance means owning the experience of suffering as a catalytic reminder. Acceptance frees you to appreciate all that you do have, rather than what you don't have. Some of the happiest, most content people with EI and CFS are also the sickest ones who have made peace with what is. They live fully from minute to minute, being as present as possible with the richness or despair. Laura says, "At times my heart breaks open. It happens over and over, there's no protection from this. In those moments when I am not attached, I am so rich, so full of wonder that I can't even remember any despair."

Summary

The more you can be in the moment with your pain, with your sorrow, with your suffering, the more you then have the opportunity to change. Being present in the moment, pain and suffering have less of a hold. There is nothing to do except to let it be and notice it. Attending to your experience of the moment allows suffering to pass through you rather than lodging deep inside. We have discussed depression, grief, stress, pain, and suffering and ways to cope. Keep in mind that these troublesome matters will never completely disappear but it is possible to see that how you respond is a matter of choice, a matter of your own creation. With a shift in understanding you can embrace and change your life.

Endnotes

[1]J. K. Kiecolt-Glaser and R. Glaser, "Psychoneuroimmunology: Can Psychological Interventions Modulate Immunity?" *Consult Clin Psychol* 60 (1992): 569–575.
[2]"Immune Activation," *Fibromyalgia Network* Oct. 1994: 5.

[3]Richard Gerber, *Vibrational Medicine* (Santa Fe: Bear & Co., 1988) 440.

[4]David Bell, *The Doctor's Guide to Chronic Fatigue Syndrome* (Reading: Addison–Wesley, 1995) 53.

[5]Michael Murray, *Chronic Fatigue Syndrome* (Rocklin: Prima, 1994) 166–167.

[6]Ginger Julian, "New Science Sheds Light on Immune Deficiencies," *HEALTHwatch* 5.3, Fall 1995: 8–9.

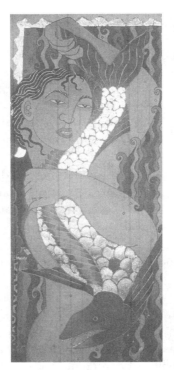

Chapter Thirteen

Mending the Mind

*O*uter work on the body and personality can open pathways into the core, the inner spiritual self. Working on repairing the physical body may make you feel better, but what is really needed is a more balanced perspective toward all of life. This chapter includes mental and spiritual practices that can help align your psychospiritual experience for greater physical healing. Throughout Part IV of this book you will be examining your symptoms and beliefs and how they have served you. You will also learn about visualization, meditation, and attention to the moment, all invaluable tools to enhance your growth.

In the process of finding balance, the only thing you may have control over in these illnesses are the choices you make as to how you feel about yourself and how you perceive your experiences. Essential to your recovery is that you establish a loving relationship with yourself. What does this mean? Where do you start? It means cultivating and listening to the inner voice that advises and guides you in this process. It's this loving voice that guides you when you go astray and, when at your worst, it reminds you that you're okay. It is a voice wise past knowing that will help you to cultivate a healing relationship with all parts of your being. The information in this chapter will invite you to open your heart to yourself.

Symptoms

When Leslie was ill with CFS, if she acted in any way contrary to her true feelings she would find herself in bed. "If I was doing something that didn't mesh my true needs, something that wasn't best for my physical well-being, I'd get a corresponding symptom." There is a hidden purpose to your symptoms: they are messengers that can offer important information.

Your illness is, in part, an expression of your distress and a representation of your attempts to relieve that distress. There can be many unconscious reasons why symptoms develop. Some of these reasons, paraphrased from the work of Leslie LeCron, well-known psychotherapist, include the following:

1. Symptoms may be a symbolic physical expression of feelings you are unable to express.
2. A symptom may arise as a result of a highly emotional past trauma which has become manifest in physical form.
3. Symptoms can result from the acceptance of an idea implanted earlier in life. The image you form as a child, shaped by your parents, teachers, and friends, can impact your physical and emotional self in later life.
4. A symptom may spring from an unconscious identification with an important figure, such as a parent who has been ill or who has died.
5. Your symptoms may be the result of inner conflict, an unmet need, or a forbidden desire. The presence of disabling symptoms helps prevent you from acting on those unacceptable desires.
6. Symptoms may come from an unconscious need to atone for wrongdoing.
7. Your symptoms may benefit you in some way such as giving you the opportunity to receive attention or by forcing personal growth.

When Audrey had CFS, she attended The Cancer Institute in Menlo Park, California, and on the first day she was urged to beat on pillows to express her anger. She resisted, saying, "You don't understand. I don't have any energy to do this. That's what my illness is about, not having energy." Eventually persuaded to give it a try, "I beat on pillows with my fists, flailed, and screamed at the top of my lungs. It was amazing: when I got done, I had more energy. Keeping my anger in check was using up a lot of energy. So I got it!" Accessing the energy behind the anger told her more about what this illness actually represented, namely, repressed and denied feelings.

Denial and suppression drain energy and life force and this disowning can create fatigue as well as all of the other symptoms of EI and CFS. Trapping emotions in the body rather than giving them voice can culminate in symptoms that force you to pay attention. "Allergic reactivity is at its worst when I'm irritated with my circumstances and refuse to speak up," notes Elaine, who has EI and CFS.

Efforts to deny emotions drain enormous amounts of energy, diverting what could be used toward healing. It's an inevitable, losing battle to suppress symptoms or suppress emotions; they will do what they please with you, regardless of what you have in mind. Some forms of disease can begin as a thought that is fueled by a negative emotion such as anger, fear, or greed. Those emotions then become repressed and cause energy to become stuck within the body, blocking the life force. Physical symptoms spring forth long after the imbalance has been created.

For EI and CFS to show up as illness there must be layers of interrelated factors seeded long before illness grows to full bloom. Symptoms—often messengers of a process that started a long time before—may be the symbolic expression of disowned feelings, a place of withholding, a memory, a fear pointing to a place where you have lost sight of your essence.

It's easy to be engrossed in curing your symptoms, thinking that to resolve them will cure the illness; but this is not true healing. Symptoms are merely a symbolic presence in the body and are not the actual problem; they just indicate that a problem exists. Symptoms are catalytic agents of change, alerting and educating you of the need to alter the direction of your life.

Discomfort compels you to change. The more you stay in communication with your symptoms, the greater is your opportunity to expand your awareness. This can be understandably difficult to do when you are so miserable or flooded with allergic reactivity that there is no energy left over to be expansive and awake enough to reflect and assimilate information. Awareness is constricted when you are depleted.

It's easy to become wrapped up in the symptoms of EI and CFS; they are treated with such reverence and fear, giving them much power and control. Giving them power holds them more firmly in place and intensifies the unpleasant experience. Perhaps you assume that since your discomfort is so bad there must be something far worse underneath. Thus, the natural reaction is to tighten your body and defend against discomfort, but this causes you to close down, locking sensations into your body.

There can be brief openings that remind you that you do have a choice to release their hold over you. You may not hear the voice of choice the first, or even the hundredth time, but at some point you may feel so broken down by your suffering that all you can do is allow the symptoms to speak to you.

Understanding what is going on regarding your symptoms can reduce fear, but that alone does not bring relief. Fear is alleviated when you accept the symptoms by just being present with them, allowing what is, to be. Entering into the physical sensations you can experience a sense of release, of free-fall as you release control. It is in the final moment of free-fall, just before crashing, that you may notice your symptoms to be carved into your physiology through choice.

As with pain, by softening into the discomfort, breathing into the moment, symptoms change. You will then find that you can impact the intensity and shape of the discomfort through your thoughts. Take a deep breath here; loosen the muscles there; and allow a bit of forgiveness for yourself. As you gain awareness, you will be able to pay attention to physical signals, uncover what is needed, and take charge to resolve distress. The more you experiment with your ability to change the experience of symptoms, the less you will be at the mercy of runaway emotions.

Acceptance of Symptoms

"On vacation my family asked me to refrain from announcing every time I was uncomfortable and reactive. Humiliated by their seemingly insensitive request, I decided to suffer in silence. During the trip I still noticed the odor of the new car's vinyl, and the car exhaust, and the disinfectants in the hotel, but I felt better than I had in years. Maybe just noticing, rather than judging and fueling myself with the fear of reactivity enabled me to feel better," muses Jamie, EI and CFS sufferer. When you see that you can choose how to hold an experience, it's even possible to decide against the interaction of toxins and your nose and body to minimize symptoms. Internal emotional states can affect physical reactivity.

How you think and feel about yourself, as well as how you feel about substances in your environment can make you feel worse and heighten reactivity. Negative thoughts can be picked up like a virus and transmitted through your body. Emotional states can hold toxic contaminants in place to the extent that holding onto rageful feelings can take days or weeks to detoxify.

Something shifts when you allow yourself to experience symptoms without all of the emotional overlay. When you do this, blocked energy is allowed to flow. There is powerful energy behind symptoms; they are a marvelous mechanism to get you to pay attention. They tell you to slow down, or inform you of changes that must be made, or of things that you may have trouble hearing unless the message is more than just a gentle tap on the shoulder.

When you recognize that suppressed feelings may be causing your discomfort, you can elect to express yourself or physically extricate yourself from the situation that's irritating you. Some believe allergic reactivity to be of great benefit, acting as an immediate reminder to wake up to your inner process. Without physical symptoms these feelings would continue to be suppressed.

Remember, symptoms are not the enemy, but rather the warning that something is not right. They are not necessarily telling you to rush out and seek medical care, or that you need to fix them; they are guiding you to reflect inward to find places of imbalance and disharmony. When you reframe your relationship with them, symptoms deserve your respect.

True Healing

Patricia Lynn Mann, recovered from severe EI and now the Founding Director of the Center for Sound Healing in Carmel, California, says her recovery was accomplished using a holistic approach. "As a nurse, I attempted to heal my physical body, but as I went through the years and did not recover I had to pay attention to what was happening on the soul-spirit level. . . . No one modality was sufficient to heal me, each level of mind, body, spirit, and emotions had to be addressed."

What interventions helped Laura get well? To ask her landlord, he'd say living in a safe house. Her dentist would testify that removing mercury from her fillings helped boost her immune system into recovery. Her physical therapist would claim that increased strength through exercise did the trick. Her homeopath would assert that his remedies allowed her body to heal at deeper levels. Her close friends would say that divorcing her husband made her healthier. Perhaps the clean air near the ocean has been the answer.

Like Patricia, Laura believes her healing to have been a combination of all of these levels of intervention. "Healing has been about growing into myself and learning to be comfortable with who I really am." Most of all, she credits spiritual awakening with having the upper hand in coordinating the process of her recovery.

The reason so many healing efforts fail can be found in the multidimensional nature of these illnesses. Healing one small part, while it may help a little, cannot take place without healing the whole. True healing has less to do with curing or alleviating symptoms and everything to do with finding balance, growth, and change from within. Coming into balance does not guarantee that a physical cure will take place. A healthy body may not be what is meant for your unique journey.

To be healed does not necessarily mean that the human organism has conquered a physical ailment. It is important to stress a larger definition of health here: the true measure of health rests with how rich and full your inner life is. Attending to this, it's possible to be healed despite the ongoing experience of illness. For some, healing means learning how to trust themselves, learning how to have fun, or expanding the notion that they are more than their physical body, and opening to a world of new choices.

It's not being well that counts, it's the journey you take to get there that matters. Healing in the true sense is found in the willingness to merge your head with your heart. It means learning to live from the inside out, matching your true highest needs with the practical everyday world. Being attentive to health-related issues is not enough. In order to move along in the healing process, you may have to change an aspect of your life that seemingly has no relationship with your physical health.

Judy ended a longtime unhealthy friendship and Gloria took a leave of absence and eventually quit her teaching job. During those first 6 months, Gloria's healing from CFS took place not just on a physical level. Her fragmented emotional life had a chance to detoxify and repair as she gave herself permission to do silly, fun things that she previously had brushed off for not having the time.

As her dreams became more congruent with real life, she stopped waiting to have enough money, or enough energy, or to get well; she was just living fully in the here and now. Each day she'd take stock, noting her physical condition and what she was capable of. Then she'd decide what adventure she wanted to pursue. One day she went to a wholesale florist to feast her eyes on a magnificent shipment of tulips. On another occasion she had an extra hole pierced in her ear. Still another sunrise found her collecting shells at a beach.

Experiencing joy can enhance and facilitate healing, enabling you to feel that you have choices. Having options makes it difficult to define yourself as a sick person. These days Gloria takes fewer vitamins and eats more exciting foods. She is relaxed and happy, less worried about exhausting herself and more concerned with enjoying life as fully as possible. You too can stop defining yourself as a sick person. The next time you wake up feeling rotten, stay home from work, but drag yourself out of bed and create an adventure you've always put off. In addition to feeling more energized, this experience can awaken you to a world of possibility.

What healing is about is discovering who you are underneath all of the rules and expectations and learning to love and accept the person you discover. By accepting the condition you are in and trying on new ways of being, thinking, and doing, you can have a full life. Healing can give you permission to reshape your life into anything you choose.

People with EI and CFS often say they are "very close" to being well. Though optimism is an important outlook to hold, wellness is not a fixed state. It can be particularly difficult for those who are newly ill to accept the changing shape of wellness. It may take years of illness to loosen attachment to the prize of recovery. Just when you think you are on the verge, you may discover you're merely looking at the tip of the iceberg. It is easy to become frightened and discouraged as you trudge over the rise at the top of the hill only to find more, higher hills.

Actually the process of deep healing only begins when you are the most disheartened. When you get to this place, something is about to fall away to be shaped anew. Allow yourself to become curious and push past obstructing discouragement, fear, and hesitation. When you think you are done healing, you can always push a little further and learn a bit more; the process is never completely done. You may arrive at a plateau of wellness only to unmask another level; like peeling away the layers of an onion, you discard a layer, only to find another underneath. At times all you can do is wait until the next layer reveals itself. And, as with peeling an onion, there may be tears in the process.

EI and CFS are illnesses that are about patience. For some, this is the hardest part, to be patient with the healing process. It may help to remind yourself that these illnesses may be the result of a lifetime of imbalance, making it impractical to expect to repair the damage by seeking a quick cure. Jamie was willing to give herself a year to get well, and even that seemed like a long time. So far, it's been 6 years and she supposes she'll have to allow as many years as it takes. It isn't possible to will the process of healing along faster than it's already going. It is not possible to become well faster than your body is ready to do so. You cannot will yourself onto another phase of mental or physical health, it has to happen of its own accord.

The essence of the process of healing is allowing. True, it is up to you to do everything you can to help, but you must also find a balance between action and the state of allowing things to unfold as they are meant to. Pushing the process faster than is meant to be may get in the way of recovery. The body has natural intuition, knowing what it needs to do in order to become well. It is a great relief to recognize this innate knowledge.

The very center of your being is wellness, which is present even when your body is badly damaged or ill. The healing process has its own innate intelligence and information unfolds as you are ready for it to unfold. The best you can do is keep your heart open and available to the clarity that comes and trust the process. You can, however, assist by uncovering factors that get in the way of your health and factors that increase your well-being.

At times you may feel better, becoming excited at the promise of blossoming wellness. When you feel energized, it is easy to rush around in an effort to accomplish all of the things you haven't previously had the energy to do. Fearing that your energy will dissipate, you don't want to waste a moment. Frantic efforts to make up for lost time can make it easy to miss out on enjoying the experience.

Escalating and behaving in a pressured way can bring about what you fear most. Rushing along one step ahead of illness can exhaust you, inviting illness to take hold once again. Even if you crash, you can still feel encouraged because, most likely, you won't decompensate back to the start of your journey. Each time you decompensate, the illness holds less power over your life.

Beliefs

David, the former CPA with CFS, used to get severe migraines when he was exposed to perfume. On these occasions he would retreat to bed. This went on for years until he realized how furious he was at the invasion of his sensory space by an odor he didn't like and that he was not in control of his environment. Perhaps he was allergic to the perfume scent, but the role of his negative emotions cannot be ignored. Once he was able to link his unexpressed anger with his migraines, they dissipated. By the way, some take feverfew, a natural herb of the wild daisy family, to control and eliminate migraines.

Jamie used to be highly allergic to cats. Contact with them made her head blow up like a balloon, her eyes would water, and she'd have trouble breathing. Despite this problem she agreed to take care of a friend's cat, Rass, for several months while her friend was away. At first it was impossible for her to be anywhere near Rass for more than a few minutes without gasping for breath. The more she grew to love Rass, the less reactive she became. They became inseparable; every spare minute Rass was with her, snoozing on her belly and cuddling in her arms.

One study of heart disease patients at the University of Maryland found the mortality rate among people with pets to be one-third of the rate of people without pets.[1] Aside from the loving presence of the cat having a positive influence on Jamie's health; the relaxed state caused by the interaction had a dampening impact on her allergic reactivity.

The relaxation and harmony experienced from Rass's warmth, and the sedation of stroking him became more important than guarding against a reaction. During those snugly times her body was at peace, completely worry- and stress-free. Jamie wasn't thinking about protecting herself; she wasn't angry about her health situation, she was completely in the moment. Her relationship with Rass brought recognition of the interplay between emotions and physical experience.

When you feel content and full of hope, your body is relaxed; as a result, stress hormones don't surge and your nervous system is not on alert.

Things hurt you if you think they can. This means it is possible to decide against reactivity and extreme fatigue. It is accepted that negative emotional states adversely affect the immune system and that positive emotional states have a beneficial impact. Studies of cancer and cardiac disease patients have found that optimistic patients recover more rapidly than pessimistic patients.[2] This applies to people with EI and CFS as well.

Audrey believes she became well when she gave up the role of victim, electing to empower herself. "Empowerment happens when there is a shift that says, 'I'm in charge here.' At the [The Cancer Institute] they teach people how to visualize in order to increase their white blood cells. This visualization practice often manifests in a clinical report that shows increased production of white blood cells. Such incredible powers of the mind to make these things happen! I believe we create our own reality. If you think the universe will take care of you, it does. I used to get angry at people who said that, now I know from firsthand experience it's the truth."

It is common to believe that personal experiences shape your inner beliefs, when in fact your beliefs hold tremendous sway over your life experiences. Your beliefs are constantly sending your body messages that shape your health. These beliefs powerfully circumscribe how you deal with illness, affecting how you feel about what happens in the experience.

When you are ill, there are a whole series of beliefs that define who you are and how you are destined to live. Prolonged discomfort and discouragement can make it easy to validate unhappy, critical thoughts. If you believe you are to blame for your illness, then life shapes itself accordingly. If you believe you are responsible *to* your illness, then you create more viable options that move you toward healing. Once you realize the impact of beliefs on your health, you can cultivate optimism, choosing in favor of activities and beliefs that support this state.

Forming new, optimistic beliefs can be like making contact with antigens—you may be in the habit of reacting to and rejecting them before they can be fully felt and understood. In the same way that antigens limit your contacts and activities, resistance to changing your beliefs creates boundaries that can limit your experiences and creative potential.

Yet, those who walk the fine line between acceptance of circumstances and recognition that they are able to choose an outlook that supports their health are typically the most emotionally balanced, remaining optimistic during the ups and downs of illness. Theresa, who is acutely chemically sensitive, is nearly completely housebound, yet she has a positive outlook and is content with her life. "My life is extremely rich and full, despite my limitations. I refuse to succumb to the power of negative beliefs."

Audrey also believes it is possible to visualize herself into health through emphasis on positive images seeing herself actively involved in the process and experience of her healing. The first step in building a positive attitude is to take responsibility for your mental state and for your circumstances. After that you can take action to change the things about your life that you wish to. At any time, even if Audrey doesn't like what is going on, she feels a sense of control and hope. Because she has chosen to take charge, she is no longer buffeted about by outside forces.

Thoughts have a self-fulfilling aspect to them, creating a certain kind of energy that magnetizes the positive or negative to you. The more you allow spaciousness for life-affirming positive thoughts, the less room there is for critical and unloving ones. A surprising side benefit when you stop running negative tapes on yourself is that you will feel less inclined to have negative thoughts about other people. This makes it easier to like and appreciate those around you and to have fewer negative interactions.

Despite illness, you are not limited by your health unless you think you are. You are much more than the illness. What your healing must do is expand the size of the box housing your beliefs about life, yourself, and all the rest of what you think you know to be true. In order to change, you must have the courage to enlarge the container that holds your life. The box becomes larger as you examine your beliefs and start to let go of old ideas of who you think you are, while remaining open to the unlimited possibilities of your greater self.

The box expands as you observe your body, which can yield valuable information about your beliefs. Physical symptoms are often about unmet needs and beliefs. Your thoughts create magnetic impulses and chemical substances that impact and change your physical form. Every time you alter your beliefs, these impulses impact your physical being.

Challenge old beliefs by asking if they serve a useful function in the present. Are your thoughts congruent with your deeper, true self? Do you cling to them because they are familiar and comfortable? Or because you are afraid to go against the grain? Or are you a mental and emotional "couch potato," unwilling to think and act for yourself?

By fearlessly examining your beliefs without attachment and self-condemnation, you can awaken to how they limit you. Once you recognize that they no longer serve, you can change them, experimenting with new ways of being. Examining your beliefs offers an opportunity to recognize how negative thoughts can pollute your body and which ideas help as well as which ones harm you.

"Getting well had everything to do with my willingness to step into my own power," notes Jamie. "For so long I was afraid to express my needs and my anger directly. Once I started asserting my needs, I also had to come to terms with the fact that I am a wonderfully powerful person. Before that, I was fighting against myself." Holding your own power in check can erode you, but it can only stay squashed down for so long. If it doesn't get expressed in ways that feed you, your wholeness will come out in other ways, possibly less constructive.

Examining and consequently transforming belief systems and attitudes will enable you to see how you have compressed your life. When you realize that the size of the box that you have chosen to occupy no longer fits, then a life of staying behind the scenes, serving and helping others to the neglect of yourself, will no longer seem honest. Being dutiful and good—repressing your true needs—may be revealed as the source of much anger and "dis-ease."

As the size of the box that is your life expands, you may notice a budding sense of openness and appreciation for new and different points of view. Your whole life has the opportunity to be more congruent and true as you permit yourself to experience the pleasure of these changes, making it easier to let go of old ways that no longer serve.

Healthy Verbalizations

You may also want to consider the language you use; the words that you speak not only reflect your thoughts, but also create energy patterns that can attract certain types of events and people into your life. Words are either empowering or disempowering and whatever you give attention to through thoughts or words takes on energy. Positive, affirmative words beget positive, life-affirming thoughts and energies. Negative words depress and disempower you.

The language you use reveals underlying belief patterns that indicate how well you respect and care for yourself. The way you speak indicates the owning or transfer of responsibility. Using the word "should" suggests that someone else makes the rules in your life. Statements such as "She *makes* me angry," or "I *can't* come to visit," or even, "I *would* be happier if I had a better job" are all ways of disowning responsibility, suggesting that you are controlled by outside forces. The use of these terms is reinforced by thought-forms that can cause you to feel out of control, or to take a victim stance, or to blame others.

Owning and holding onto the image of yourself as weak or disabled can also be reinforced by your choice of words. Describing *my* aches and *my* pains creates and holds the sensations into *my* physical form. You're possessively claiming them into your body by saying they are "mine." Expressing negative, helpless verbalization will also prompt others to hold this image of you, sending you illness-based energetic thoughts. Their thoughts continue to define you as a helpless person, creating energy that may keep you stuck long after you have moved on to something else.

Understanding that words have a self-fulfilling quality, empowerment and choice can be created by using certain strong, self-supportive words. Entertaining affirming words instills you with greater energy that your body can use toward healing. By saying "I *am* healing" or "I *am* in charge," positive physical states are stimulated that cause the cells to awaken. Speaking and thinking in this positive manner creates an attitudinal shift. By consciously using empowering words, you are calling a halt to seeing yourself as a helpless victim, which then enables you to get on with your life.

Visualization

In the book *Getting Well Again* (Los Angeles: J. P. Tarcher, 1978) by Dr. Carl Simonton and his now former wife, Stephanie Matthews-Simonton, it was reported that several patients with untreatable cancers had recovered with the use of a simple visualization technique. Affirmations and visualization are powerful tools that seek to invest the mind with the ability to create a more desirable life.

In visualization, you attempt to experience yourself in a new state, effected by shaping your thoughts and releasing energy blocks that represent destructive, disempowering beliefs. In a state of deep relaxation, you direct your mind to create pictures that can help you heal. In this way you are learning to control and direct your unconscious energies, bringing amorphous potential into the realm of the possible.

The benefits of relaxation include much more than relief of tension. Being able to relax on command heightens the confidence that you can control emotional, physical, and mental states. This means you can control how you react to the worst of situations. Relaxation can make it easier for you to identify sources of stress and tension. In addition, relaxation interrupts habitual negative thoughts, clearing your mind and opening you to creative ways of problem solving.

You don't actually have to "see" in order to visualize effectively; all you need to do is imagine that you are seeing. Don't try to summon images using conscious control. The goal is to use the conscious and the unconscious mind in concert to replace harmful beliefs with life-affirming ones.

Visualization need not to be confined to the visual. You may have other senses that are more finely developed: images can come through intuitive feelings, or sound, texture, or smell, instead of by creating and holding pictures in your mind. You may be able to determine which of your senses is the strongest by asking yourself how you dream: do you dream in vivid pictures, or does sound guide your images? Everyone has a more finely developed sense that leads to contact with the unconscious. And don't worry if your images aren't bright and colorful. Close your eyes now and note whatever occurs. Do bright colors dance before your eyes? Does a scene come to you as on a movie screen? Is there a voice that tells you what is going on?

Developing an Effective Visualization

The visualization technique that you use can be tailored to your own needs, but it may be of most benefit to ensure it contains the following ingredients:

1. Define a state of being, either physical, emotional, mental, spiritual, or a combination of these, which you would like to examine or change.
2. Using as much self-honesty as possible, examine the attitudes and images related to this state which may be disturbing you.
3. Clearly and specifically identify the state that you would like to move toward.

    a. Establish clear, strong images that show the current situation being transformed into the desired one.
    b. Use verbal affirmations that support the visual image, such as "I am healthy and whole" or "I am alert and open to change."

4. Use images and words that have a somatic impact that can be felt physically, such as "My body is vibrant and full of brilliant yellow light." Include as many senses as possible in the process of savoring the positive state.

5. Seek an optimistic stance that enables you to feel the pleasure of the experience and in your accomplishments.

6. Maintain this procedure at regular intervals, at least once or more, throughout the day.

You may be able to uncover the meaning of your symptoms or your illness through imagery. Imagery can include dialoguing with your illness in order to increase understanding. Answers may come in clear form or in symbols to be revealed later as you attempt to understand. Your symptoms may be guides leading you back to your forgotten self, trying to assist you toward reintegration.

In the relaxed state of visualization, illness may take on new meaning, allowing greater understanding to give way to increased acceptance. When you accept, you are no longer at odds with the war taking place in your body. Practicing visualization on a daily basis helps form an alliance, as all levels of body, mind, and spirit work together to uncover what is needed in order to heal. When those needs are met, symptoms may hold less of a charge or disappear.

Symptom Visualization Exercise

Studies in the United States and England have found that 50 to 75% of all problems that manifest as pain or illness are emotional, social, or familial in origin.[3] Examining the impact of your emotions and how they play out in your body in the form of symptoms is critical to your physical health. The following is a two-part, deep relaxation exercise that can assist you in mobilizing healing imagery.

Symptom Visualization Exercise Part One. Find a comfortable, quiet place, positioning yourself sitting or lying down. Use deep breathing to achieve a relaxed state, noticing the images that arise as you focus on the ebb and flow of physical sensations and symptoms. As the images play their way through your mind's eye, begin a dialogue with your inner advisor as to the cause of various symptoms. Your inner advisor is a symbol of your inner wisdom and the cumulative information derived from your life experience. This inner advisor can offer information regarding any area of your life, serving as a liaison that links the unconscious part of your mind to the conscious. The way to access this advisor is to simply ask and then stand back and allow the information to flow.

Ask your advisor to explain how this illness has helped and served you. Ask the illness what it's doing in your body. Ask a specific symptom what it needs from you and how it's trying to help. As you focus on the sensations and emotions that arise, notice if there is a shape, texture, or color. Observe carefully without changing the information that floats up.

When the images have clarified into feelings, tell the image how you feel about it, speaking directly and honestly. Next, allow the image to have a voice and listen to what it says. Though this may intensify discomfort, allow the virus or allergic symptom to articulate as fully as possible. If you have trouble understanding the answers, ask for clarification, and keep asking until you feel satisfied.

Surprisingly, some symptoms such as allergic reactivity may be assisting you to find the energy needed to mobilize you out of a particular environment. When you notice feeling poorly, travel back in your mind to the point in time where you lost energy and evaluate what you were doing when this occurred. Recognizing situations and factors that cause you to feel poorly will give you sufficient information to steer clear of circumstances that exhaust and deplete, while supporting you to create more experiences that vitalize and energize.

Are you suppressing feelings, or consenting to do something you have no interest in doing? Are you needlessly risking toxic exposures or toxic interactions? Have you been using your sensitivities to be a little bit superior to all those "blockheads" who don't know what is harming them? Does the drama of reactivity give you a temporary boost, but ultimately deplete you?

EI and CFS have a lot to do with the inability to filter out the emotional, environmental, social, as well as spiritual influences of the external world. Experiencing symptoms may enable you to detach and distance yourself. Symptoms may help by forcing you to withdraw to protect yourself and recuperate. Some of your most severe physical symptoms may occur in the places of your greatest vulnerability. If it is true that symptoms are actually messengers, then each physical site or quality of a symptom carries with it a special message in the form of the disease.

As you explore these images, you may meet with anxiety and resistance. It is not uncommon to fear that your symptom may ask you to give up something dear to your heart or something hard to let go of. If this is the case, remember that you do not have to comply with the message. You may also find that what is needed is easy to satisfy and that the relief of compliance exceeds your expectations. If a traumatic insight bursts forth, pay attention to your fear; if it is too strong, you may do better exploring this area with professional assistance.

Symptom Visualization Exercise Part Two. Once you feel complete with the preceding information, you may elect to move to the second part of this exercise, which has been adapted from the work of Dr. Sherry Rogers, EI specialist. Imagine yourself in a hot air balloon hovering above the ground but not able to take off. The ballast that keeps you from floating up into the sky consists of several sandbag-like containers full of your worst allergens: pollen, plastic, petroleum products, foods, and so forth.

If fatigue is your main problem, imagine that the bags contain physical stressors and mental and emotional factors that exhaust and deplete you. In your mind, begin to allow yourself to be near these allergens and stressors for brief periods. Recognize your resistance and repulsion at making this contact, but continue to move forward to increase contact with these substances. As you do this, intentionally visualize your cells as calm and relaxed; no need to react to anything you might believe to be harmful.

As you are able to tolerate being around a particular allergen or stressor, toss that corresponding sandbag over the side. Notice your body becoming stronger and more resistant as the balloon becomes lighter and floats a little farther off the ground. See your organs and body systems actively removing sources of illness. As you toss more of the sandbags over the side, you will float with greater freedom, finding that fewer sensitivities or matters drain you.

When you complete this exercise, take time to write down anything that was significant. Describe the images of the symptoms in detail and how images in the first portion of the exercise relate to your experience of illness. Note any feelings you had about those images and what they were asking you. Did the images give you any relief? Is something more required? Are you willing to negotiate and make changes?

Writing about the experience may make you aware of connections and information emergent from the imagery. When you ask the unconscious for advice, it may respond in surprising ways in the weeks that follow: through dreams and flashes of insight, as well as through synchronistic experiences with people, books, and TV. In order to optimize the use of your visualization work, you will need to ask at some point, "Now that I have made a shift in awareness, what do I plan to do about it?" In some cases the imagery itself will be enough, in others it will only direct you to where you need to go.

You can also carry protective imagery with you throughout the day by mentally surrounding your body with a semipermeable meshlike membrane extending at least an arm's length out from your body. This membrane will filter out unwanted debris, toxins, and emotions, yet still permit good energy to touch and heal you. Try this two-part exercise once a day, spending about 15 to 20 minutes. In a month evaluate what's changed about your perception of the symptoms, noting if you have been able to reduce or alter their impact.

Meditation and Mindfulness

David, who had CFS, says his daily practice of Transcendental Meditation saved his life and sanity many times during his illness. Varied and diverse healing practices point to the healing benefits of meditation in helping unstick the body from physical or emotional illness. Meditation moves the body and mind to a higher rate of vibration, allowing healing energies to take over.

A major problem with EI and CFS stems from the inability to control the actions and directions of the mind. Daily practice of meditation quiets the mind so that it can watch itself without judgment. As you come through the stillness of watching, it is actually possible to feel more energy.

Scientists at the Maharishi European Research University have found that long-term meditators demonstrate more balanced brain wave activity between the left and right hemispheres of the brain.[4] Other research has shown that certain meditative practices which emphasize special breathing techniques are beneficial to people with respiratory illnesses such as asthma.[5]

There are many different systems of meditation: one involves the use of specific types of visualization to promote healing, another involves following the breath, another includes repeating a mantra, and still another involves tapping into levels of higher consciousness. Losing yourself in reverie or going for a walk can be meditative. Biofeedback is a therapeutically used form of meditation that teaches you to interrupt disturbing emotional or physical conditions by consciously learning to relax. Progressive tensing and relaxing of muscle groups can promote a relaxed meditative state. Guided or taped meditations can emphasize a particular issue that needs to be addressed. Stephen Levine has written an excellent book, *Guided Meditations, Explorations, and Healings* (New York: Doubleday, 1991), which includes a variety of useful guided meditations for developing healing awareness.

Most of these practices require that you set aside quiet reflective time in which to attend to subtle inner information. This means occupying the body, being present with your feelings, and noticing information that drifts into awareness. Through meditation it is possible to uncover the true meaning of your physical illness. The answer may reside in details about problematic emotional and spiritual dysfunction which can be corrected, enabling the illness to abate.

If you resist the idea, thinking that you must have discipline to meditate, consider that you may already have carved a space for meditation in your life in the form of resting. When you are ill, there are plenty of opportunities to take up this practice. The illness may have forced you into isolation or you may spend enormous amounts of time resting, to the extent that your attention has had ample opportunity to become keenly attuned to your inner life.

You may elect to use time spent resting for meditation. Instead of seeing this time as a waste, there is much you can do to enrich your life from a supine position. Since meditation is one of the most highly touted interventions for persons with physical illness, it provides an excellent opportunity to heal.

Meditation can be used to amplify the process of your awakening by tuning into your own needs. Resting coupled with long periods of silence can give way to important ideas and new ways of perceiving your experiences. Awareness can help you make the shift toward increased acceptance and understanding. Insights and creative freedom may become available because the mind is not weighted down by its usual conditioning. Meditation as a daily routine may refresh and energize you to the extent that you don't need to rest as much.

Creating a place for quiet increases awareness of the internal witness who can choose from one moment to the next to engage or disengage in life's dramas. This witness is just a higher aspect of yourself which observes your reactions to your thoughts. Witnessing without judgment creates an entirely new relationship to life, helping you to see that you can choose from moment to moment. Through meditation you can sort out the difference between the emotional, reactive self and the self of clarity and acceptance. With nothing to fix and nothing to do, life only need be accepted as it is revealed. Thoughts are seen for what they are, only having the power you give them.

Life itself contains constant small moments of meditation. You can convert simple everyday acts into a spiritual or meditative practice by being present and engaged. Walking, eating, driving, washing clothes, even resting become your practice. The relaxation and open-mindedness of gardening allows Josh the opportunity for increased clarity as to how to resolve various conflicts and concerns.

Mindfulness and Illness

A tremendous amount of energy can be expended pretending you are present when you are not. You may spend the bulk of your life as a ghost vaguely inhabiting various areas of your body and mind. The shape is there, yet you've abandoned what's inside. Just once dare to fully connect the inner with the outer.

You can do this by taking a mindfulness retreat for a day. If you can, clear your calendar and take one day off, spending it alone without talking, answering the phone, watching TV, reading books, or writing. On this day, do everything with your full attention, noticing each act without distraction. Try to be conscious of every breath and every minute. Notice how your food tastes after you've given its preparation your undivided attention. Notice how your throat feels, is it aching to speak? Will you evaporate if you are not heard? Notice the moments when you feel frightened and empty having none of the usual sources to grasp onto for support or entertainment.

As the day progresses, allow yourself to fully experience how you feel about your illness. Sweep with awareness up and down inside your body, focusing your attention as emotions and sensations arise without judging them. Guide your awareness back to the moment; gently breathing peace into areas of physical tension and discomfort. The more you allow yourself to just experience each moment in its wholeness, the more you will arrive at a level of detachment, expending less energy trying to resist and fight the enormity of illness.

Appreciate what is, savoring what you have. Take time to fully appreciate the wealth of what you have rather than resenting and resisting what has happened to your body and your life. Notice who it is that inhabits your body. Who are you really, aside from all the external fluff? Permit any and all feelings to surface. Rub up against those dark scary places, and allow yourself to bask in your own bright light. Feel each moment melting into the next. As you let go, notice with wonder and fear how alive you are. The more alive you are, the less room there is for illness.

Punctuate the end of this day by lighting a candle, saying a prayer of thanks, or writing of your experience. Thank yourself for providing the unique opportunity to change your relationship to the moment, an experience that can be very freeing. In the days that follow, carry the knowledge of this experience forward as you go about your activities, being fully present in the rest of your life. Practice mindfulness in everything you do. Do not hurry your movements by rushing onto the next experience; give every act your full attention as if it is the most important thing in your life. When you are completely present, you have the ability to fully feel your illness or completely free your mind from it.

Creativity as Healer

"One of the biggest things I have to thank my illness for is my newfound creative self-expression. If I hadn't been ill, I might never have tapped into it. The more creative I am through my writing, the healthier my body has become. If I have one piece of advice for those who are ill, it is to find what you are passionate about and do it. Immersion in creativity has become the most blessed and richest part of my life. It has enabled me to become more myself," enthuses Josh about his work as a freelance writer. The key to finding meaning in your life is to identify your passion and follow it.

At first it may be difficult to define what it is that you feel passionate about. The main way to gather this information is to make room so that you have an inner life. In order to create, you cannot be other-focused, it must be identified from within. The more you make space for creative, pleasurable activity, the more you will be able to find your passion.

Meditation can be one way into creativity, showing you places where you are holding your life in check or are suppressing your needs. By releasing you from self-limiting ideas of who you should be, meditation enables you to find the courage to step out of the mold to try on new ways of being and doing. As you sit on a regular basis, you will inevitably open to higher levels of awareness which can help you to tap into your own vistas of creativity.

If illness is about the disconnection between the body, mind, and spirit, creativity is the way home. Tapping into creativity inevitably opens you to spirituality which can enable you to find your way home. The heart of creativity is about the mystical union between yourself and the universe, finding the two to be one and the same, completely whole. You are a creator whether you believe this or not; the potential resides within every person who ever breathed life.

All that is needed to embrace the creator within is to believe that it is possible for you to join hands with your creative spirit. Once you establish that, creativity is about your infinite potential. An important tool used to tap into creativity is to notice synchronistic events as they tumble into your life. As you consider your creative potential, openings in the form of events, people, and circumstances will unfold, offering you opportunities to tap into your creative aspect.

Creativity is not necessarily about being the best, or about being able to make things with your hands or with your mind. It happens when you are able to focus on the here and now, allowing the flow of harmonious, balanced energy to move through you. Whether it's writing, painting, or finding a more efficient way to organize your desk, or frosting a cake, or learning a computer program, your healing has everything to do with expressing and manifesting your heart's desire.

It isn't necessary to be enormously talented or skilled in order to be creative. In many ways it doesn't matter what you make; what matters is the way you are changed by the process. Creativity is an experience, ordinary or extraordinary, which opens you to the world of unlimited possibility, connecting your inner with your outer life.

For some, creativity will flow easily once the intention is established. For others, it will take work and require much time. In order to tap into your creative potential, you must make a commitment to explore what this means for you. How about keeping a journal of your dreams? Recording your thoughts, feelings, and dreams will help chronicle your journey and offer insights into many aspects of your life. As a way to measure your progress keeping a journal is also an opportunity to open to creative self-expression. Judy used *The Artists Way* (New York: G.P. Putnam's Sons, 1992) by Julia Cameron, a 12-week program to help find her creative voice. Faithfully writing "the morning pages" helped her to move through fear and guilt about her illness. Writing filled her with energy and made her more honest in her interpersonal relationships.

Write to Life

By writing your way through conflicting and draining emotions, you will decrease their power over you. Putting down your worst thoughts and fears can help release them, enabling you to regain balance in order to move on. Writing also offers an outlet, preventing you from dumping your feelings on those who are important supports. Putting thoughts to paper is one means of exploring, embracing, and bringing clarity to your feelings. Most feelings are amorphous until they are named and writing helps to identify them so that they can be faced and handled. Working to increase your mental clarity and to organize your thoughts can help open you up.

You may see yourself as too sick and too depressed to write, but doing this on a daily basis will force you to exercise your brain and not give in to physical discomfort. Writing can help you to focus both on and off yourself and offers the opportunity for potent detoxification on many levels. Setting aside a few minutes a day, every day, to write, you may have to push through your fatigue, a myriad of distractions, and your resistance.

This time for yourself can be the thing that pulls you through the rough spots, making it possible to make sense out of confused emotions and unhealthy states. When you start, there may not seem to be a creative, expressive bone in your body; but, over time you will begin to notice greater clarity of thought. If you cultivate it, that clarity can even trickle into your everyday life. At first, you may feel stiff, shy, and self-conscious about applying words to print. Keep at it; eventually you will be able to see where you have come from and note the incremental changes in your skills. These small changes will have a cumulative effect over time. Why not give writing a try to see where it goes, all you have to lose is yourself.

For years Laura entertained fantasies of being a writer. Mostly these thoughts snuck up during sleepless nights, flooding her with fantastic, eloquent thoughts that longed to be expressed. In those wee hours, filled with uncontrollable energy, she'd get out of bed and commit these heady, inspired ideas to paper. Effortlessly scrawling, she'd yield herself to waves of bliss that washed over her entire being. In those moments she was the most connected to her true nature, she could be and do anything, she was completely well and allergy-free. In those dark hours she understood with utter certainty the greater plan for her life—she had to write.

These episodes always entered her life unbidden, without any apparent context to explain them. Her everyday waking self could not will these experiences into existence and dreams of writing had no context to her everyday life. Yet, in the days to follow she would feel true and whole, unlike her sickly, fragmented everyday self. Inevitably, her rational self would kick in, doing it's best to squeeze her life back into the old familiar mold. How could she presume to be a writer, she'd wonder. What made her think she had something to say? After running a few negative, constricting tapes, she'd squeeze back into her old familiar self and dismiss her dreams.

After many years of these rounds of expansion and suppression, a stronger voice began to emerge. Why should she prevent herself from doing something that felt so right? And even stronger, "You can do anything you choose to do." It became clear that she had to find out.

Your own dreams are nudges, the feathers of the soul seeking to take flight into reality. Once you stop disowning and denying your creative, true self, you'll experience a new world of possibility. What's important is to actively seek to bring your dreams into everyday life in order to make them happen.

Summary

Do you feel any different than when you started this chapter? Hopefully you will see that you can create an entirely new relationship between yourself, your illness, and your health. What might seem like an impossible task, to change old ways of being and doing, may involve nothing more than faith in yourself that you deserve better, and setting your intention on that.

Endnotes

[1]Alan Beck and Aaron Katcher, *Between Pets and People* (New York: G.P. Putnam's Sons, 1983) 20.

[2]William Collinge, *Recovering from Chronic Fatigue Syndrome* (New York: Perigee, 1993) 96.

[3]Martin Rossman, *Healing Yourself* (New York: Simon & Schuster, 1987) 21.

[4]Richard Gerber, study by P. Levine *et al.*, "EEG Coherence During the Transcendental Meditation Technique," *Scientific Research on the Transcendental Meditation Program* Vol. 1, Orme, Johnson, and Farrow, eds. (Livingston Manor: Maharashi European Research University, 1977) 187–207; *Vibrational Medicine* (Santa Fe: Bear & Co., 1988) 402.

[5]Gerber, 402.

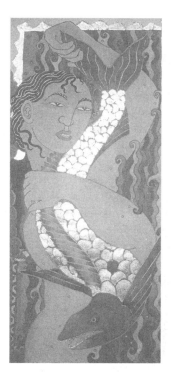

Chapter
Fourteen

Releasing
Attachment

*M*any things besides a rebellious body can keep you ill; there are attachments of all kinds that can interfere with the recovery process. Attachment can take the form of an unhealthy relationship or even a fondness for some aspects of the experience of illness itself. Adhering to useless, outdated survival programs, such as thinking that you have to hold onto that high-paying job, even though it's making you sick, is another form of attachment.

Attachment takes many forms, but denial, resistance, and guilt are at the top of the list. These states all serve useful, protective purposes to some extent, but carried to extremes they interfere with your physical and emotional welfare. Denial is a tool that enables you to control things around you in an attempt to avoid coming to terms with your true feelings of rage and despair.

For example, it may be that you cannot give up sugar, even though you know it makes you sick. Constant consumption gives you an emotional lift, preventing you from dipping into darker emotional states. Continuing to consume sugar then also requires that you expend tremendous amounts of energy keeping your emotions at bay when this energy could better be used toward healing.

It may be that you are afraid to examine how you feel about being ill, i.e., you deny the problem by not looking out for your welfare or by failing to care for yourself. Many go to great lengths to sustain denial, refusing to face their terror and despair. Resistance is a way to harden against the experience of fear. Resistance keeps you in a contracted state and happens when the box that contains your life becomes very small.

Ironically, the more you resist what you fear, the more it is solidified into form. When you are willing to fully accept your health problems and feel the deep pain that arises, you will release your resistance. Accepting what is opens the floodgates toward healing, and in the process of feeling the full potency of your weakness and vulnerability you may uncover your strength.

When you release your resistance, the floodgates may also open into feelings of guilt and shame. Remaining stuck in these states offers the opportunity to avoid taking responsibility for your actions. To some, guilt may look like the acceptance of responsibility, but guilt is simply a way of immersing yourself in self-punishment in the process of attempting to justify behaviors you cannot accept. On some level, guilt is a way of doing penance, attempting to expiate yourself from wrongdoing. How can any force from outside condemn you when you are so eagerly heaping punishment on yourself? Surrounding yourself in shame and guilt merely creates a smokescreen that keeps you from getting about the business of your life.

Resistance and holding fast to fear and attachment are the places where you say "no" to life. You may be playing it safe by staying with the old familiar, "safe" scenarios in order to protect yourself from harm. Ironically, by keeping your life in check this way you create a life full of "no's." By exploring the places where you are stuck, the sites of your "no's," you then make yourself available to your "yes" to life.

True healing means saying yes to everything, the good and the bad, your illness and your health, your anger and fear and sorrow, and your denial. As the disowned parts of yourself come home, you will once again become whole. In this chapter we will talk about changing your relationship with yourself in order to achieve integration and wholeness. But you will also be asked to examine your relationships with others and the uncomfortable possibility that you may unconsciously be a coconspirator in your illness.

No-Fault Secondary Gains

In addition to Dr. Carl Simonton and Stephanie Matthews-Simonton's visualization work with cancer patients, they also reported the most common benefits of illness as revealed by cancer patients. These benefits include:

1. Illness offered the opportunity to get out of dealing with difficult situations or problems.
2. Illness allowed the person to be the recipient of attention, nurturing, and care.
3. Being sick enabled the person to regroup and develop new ways to solve problems.

4. Illness prompted the changing of unwanted behaviors and helped the individual find the incentive toward personal growth.
5. Illness also offered the opportunity to avoid having to meet the demands and high expectations of others.

With the work of the Simontons in mind, consider the possibility that you may actually be benefiting in some way from your illness. If you elect to explore the subject of secondary gains, you must approach this task with great sensitivity, because it is easy to use this information in such a way that you will feel guilty or responsible for becoming ill.

So why would you be interested in looking at your own attachment to your illness, risking blame and shame in the process? You might opt to do so because this information can be vital in helping you to move from being a victim toward self-guided mastery. By asking yourself the uncomfortable question, "In what ways does my illness benefit me?" you may uncover information regarding your unconscious participation in your illness. Examining your attachment to your illness, without judgment, will help you to see the places where you are stuck. In this way, you can identify other ways to reap the benefits without having to stay ill to get your needs met.

"When I was in the first grade, I was home ill so many times I had to repeat that year. It's clear that a pattern was set very early on; being sick was a way to get love and attention. Now the question is, can I get these same needs met without being sick?" muses Audrey, who is now well from CFS. When David had CFS, he came to enjoy the simple life-style that his illness imposed. As he began to get well, his old, too busy life would take over and he'd find himself missing the simplicity of the life he had when ill. Consequently, he would become ill all over again. Recovery for David has meant understanding that he doesn't need to stay ill in order to maintain the life-style he prefers.

In many ways, illness serves to fulfill unmet needs. Being sick may enable you to leave a stressful situation that has reached an impasse or it can provide a convenient excuse to justify opting out of social and work obligations. Illness may force you to attend to your own needs, enabling you to ask for things you might not ordinarily request, such as love and attention.

It's even possible that the secondary gains of illness can be too rewarding to give up, making it difficult to get well. For some, the extent to which the illness helps to meet unmet desires may reflect the degree of effort you will put out to stay ill. It is important to note that getting your needs met may be absolutely legitimate, but opting to stay ill in order to continue having these needs met is not. Figuring out how to meet your needs may mean you have to change from a foundation based on illness to one based on wellness.

It can be instructive to explore what the secondary gains are in your illness. Once you recognize the ways you are attached, you have the opportunity to make a shift in your relationship to them. For example, Laura discovered that some part of her needed to stay ill in order to create boundaries because she was so poor at creating them on her own. "I had a history of allowing people into my life who asked more from me than I cared to give. One friend was constantly calling at all hours for advice. I felt invaded by her to the extent that I automatically felt fearful when the phone rang and I was exhausted after every conversation with her."

Just as parasites invaded her bowel, and candida and environmental pollutants took over her body, she allowed her life to be invaded by this person. Afraid to claim her power by setting limits, many other relationships also depleted her. Consequently, being sick gave her an acceptable excuse to say no. In Laura's case, being afraid to speak her truth had something to do with squelching her power. Rather than speaking up, she was, to some extent, hiding behind the skirts of illness.

As Laura began to set limits, she noticed feeling more honest and less conflicted inside, plus feeling energized when she spoke up. Once Laura stopped giving herself away, it was no longer necessary to defend against parasitic relationships. No longer needing to protect herself, she had more energy to enjoy her friends. If you want to have more energy, you must learn to accept and manage your power. Saying no can electrify your body with energy. Are you ready for that? As you come to see yourself as powerful through the use of visualization, relaxation, or greater clarity and consciously choose to focus your mind, you will be more capable of setting limits and expressing your needs.

How Sickness Helps

As noted, illness may offer refuge from life or it can make it easier to set boundaries that you are loathe to set on your own. It's always easier to bow out of an engagement by telling someone you don't feel well, rather than saying no. Reclaiming your power by setting limits and speaking from a place of truth rather than from wimpishness forces you to be less dependent on having the illness set boundaries for you. Learning to say no may make you less popular, but illness is an enormous price to pay for your lack of assertiveness.

It is possible that your support systems may feed you in ways that cause you to hold onto the role of being sick. Judy notes, "I was always the identified patient in my family which diverted the focus from my parent's relationship problems, particularly from my father's drinking. When I decided to take charge of my life, I blew apart many unspoken, hidden family myths. Because everyone was so attached to the myth that I was the sick one, it became extra hard for me to get well." Like Judy, it's possible that your family may have an unspoken investment in your staying ill in order to avoid having to directly examine those disturbed relationships.

Overidentification with another family member can also prompt illness. Jamie's father was ill most of her life, to the extent that family life centered on his cancer and later cardiac problems. Jamie became acutely ill with chemical sensitivities shortly after he died. Years later she was able to see that she entertained the magical thoughts that being well meant forsaking and forgetting him. Jamie believes that her body absorbed the imprint of his memory, carrying the torch of illness forward so that he would not be forgotten.

Illness offers the excuse of getting longed-for desires met without ever having to face them directly. You may want to be taken care of, thinking this is what it means to be loved. As a child you may have used illness to manipulate your parents in order to get special attention. You may be using illness now to manipulate others in order to get your needs met. As a grown-up, this tactic, using the illness to get what you want, ultimately harms you.

Once you get well, you may no longer be treated as special; there will be no volunteers to do the cleaning or the shopping, or people who will give you extra consideration and attention. Doubtless, you will be thrilled to be restored to health, but you will then be expected to do your part and will receive less attention to boot. For those who are really attached to the escape that illness offers, it's no big surprise when illness returns. Though it may not be a conscious act, your privileged status as a sick person may offer you more of what you want. If you find this to be true, it's your task to discover ways to receive this same quality of caring and love without the overlay of illness. Care and consideration are your right, but you don't have to create greater suffering in order to get what you want.

A simple exercise is to write down all of the ways that your illness helps you. Don't think too hard or else you will censure some of the most useful information. Write whatever comes to mind and keep writing until you're done. When you're finished, compare your list with the following one, as there may be some issues you didn't think of.

Exercise to Explore How Illness Helps

- Being ill enables me to stay home.
- I get to whine freely. (Whining is something I may do when I assume I won't be heard.)
- It keeps me from having to meet social obligations.
- Being ill provides me with a handy excuse when I can't think of how to say no.
- It removes me from the stress of upward mobility.
- Illness reduces the amount of external pressures in my life.
- It enables me to control a small portion of the out-of-control world.
- It may give me attention and love that I might not receive otherwise.
- It gives me a chance to be taken care of.
- Perhaps it is a way of punishing those around me who I feel to be unappreciative.
- It forces me to take life slower, enabling me to enjoy it more.
- I am able to reduce toxic exposures.
- Being ill gives me a constant companion, filling the void of emptiness.
- It can make me more interesting.
- Being sick means I don't have to pay back the kindness of others.
- When I am ill, I don't have to form or invest energy in building relationships.

You may be surprised by what this exercise reveals. It can expand your understanding of the factors that are involved in staying ill. Examination of the secondary gains of illness makes it possible to see how your particular illness may serve you.

Ambivalence

Let's face it; there may be a part of you that may not want to get well. You may not want to be in charge of your life. It may be easier to avoid career decisions by continuing to collect unemployment. It may be easier to use the illness to punish your partner for having an affair. If you are unflinchingly honest with yourself, you will recognize your own ambivalence. Once you recognize that there may be a conflict, you can make changes or not.

Recognition brings you to the first step in acknowledging ambivalence; now you must engage in an honest dialogue with yourself about what you really want from life. Examine your regrets, allowing yourself to hear all sides, even the perspectives you have suppressed or those that may embarrass you. If you've been sick for a long time, there is a good chance you are dissatisfied with a great many aspects of your existence. Give yourself permission to notice all aspects of your dissatisfaction, giving each area equal air time.

Examine your regrets. Have you selected the wrong career? Or, worse yet, the wrong mate? Do you wish you had more friends? Do you regret some important choices in your life? Perhaps it has been easier to stay ill than to examine these issues. Ask yourself if this is the case. When you have taken a complete inventory, consider what one small change you might make that will enhance your life and figure out how to implement it.

Once you take this step, however small, you will be engaging your immune system to work for you. The more small steps you can take, the more these measures will activate your immune function. It's impossible to get your immune system to protect you if you don't have a general internal consensus that this is what you want it to do.

When you are ill for a long time, you may have become attached to the idea that you are a broken machine that needs to be fixed. Many with EI and CFS grope frantically, going from physician to health practitioner, trying out all kinds of interventions in an effort to be safe. As a result, you may have become more interested in the safety and security of having some external force fix you rather than finding your own internal freedom and health. Thinking that you are broken is an attachment, a kind of shackles. You are whole right now; you don't need to be fixed or well in order to be complete.

You are not limited by the boundaries of illness unless you think you are. Each negative concept that you hold about your illness is an attachment to drama. What you are really doing is becoming attached to the fragments of clouded emotions that give these aspects the power of truth. If you think these little pieces, these dramatic aspects, define who you are, it's understandable that you might be reluctant to give them up. After all, who would you be without them? What would you then make of your life?

Attachment makes it difficult to let go of the way you see life, even if those ways don't work. You may keep trying to do the same things, making the same mistakes over and over, even when they don't serve, and in fact hurt you. Preferring to think of yourself as a good person, you may go out of your way to be liked even when this means subverting your true needs. It is easy to be attached to this image of who you are to the extent that you neglect to put your needs first.

These lessons, the places where you need to change and free up attachment, will keep coming up until you master them. If you suffer from repeated relapses, returning to the world and forgetting all that you have learned, this may mean that information has not have been fully integrated. Your symptoms may keep occurring, often with greater consequences and intensity each time until necessary changes are made.

Mostly your attachments cause suffering when things don't happen as you wish they would. Becoming attached to being well causes suffering because you are not. You may be attached to who you think you are or who you are not. You may be attached to giving meaning to illness when there is none to be found. Attachment may take the form of excessive drama and emotionalism. In some respects, attachments give meaning to what might otherwise be an empty existence; yet these attachments also keep you from living in the here and now.

Attachment Release Exercise

Christopher Tims, a teacher of metaphysics and healing, has an exercise that can assist you to examine and release your attachments. Begin the practice that follows by making yourself comfortable in a quiet place. After you get situated, bring your attention to your third eye, situated about an inch above your brow, in the middle of your forehead. Next, bring to your mind an image of an open, large, old wardrobe trunk.

When you have this image firmly in mind, create an imaginary beam of light emanating from your third eye, allowing that light to flood into the trunk. As you do this, permit the beam of light to carry all of your ideas and concepts of who you think you are and who you aren't as the beam fills the trunk. Permit all of your ideas of what your mind is and what it isn't to flow through the beam of light into the trunk. Allow all of your ideas and all of your attachments to flow from your third eye further filling the space. With this beam of light, project all of your notions of the "Divine," all that the "Divine" is and all that it isn't, into the container. Continue to permit all of your beliefs and notions about life, about right and wrong, about good and evil to fill the box.

At some point the box will seem to be full; when you are done, close and latch the lid. You may then wish to visualize yourself tossing it out into the ocean to be carried away with the current, or you may elect to mentally detonate it. Or you may elect to write your name on the lid and just set it outside, with the intention of taking it up at a later time.

Throughout the day, every time you notice yourself feeling disturbed by events or attachments that come your way, beam up that light and put the disturbance, that attachment, into the trunk. You can beam your "stuff" into the trunk any time you wish, during daily meditation, or when you experience a glitch in the day. This exercise will call attention to how heavily you burden your aliveness with attachments and provide a vehicle for their immediate release. You will never be done freeing yourself, there will constantly be new attachments, but the more you recognize them, the easier it will be to set them free.

By understanding the transitory nature of all types of emotions and experiences, you are released from their hold over you, freeing you from the grasping and struggles that can divert much of your life experience. Every second that you are alive, you are infused with the infinity of choice. You can alter how you perceive or how you hold onto hurt, and what you elect to give back to the world. Coming to terms with your attachments brings you the freedom to choose to stop identifying with self-limiting ideas.

When Jamie's husband told her he thought she treated her illness as if it were a hobby, she was hurt, but the truth of that statement could not be denied. "I was deeply attached to seeing myself as a sick person. In order to get well, I had to set free my attachment to being ill, becoming fearless in doing what is required of me in order to be healed." The process of healing asks you to fully engage, not just go through the motions. As you let go of old useless beliefs, deeper levels of information will be revealed.

You must be willing to let go of old dysfunctional ways of being and doing. This may mean learning to say no without feeling guilty. When you no longer have the pretense of illness, you will have to find ways to set limits that will be more congruent with your inner needs. You will heal as you learn to live in greater connection with your heart's desire and are willing to speak the truth. To stay well, absolute honesty will be required in order to live congruently in the world.

As you become more congruent, it will no longer be acceptable to use the illness as an excuse for not having the life you wish you had. The credit for true healing belongs to you for embracing life-affirming thoughts and actions. This change can evoke the physical event of healing, but also deeper, more substantial change at an inner level.

Phobic of Life

It makes sense to stay at home if you run the risk of toxic exposures or of being depleted by the outside world. But there is a pathological state that exceeds the need for physical self-protection. This state includes a fear of life itself. Many who have become ill with EI and CFS are afraid to venture out in public to go anywhere or do anything other than the most routine chores. When they do, they quickly retreat to the safety of home again. In this way, the container that holds their life has become very small.

True, many learn to live within this box with great courage and clarity. But for some, this box becomes a refuge, a way of controlling the uncontrollable, a way of hiding out from life. Efforts to control your surroundings in order to avoid toxic exposures can constrict life to such an extreme that you may close out the experience of living.

Living a small, narrow life need not be. By using healthy discernment you can determine which physical self-protection efforts are actually helping protect you and which are cutting you off from life. At times, risking toxic exposures can be more advantageous than avoidance. Attending a special family event, your son's graduation, or watching a parade can be more important in feeding your soul than the adverse impact of exposure to toxic fumes. It's a balancing act to determine which activities will feed you and which will harm you, but some people who are ill needlessly opt out of the world altogether.

You may find that you react to the excessive demands of the external environment in adverse ways which may make you try to control it by withdrawing. Perhaps you react to demanding relationships in the same way that you respond to external forces that trigger allergic or stressful symptoms, by withdrawing.

In some cases this may be the result of phobic states. A phobia is a persistent fear of an object or situation that your rational mind knows you shouldn't be afraid of but you can't help it. The purpose of your fear is to give warning and protection against dangers. Living with EI and CFS can cause you to fear that anything and everything will harm you. It happens when you have trouble finding and creating safe spaces for yourself. Staying home may be an attempt to control the uncontrollable, keeping a myriad of fears in check.

However, when the urge for self-protection reaches past what is considered to be ordinary and practical, it can stunt your life. Since phobias are originally created by beliefs, creating a shift in your beliefs can help dissolve them. In good time, if you keep making yourself available to examine and change the beliefs that no longer serve, you can challenge your fears and free yourself from these unnecessary impasses. This is where psychotherapy and possibly the use of antidepressant medications can help break the cycle of this harmful habit.

When you express your needs, you are controlling and directing your energies to best advantage and you no longer need to control events and people around you. As you become proficient at owning and expressing your feelings in more direct appropriate ways, you are taking charge of your internal and external experiences. As your internal world becomes more congruent and aligned with your truth, you are no longer a victim, suffering at the whim of external forces. You no longer need to perform the impossible, i.e., controlling the actions of others, and controlling forces outside your grasp.

Healthy Boundaries

"I often catch myself going over the line between being a caretaker and being a caring person. This may be one of the reasons I don't go back to teaching, because it throws me back into the care-giving arena." Gloria notes that across the board, people who have CFS and EI seem to have trouble maintaining their boundaries. Besides the damage caused by toxins in the environment, the agitation and disturbance caused by interpersonal relationships actually seems to manifest for some as physical harm.

What is a healthy boundary and how do you create it? A healthy boundary is created by determining that one thing is safe or okay, but another isn't. Firming up your boundaries means learning to identify and be true to your needs. Just as there are different immune pathways to send out commands against pathogenic invaders, you can learn to say no to protect yourself from interpersonal invasion as well.

When you fail to establish firm boundaries for yourself, it's likely that the protective command doesn't get sent out to the rest of the body to protect you when it's being invaded by toxins and pathogens. When that command doesn't go out, the immune system doesn't take you seriously. As you establish firm interpersonal boundaries, the body is more competent at holding its own against environmental stressors and mobilizing its immune forces.

Why are some people better at establishing interpersonal boundaries than others? It is believed that coming from a dysfunctional family prevents the development of a healthy sense of boundaries in childhood. The emotional stress of holding painful childhood memories at bay leads to chronic low energy and incompetent immune vigilance in the adult. Since these boundaries were never established in childhood, the adult continues to be assaulted and beaten down by out-of-control forces. Inevitably, the body absorbs all of these messages as judgment and rejection, translating them into poor health.

This lack of firm boundaries is easy to recognize in people around you who seem to absorb the energy of rejection, pulling it into themselves in the form of shame and guilt. Yet, what is obvious in others is hard to translate for yourself, to know how to modulate your own energy in order to prevent this from happening. As you recognize and establish firm boundaries for yourself, the body becomes more competent at holding its own against environmental stressors and mobilizing immune competence.

Boundary Language

Let's look at how you can be more proficient at setting firm boundaries. Examining the verbal and nonverbal messages you give others offers clues toward boundary strengthening. Tone of voice is the first line of defense in standing up for yourself. Drawing a fuzzy boundary instead of a distinct one conveys the inability or unwillingness to stand up for yourself in order to enforce what you've said.

How boundary statements are made sends a message as to the strength of your intention. Ending a sentence with a high, questioning note is disempowering. Pulling back when a statement is made implies that you aren't willing to stand up for yourself. Posture, eye contact, and tone of voice help or hinder you in achieving the desired effect. Those nonverbal messages offer information that indicates that beyond a certain point you are not willing to back up what you say. With practice, the voice can carry a firm, strong edge, giving a clear message that delineates firm, clear boundaries and penetrates into the awareness of the receiver.

Many of us were brought up in the school of communication that says, "I am standing firm on this one, but if you're going to reject me I'll back down." The effectiveness of your limit setting depends on how much of yourself you use to say no. When your words and body language fail to match up with your intention, it's difficult to get what you want.

Congruence is power. Using all of your resources, mental and physical, to communicate creates greater personal power. The responsibility for clear communication depends on you; others just take your cues and run with them. The price of incongruence is particularly noted when one part of you really wants something, but another, insecure, indecisive part gets in the way. Beginning a sentence, "You may not want to, but I'd like to go to the movies," sets an expectant tone of failure. State your wishes clearly.

By speaking clearly, from a place of truth, you may have to face your fears of rejection. Being grounded, centered, and congruent, you will be less likely to personalize any rejection that comes your way. When rejection isn't personalized, it will be more comfortable for you to stand up for yourself.

No longer giving yourself away calls a halt to taking blows of rejection and judgment into your body. No longer giving yourself away means setting limits, standing firm, and taking responsibility for the consequences.

You will stop losing energy by first filling yourself up. The way to become full is to be good to yourself—treating yourself with loving-kindness. Treating yourself in this way will cause others to treat you with respect as well. It's unlikely that others will treat you with respect if you treat yourself poorly. Treating yourself better, you are less damaged by outside forces and by other people. Aside from having more energy, you will attract healthy individuals and feel more satisfied with life.

Changing the Score Exercise

For the next 2 weeks, try to refrain from beating yourself for any reason. In this process, examine your life without judgment, noting where you hold onto negative thinking, but don't give in to those negative thoughts. During this time, decide you are not going to accept that habitual negative self-view, but instead make yourself available to the emergence of something new.

Consider loving and liking within yourself and how it translates into action. Sort through your feelings without any predetermined guidelines, noting places where you hold judgment and where you are kind to yourself and others. Part of the task is to recognize your limits, including who and what you like and don't like, without self-punishment. It's okay to recognize when you don't like someone or something. This doesn't mean either of you is bad, despite the informal rules that say you have to like everyone.

Noticing and accepting both internal and external forms of disharmony means you don't need to follow the rules to be like anyone else. Increased recognition of the presence of natural disharmony offers the opportunity to work through conflict. At some point, recognition of your limits and how you feel about all kinds of matters will create a shift.

By assuming a fresh, new perspective about old habits, that old mode of self-relating will be cast aside. In the process of filling yourself up, a new path is forged without the need for approval or liking from anyone but yourself. Being true to yourself will create a new definition of self-love and liking that will translate the awareness of your personal boundaries into everyday action, bringing truth into every part of your life.

Creating Healthy Relationships

"As long as I took responsibility for others, people would always allow me to do so. It was a big challenge to allow others to be responsible for their own lives. Though I still grapple with the overwhelming need to be a caretaker, I had to come to terms with the fact that this care giving behavior had done a lot of damage. It was a monumental thing to recognize that I wasn't going to survive if I continued to try to take responsibility for other people's lives and that they wouldn't be able to grow and survive either." Gloria, now well from CFS, muses, "When you recover, you assume that all your relationship problems will be over. That's not the case, there's ongoing work to be done."

It is not uncommon for people with EI and CFS to lack the mechanism necessary to filter out unhealthy relationships in their life. Illness has helped to compensate for this lack, serving as a filtering device, to keep people at arm's length. Returning to health may require that you transform old relationships into healthier ones, and this has everything to do with creating and sustaining healthy boundaries.

In order to change these long-standing unhealthy dynamics, you will have to disconnect from unhealthy dependency needs, rerouting them into greater self-sufficiency. This can be a scary proposition because the comfortable refuge which that relationship offered may be in jeopardy if you change. Gloria gave herself away; not knowing how to be a real friend, she tied people to her with generosity and overzealous consideration, hoping this would make people beholden to her.

Little did she know that by attracting unwanted people, she was creating scenarios that depleted her because she felt so inadequate and unlovable. Inevitably she found herself becoming resentful and disappointed; after all, who could keep pace with Gloria, the ultimate, all-giving friend. As she became healthier she began to recognize that her efforts to develop healthier, more supportive relationships reflected an improvement in her own internal health. In time, she realized that having people disappoint her elevated her own standing with herself.

Creating a sense of supportive community allows you to have a safe place to heal. This may be difficult to do if you have felt rejection from family, friends, and community because of their lack of support and understanding regarding your illness. It is, however, possible to find this support and security in those who know firsthand what you are going through, namely, support groups and individuals who are ill. These people can support your journey into self-love. Without judgment, they will receive you openly with acceptance and understanding needed for you to heal.

Illness will force you to examine your relationships and ask you to surround yourself with emotionally healthy people who heighten, rather than deter, your progress toward recovery. Attracting healthy relationships happens when you set about to have a healthier relationship with yourself. Becoming conscious of how you want your life to be will bring people of like mind into your sphere.

Evaluating Your Relationships

Ask yourself who your friends are. Are you satisfied with the give and take of those relationships? Do those relationships feed you or do they weigh you down? If they do not satisfy, what can you do to create appropriate change that makes them rich and rewarding? If you don't have many supportive relationships, what can you do to attract healthy people into your life?

Instead of seeking eccentric and unusual friendships, look for people who support your best self. These days Gloria chooses more normal, traditional, and yes, boring people, rather than those who are exciting and neurotic. She notes, "Neurotic people may have great adventures and great highs, but my recovery depends on choosing in favor of happy, stable, sensible relationships."

If you have to shut down in order to be with someone, it's a signal that you should avoid contact. If watching someone stirs up uneasiness in you, it will probably be an uneasy relationship. There are some relationships that may be so detrimental to your well-being that you may have to muster the courage to call it quits.

Sherry, the mother with EI, describes one close friend whose life was in constant chaos and distress. Time spent with this friend left Sherry depressed and exhausted for days after. Coming to terms with her own chaotic inner life enabled Sherry to see that this unhealthy relationship reflected her own internal disturbance. When she recognized this, she saw how destructive this friendship was to her health.

"It was impossible to change the well-worn, habitual groove of our friendship." With a sigh she says, "One of the most important, but difficult decisions I have had to make was to terminate this friendship, letting it go with love." Though this was a painful step, she no longer received hysterical calls about her friend's latest fight with her husband or the chaos of her life. Letting go of this relationship marked Sherry's coming of age, her decision to consciously establish and hold to healthier boundaries.

If a particular relationship is not working for you, it may surprise you to realize that you can stop participating. If you have someone in your life who depresses or depletes you, ask yourself: "What is keeping me tied to them?" The honest answer may shock you. Regardless of the past good times and memories, you don't have to remain permanently glued to the misery of another.

It is bittersweet to find the courage to leave a dysfunctional relationship. Once you decide to end it, be prepared to stand by your words. You may need to say no, holding fast to that boundary over and over again. Even recognizing the harm caused by that relationship you may miss them; their absence will leave a void in your life. The loss of this relationship can be offset by the recognition that you are actively creating greater harmony in your life, moving on to healthier nurturing relationships.

The more you are able to put yourself first, removing censured self-expression, and living on track with your true needs, the more your inner harmony is able to merge with outer reality. Giving up superficial games as well as relationships that exhaust and distract you makes it easier to get on with your life.

Changing Old Relationships

Gloria says it is hard for those in recovery from CFS or, for that matter, any illness, to change habitual patterns of relating in old, long-standing relationships, particularly with family. When you change in the process of becoming well, the people who know you best may have the most difficulty accepting the new you. Unwittingly, certain lifelong behaviors, reactions, and opinions continue to be expected from you, to the extent that friends and family may persist in trying to maintain the status quo, keeping you locked into the old familiar mold. With new relationships, no one has preconceived expectations that can tie you down. It can be easier to try on new ways of being in new relationships, rather than to remake old ones.

Your relationships may not always support honest expression, making it difficult to express uncomfortable or negative emotions. Particularly in the family but in friendships as well, there can be an unspoken agreement to keep these feelings hidden for the sake of superficial comfort. This unspoken dynamic may be so ingrained that it is not recognized as such. However, years of suppression can result in depression, illness, and codependent behavior.

If you are ill with EI and CFS, you may be the "identified patient" in your family to the extent that your body manifests unspoken, dysfunctional family agreements. Your illness may be the external expression of a suppressed family dynamic, serving as a barometer that reflects unspoken hostilities and tensions that rest below the surface of seemingly comfortable lives.

Becoming well includes learning to express, rather than to suppress, feelings. This is particularly difficult when there are long standing agreements not to honor or recognize certain feelings. It is hard enough to change your own habitual behaviors, but change in the face of familial resistance can pose an extreme challenge. There can be fierce resistance born of fear that makes it hard to change the old dynamic between yourself and others. These people approach you with conclusions as to who you are, thereby limiting the relationship.

When you change, any imbalance in an old relationship becomes more pronounced, unless it is faced and accepted. People around you may have no sense of their own resistance, but the changes you make can greatly disturb long-standing relationships. While this shift can be healing and exciting for you, it may be met with tremendous resistance and fear on the part of others. The new persona you have outfitted yourself with in order to become well has a domino effect, prompting everyone else in your life to make shifts in relation to your own changes.

As you discover new and different ways of being and living, all relationships undergo a shift. As you change, your relationships cannot help but change as well: anything that affects you will inevitably alter the lives and habits of others in your life. The fact that others resist your efforts to change should not provide you with the excuse to give up. Suppression of what you need to do to get well can mean a return to illness.

To keep you steady on your path, remind yourself that unhealthy dynamics found in your relationships may contribute, for better or worse, to your health. Recognizing this may make you unwilling to continue unhealthy interactions. At times you may find you have reverted back to old useless ways of relating. When this happens, you may do best to notice the old traps, stand back, and with loving-kindness allow new ways of being to emerge. As you change through healing, all you can do is hold your heart open to those you love, but it isn't helpful to stop your own healing progress to protect them. This makes for exciting, but scary times that require that you let go and trust the process.

You may want to ask others to participate in changing the shared relationship. Communicating the changes that have come to pass in your life can make the transition in your relationship more smooth. If you need to, ask your friends and family to give you room to change and suggest that you set each other free from the habits of the old relationship. If you have such an agreement, you can mutually assist each other to free-up old patterns and expectations. Changing your relationship to yourself and with others is required in the process of becoming well. Change renews and enlivens your relationships. Without change, relationships become meaningless and eventually die.

Summary

This chapter deals with learning to address the attachments and conflicting emotions that you may uncover in your recovery. How to build and maintain healthy boundaries becomes an issue when you lose contact with how you feel. If you haven't developed a keen sense of how to protect yourself when there is danger, you may end up completely withdrawing, perhaps becoming phobic of life.

Healthy boundaries and healthy relationships become less problematic when you begin to take care of yourself. Learning about your boundaries doesn't mean retreating; when you bump up against an edge, instead try to hang out there to discover the window of opportunity. When the boundaries of the box in which you reside become too tight, you will either shrink yourself to fit the environment or hopefully shed the environment in order to expand outside.

Part Five

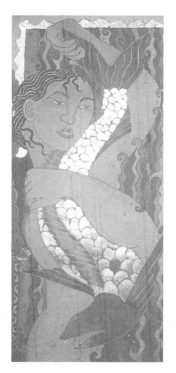

Sustaining Your Healing

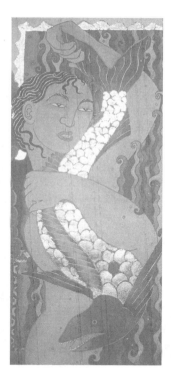

Chapter Fifteen

The Challenges of Health

*a*sk yourself again and again, "Who is getting well and what are they doing to get there?" This is a most important tool to guide your own return to health. What is meant by "well" is those who have achieved greater physical and/or emotional well-being. This question emerges again as we move into this chapter, which is about taking responsibility for your life as well as taking decisive steps to protect yourself in the process of reentry into everyday life. When you begin to feel better, you may wish to challenge yourself to connect with the environment and the outer world in new ways; eventually sharing what you have learned by making a contribution to others in the process.

People who are becoming healthy as well as those who are able to live in harmony, despite ongoing illness, seem to be those who take responsibility for the choices they make while responding to circumstances they cannot control. Rather than blaming circumstances, external conditions, or the behavior of others for any of their problems, they seem to make conscious choices as to how they cope with their experiences. People who are "well" are those who have decided to take responsibility for they way they hold their illness; consequently, they move from a passive, victim orientation toward one of personal empowerment.

Many with EI and CFS struggle with this issue because accepting responsibility implies self-blame, shame, and guilt. The implication is that since you are responsible for everything, you must be in some way to blame for being ill. Bearing the burden that you may have colluded to create your illness can be unnecessarily cruel and lead to greater disempowerment. Then there are others like Elaine, with EI and CFS, who refuse to let themselves off the hook. She holds her body accountable for all of its difficulties, including profound fatigue and the trouble she has filtering toxins. "It's a personal thing; if I choose to react to chemicals by being fearful. If I elect to react, I create symptoms; if I don't choose react, I don't become sick."

Being Response-Able

Audrey says, "Taking responsibility for my disease brings up all the issues of blame and guilt which only offers greater immobility. What is most useful to consider is that I am responsible *to* myself, while being responsive *to* the disease. This kind of thinking helps me to disengage from self-destructive thinking. My primary task, regardless of what has caused this, is to uncover what I can do to heal." Being responsible *to* your illness means learning to be kind to yourself, while taking charge of how you live in this moment and in the next.

Laura emphasizes the word "able" in "response-*able*," creating the image that she has the ability to move beyond victimhood by taking charge of the things that she can. "Whatever caused my disease, I am *able* to limit my activities when I feel poorly. I am *able* to fight for chemically free bathrooms at my college and I *am* able to choose the healthcare that is most suited to my needs." She uses the term "response-*able*" in such a way that she can choose how to respond, even to out-of-control circumstances.

Using the concepts found in the terms "response-*able*" and "responsible *to*" as Laura and Audrey have means choosing how to respond to difficult, out-of-control circumstances in such a way as to create an enormous shift in your physical and mental health. During the course of your illness, you may have been able to accept varying percentages of responsibility for your situation. When you feel pretty well, it's easier to claim 99% responsibility. At times, when your health is at a low ebb, you may not be willing to claim any part of it. It's normal for your perspective to fluctuate; taking responsibility for however much you can at any one moment means doing the best you can.

New Age Pitfalls

The awakening of interest in mind–body relatedness has sparked an ambivalent shift regarding the influence of the mind and beliefs on physical illness. Accepting the mind–body connection at face value has spawned harmful, erroneous beliefs that can deepen feelings of guilt, self-blame, despair, and confusion in people who are trying to get well. The mind–body link in New Age thinking creates a baffling paradox which, at its core, has two seemingly contradictory views.

The first holds that you are responsible for all that happens. With this notion, as supreme creator of all that happens, you are expected to harness your will and intention to create any state you desire. The other view says that it is imperative to let go of all attachment and accept the unfolding of The Greater Plan which will take care of your every need and has your best interest in mind. This view implies that you can passively sit back and allow the greater forces of the universe to shape your life. This means being able to trust that a Higher Power is in charge, even in the face of seemingly cruel and arbitrary events. Is it possible to have it both ways?

Both the New Age and the traditional concepts involved in taking responsibility for your life and for your illness are geared toward self-blame for past actions. This means that if you embrace the mind–body link, you play an important, though unconscious role in planting and fertilizing the seeds of your own illness. Inevitably, if you accept responsibility for the presence and persistence of illness, then you are at fault for creating the disease in the first place.

In illness, the question of who is responsible for what is a painfully murky issue at best. For many with chronic illness, the word "responsibility" is often synonymous with "shame" and "blame." The real rub lies in the next step. If these diseases are self-created, then why is it not possible to heal yourself as well? And if you cannot figure out how to get well, you must be terribly bad.

It's even possible to feel so guilty about being sick that it is difficult to feel worthy of getting well. Giving in to helplessness and self-blame inevitably weighs the body down, paralyzing the healing process. But there can be a degree of comfort in accepting that your thoughts, feelings, and attitudes do have an impact on illness though you don't have complete control. What is within your control are the choices you have to change your attitudes so that you can emphasize a certain amount of loving-kindness toward yourself.

Learning Balance

The key to the mystery of how much of your life is within your control is to learn balance. It is possible to accept external circumstances while choosing to be responsible for how you wish to respond to events that you cannot control. Surprisingly, change also comes when you give up trying to control external events and accept your difficulties. The inability to accept only serves to heap further suffering on what is already a difficult situation. Acceptance of what is, surrendering into the present, rather than blaming yourself for the past offers a more promising path. When you are no longer resisting what is, life takes on greater ease and fullness.

Whether or not you believe that your illness is caused by your attachments and unhealthy thinking, you can use the opportunity of this crisis for healing. Accepting responsibility for your life is a powerful force that can enable you to recover missing parts of your essence so that you can be restored to wholeness. Once you stop blaming circumstances, external conditions, or the behavior of others, it is possible to make the conscious choice to live as fully as possible despite the ongoing limitations of illness. Many who do this, such Laura who has severe EI and Crohn's disease, face ongoing physical illness, living within the limitations it circumscribes with enormous courage and grace.

Assuming blame covers all of the territory of your previous ignorance, moving backward from this moment in time, squarely placing you on the hook. Being responsible doesn't mean you must inflict self-punishment for all of your shortcomings. It also doesn't mean that you can pin your illness on the fact that you've had disagreeable experiences or on improper parenting. Illness cannot be blamed on the suppression of feelings either.

Past circumstances may have truly been out of control, and assuming you've always done your best, it's time to let yourself off the hook. Reluctance to release yourself from blame is a matter of choice, but it is important to distinguish between unconscious motives and causation. Bearing the burden that some unknowing part of yourself may have colluded to create illness can be unnecessarily cruel and lead to greater disempowerment. But it can be helpful to recognize that illness may stay rooted in the body because of some form of attachment or secondary gain.

Rather than self-recriminations and a self-critical emphasis, it is possible to create a shift by making the best choices for yourself in the moment. This means responding to the best of your ability, using the resources that you have at this time, in this moment and in the next. It means being in the here and now to face the challenges of life, not holding on to mistakes and woeful obsession with the past.

Creating a different relationship to the idea of responsibility can alter your experience of illness. When you assume responsibility, you are able to respond to forces in a manner that causes greater healing and integration. Accepting responsibility *to* the illness, rather than *for* the illness, makes it possible to move forward from this moment on. When you are responsible *to* the illness, choices are actively made as to how you elect to experience this moment.

You are now accountable for doing all that can be done to help yourself today, in this moment and in the next. Cultivating this attitude toward all of life's experiences makes it possible to work with what is to shape each moment to your choosing. It's a sure bet that as your awareness grows, you will repeatedly have to forgive yourself for some of the decisions you will make today.

There is, however, value in examining the past in an effort to prevent repeating the same mistakes today. This is best done with an open, accepting, exploratory attitude, not with the intention of heaping greater self-blame. By taking this turn you must first promise to treat yourself with forgiveness and kindness; uprooting and reexamining what is past can be a trap into a destructive spiral that merely distracts you from change. Although your illness was not intentionally created, once there is an understanding of the role of choice, it is possible to use your intention to elect to live in gratitude, seeing every experience as an opportunity to deepen your understanding and healing.

Being response-*able* means taking charge of your feelings so that it is no longer necessary to allow others to regulate and control the direction of your life. Sure, there will still be the influence of external relationships and events, but your response to those events will be a matter of choice. No longer at the mercy of external forces; it's possible to have a good day even when everything goes wrong; or it's possible to feel good about yourself when treated with indifference.

Taking this kind of responsibility means being able to move past self-limiting views. Most of us assume that inner states, in particular, anger, judgment, and fear, are simply responses to external cues. When you are responsible, it's no longer necessary to assume that outside forces are in charge. The choices you make as to how to think and feel actually determine your life experiences. Helplessness is the worst possible medicine for your immune system. Seeing yourself as a helpless victim will simply maintain the status quo. Seeing yourself as cocreator, taking responsibility for life's experiences, means you are response-*able* to make choices and changes accordingly.

As you choose to be response-*able*, it is no longer easy to deny that most of what comes your way is within your control. When you take responsibility, you will have more energy because you no longer need to work hard to blame yourself or things outside you. Difficulties will resolve with greater ease when you stop blaming and when you no longer seek refuge in your guilt.

Being responsible for your life means choosing to face your fears and offering self-forgiveness for your shortcomings. Holding onto these fears and destructive emotions is the cause of so much unnecessary suffering; besides leaving you powerless, this creates a smoke screen that diverts you from living fully. The less energy spent blaming external forces for your unhappiness, the greater is the empowerment from within.

The most definitive step taken toward empowerment is to recognize that the source of happiness resides within. It is easy to overlook this key point, looking outside yourself for the answers or to pin blame. When you take responsibility for your life, resistance melts away; there is no longer suppression or avoidance of the truth.

Though life may not include having all you desire, though your body may not achieve full health, reclaiming responsibility does mean being fully engaged in life's choices. On some level you choose everything that is created. If you have a physician who you don't like or a job that makes you unhappy, you are choosing to go to that office and take what is dished out anyway. Whether you are ill or healthy, you are responsible for the choices you make.

Reentry

Most people who have been ill with EI and CFS can look forward to a gradual return to health. While it isn't clear precisely what factors prompt recovery, Jamie notes, "I began to get well once I decided to take charge. After being desperately ill for years, waiting for someone to come along to fix me I began to examine the choices I had been making with regard to my illness. I was sick to death of being sick, so I decided to do something about it by putting my needs first and scaling back my too busy life-style."

In the process of recovery you will doubtlessly experience relapses and remissions. Over time your relapses will become less intense as your body makes positive shifts in relation to the changes you've made in life-style, health interventions, and self-help. During this time you will need to be attuned to the signals your body conveys in order to protect yourself from stress, toxins, and other forms of harm. Tuning in to these signals may become an ongoing part of your life or they will fade as your body becomes less vulnerable.

"I feel like I have been in a coma for 10 years and am now just coming out of it. I'm greedy for everything and don't want to waste a minute. To make up for lost time, I clean the house and cook while listening to educational tapes. I'm hungry for life." After a 10-year hiatus, Laura self-consciously wonders if her social behavior is appropriate, or if she is too revealing, or too needy. Away for such a long time, Laura's return to the world has been awkward.

Reentry can be a most exciting but difficult time: there can be immense hope, yet it can also be very tricky because increased wellness calls on you to exercise extreme patience and discernment. You may rest and revel at one phase of recovery, then circumstances may force you to move on to another level of health.

Sustaining wellness requires ongoing work to maintain a balance between setting limits and living fully. Gradually you will need to learn to balance the need for retreat with activity, as well as paying attention to your emotional needs and states. Becoming more attuned to your inner signals will let you know when you are overtaxing yourself and prevent you from backsliding.

When you first become sick, these illnesses may force you to restrict your life; yet in time you may come to find greater balance. At times it will be worth paying the price of loosening restrictions for the sake of pleasure. You may eventually compensate to the extent that you consider yourself to be well, yet the process of healing is not linear. Return to health does not mean your difficulties are behind you. It is a constant effort to sustain your healing, and just because you are symptom-free doesn't mean you are permanently well. Recovery is an ongoing, lifetime project necessary for all parts of you to heal at deeper levels. There is no limit as to how well you can become.

Some may get well quickly, while others take years. The rate of recovery seems to have no direct relationship to how rigorously you adhere to healing practices. Those who are lazy and not so careful to avoid allergy-producing foods and stress-producing situations may even get well faster, bypassing those who plod along and are extremely conscientious. Interventions that work for Laura may be of no benefit to you; your program of recovery must be your own.

Yet, even the solitariness of the journey can be a source of your strength. Simply being handed a list detailing the necessary steps for recovery may short-circuit empowerment. As you move to increased levels of wellness, you may become stalled at a particular plateau. This may be a reminder to address a physical problem at the level of the cause. This symptom may be caused by an internal conflict that will keep showing up until it is resolved. Or, with a long trail of ups and downs the return of old symptoms may tell you when you are becoming sloppy.

Despair and Relapse

Once you have experienced improvement, the subsequent return of symptoms can cause anger and depression, far worse than when the illness was a constant companion. Suffering a relapse may simply be an offering of information that you need to pay increased attention to self-care. Taking your precarious health for granted by eating too many processed foods, increasing exposures, or taking on too many social commitments can cause setbacks. The resurgence of symptoms means it's time to break a few dates or climb into bed to rest.

Learning to tune into your body's warning messages and recognizing your personal limitations can go a long way toward preventing decompensation. It is easy to fail to notice decompensation in its early stages, until it becomes more intrusive and demands your full attention. By the time you finally notice, it may be invasive and persistent, requiring much more effort to heal. If you have been ill for some time, you may have taught yourself to tune into areas of weakness and sensitivity, noting subtle warning symptoms that may signal a pending relapse.

People who are newly ill assume that recovery means they can return to the life-style they had before they became sick. After several relapses you may come to recognize that this outlook will simply re-create the situations that allowed the illness to thrive in the first place. Recovery then takes on new meaning, which doesn't include assuming your old life-style. Recovery means changing the way you have lived in favor of a life of greater balance. This may mean moving slower, anticipating your areas of greatest vulnerability, and attending to your emotional as well as physical needs.

As you begin to experience a more normal existence, you may be less tolerant of setbacks. Relapse must be reckoned with as a part of the process of healing, serving as a reminder not to get sloppy and return to old detrimental habits. Relapse can offer you the opportunity to reconnect with yourself when you've slipped, forgetting to put yourself first. If you choose to reframe the experience, relapse is a review course that forces you to reexamine all you have learned, giving you a chance to brushup.

Relapse calls to question everything you've been doing to get well. You may wonder why you took all of those supplements or why you've tried so hard when it really makes so little difference. A setback makes it difficult to be patient and accepting, yet each time it happens it can be easier to get through if you recall the previous times when you have returned to health.

No one really knows why these illnesses cycle through as they do. Relapse can be caused by increased stressors such as: physical exertion, exposure to viruses, other infections, disregard of dietary restrictions, fatigue, depression, environmental damage to your body, as well as reaction to medical interventions. No one knows why it is that when you try a new intervention you may experience a great burst of energy and resurgence of health that leads you to think you've found the answer, but that shift seems to inevitably wind down. Perhaps your needy body has just absorbed and acclimated to the positive change so that the benefits of the healing intervention are not so noticeable.

A day of feeling pretty well may be followed by one that mandates staying in bed. At times you recognize the ways you have overtaxed yourself; other times there is no explanation as to why you feel worse. This reflects the mysterious portion of the disease process which is completely out of your control. Most likely, it took years of imbalance to accumulate the toxins and viruses and stressors that tipped the scale into illness. Just as it takes a long time for illness to take hold in the body, the process of healing doesn't take place all at once. It may help to appreciate that your body is devoting much of its tremendous reserves to healing, which may help explain why you are short of energy for the basics.

Reentry and Balance

Though attention to your illness is necessary, it's possible to become lost in it. When you are at your worst, it's difficult to recall times when you felt normal. Some give over their entire life attending to the difficulties of illness to the extent that they lose themselves. Over time, illness has become a safe refuge or it may have made you special. It may have given you excuses to avoid living in the world. Much of your existence has probably adapted to the concept of yourself as being ill. For some, getting well means dis-identifying with being an ill person.

You may also have ambivalence as to how much room to devote to illness. Throughout the years the pendulum may swing in either extreme. At times you may choose to give it as little room and attention as possible; at other times you may monitor carefully, controlling every inch of your life, strictly adhering to the guidelines circumscribed by the illness. Being careful helps avoid toxic exposures, which, in turn, enables healing. However, carefully and narrowly circumscribing your life may also shut out many opportunities and pleasurable experiences. Hypervigilance may breed increased reactivity in some cases and maintaining continuous attention to your health can make it difficult to live a normal, sane life.

This may mean that you need to find an identity that is larger than that of a sick, reactive person. It is your right to protect yourself from exposure to toxins and allergens; yet if hypervigilance narrows the quality of your existence, it harms you in the long run. A calm, accepting approach to self-protection seems sensible. Jamie says she feels best when she goes about her life with as much equanimity and normalcy as possible.

Inevitably, there will be exposures if you venture out in the world, but it's self-defeating to become agitated, angry, and fearful at each of these events. Once again, the key is to examine the way you choose to respond to these exposures and stressors. Making positive choices can carry as much of an impact as the reaction itself.

Avoid invalid consciousness, that is, treating yourself like a delicate breakable object at every turn. Being overly protective keeps you passive, preventing and limiting experiences out of attachment to the sick-self. You can safely limit activities according to your physical needs and avoid situations that will threaten your welfare, even after you shed the idea that you are an invalid.

Theresa moves forward with her life even when she experiences symptoms. Still careful, she no longer wishes to dwell on the illness, but places her attention on living. Illness no longer has the same power it once held over her. People who are returning to health have to balance attention to the demands and priorities of the body, remembering not to give illness all of their attention, as well as not becoming swept away with the fast pace of life.

It is natural to feel fearful and uncertain when moving back into the world. Reentry can make you cautious, afraid of reverting back to old ways. Because you are no longer constantly suffering, it is easy to become lax and take your health for granted. It is important to recognize and accept that you cannot expect to take up right where you left off. Returning to a life full of doing and action can make you ill again. If the learning and growth offered through illness is not permanently embedded, you may revert to old habits. Self-abusive behavior will keep causing relapses until you are willing to make life-style and internal shifts.

Easy Does It

Cultivating a life that is more in tune with your personal needs and perhaps slower in pace will sustain your recovery. At first, it is common to move with great caution, testing every step. Take it slow; that way you won't get off balance and lose the knowledge and hard-won insights that have emerged from your experiences. Taking small steps in the process of reentry offers the most solid path. For some, returning to work full time can be chancy. Settling for part-time or incremental increases in work and activities, gradually testing the waters, will enable you to find your limits.

When you return to the world, if you are like Laura and have been out of touch for a long time, it's difficult to know how to behave. Having spent so much time alone, she feels particularly vulnerable in group situations. Impatient, wanting to make up for many lost years, she cuts through the mundane niceties with a direct approach that tends to make others uncomfortable.

The image of a female Rip Van Winkle comes to mind; she has reawakened to a world that has changed radically from the one she left. Reentry poses the problem of not knowing how to be when you are no longer defined as ill, reactive, or tired. Being stripped of this long-standing relationship to the world forces you to face the important issue of how to move forward with your life.

Sustaining Laura's health requires that she advocate for herself, asking for help in meeting her needs. She can rake the lawn, but needs someone to pick up the leaves. She can go to the movies, but only if she finds a "safe seat." If she needs photocopying, she asks the printer to meet her outside the building. At times she protects herself by donning a mask which, despite stigmatizing her as different, helps others to accept her status.

Along the way she has become comfortable telling people, "I am a person who is challenged. Though I have to do things in a different way, I can do anything you can do; I just need to find the way that works for me. This means being creative and free enough to ask for what I need." Your recovery may require that you make adjustments to your former ways out in the world and you may need to learn how to stand up for yourself.

This may mean finding people with whom you can express your needs. It may mean making your limitations clear, letting others know what your body can tolerate. Recognizing the potential for people to take offense, you must learn to express your needs with tact and kindness. It can be a new experience to express your needs directly and openly without apology. Giving yourself what you need is one of the major hurdles to sustaining recovery which will be put to the test as soon as you return to the world.

A major obstacle to recovery is that you are seeking reentry into a world that is increasingly more polluted and stress-filled. Even when you become well you must return to the same environment that made you ill; so the cycle continues, unless you take steps to protect yourself. Efforts to impress others or living with a list of "shoulds" will no longer be a viable way of life. Excessive concerns about what others think and how you measure up should take a back seat, otherwise you will reestablish a well-worn groove that will cause relapse.

When you repeatedly start to get well and go into a tailspin back to poor health, it may be that you are reverting to old codependent ways. One hilarious, but appropriate description of codependence is when you are dying and someone else's life passes before your eyes. Codependence is about putting the needs of others before your own in a perpetual struggle to find your center and sense of worthiness. Illness and subsequent recovery may offer an opportunity to help you find your center, but sustaining this requires that you no longer give yourself away.

Summary

With EI and CFS, separation from the external world may have been the only way to survive. Yet, separation may also take the form of avoiding responsibility for your life. Taking responsibility for your life will help make you whole. You have developed the issue of separation in the form of illness, but as you get healthier you will need to challenge your body to reenter the environment in healthy, self-protective ways.

Chapter
Sixteen

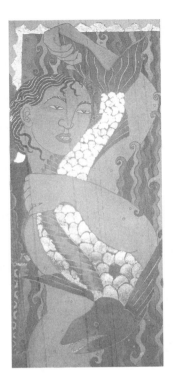

One Earth,
One Fate

Some regard that EI and CFS to be the result of our species' failure to live in harmony with nature. Our disharmony, has affected not only ourselves but also environmental conditions on the earth. "Human beings evolved over millions of years with a certain balanced relationship to the planet," says Michael Mamas, director of The School for Enlightenment and Healing. "When we started to act in ways that deviated from living in balance within ourselves, we began to affect the earth in an adverse way."

Michael Mamas believes that the individual has to evolve and come back into harmony within him- or herself in order to achieve personal healing. When individuals have achieved balance through internal healing, this will have a healing influence on the planet. The numbers of people with immune system illnesses seem to have increased directly in relation to the degree of our disconnection with the environment. This chapter is about how to reconnect in useful, healing ways with the earth.

Joining the Human Race

"There are growing numbers of people who feel that immune dysfunction is directly proportional to our estrangement from social, political, and spiritual concerns. These diseases are a reflection of the addiction and dysfunction of an entire society," notes Judy, a former market researcher, now recovered from CFS. The media, government, and industry all act to brainwash us into maintaining these addictions because addictions equal big profits.

It is estimated that 15% of the population cannot live comfortably on the earth. This number was determined in 1987 by the National Academy of Sciences and has undoubtedly increased since then.[1] It is increasingly difficult to avoid this harm, and the daily news is rife with reports of large-scale environmental problems. These include toxic spills into the ground and water, as well as air that is being loaded with poisonous fumes. Even the once clean oceans, mountains, and deserts are becoming polluted.

Seeding Change

Despite growing awareness and efforts to turn back the tide, the environment continues to become more contaminated. We are coming to the realization that the earth may not survive us.

EI and CFS are symbols for what can happen when you take the world into your body. EI is blamed on the advances of technology that are polluting the earth, and CFS reflects the impacts of the cumulative stressors of the environment on our immune system. Some regard that our destructive, polluting, greedy practices are depleting our bodies as well as the earth. Whatever the cause, these illnesses are on the rise.

The benefits of living in our modern industrialized world are becoming more subject to question as we awaken to the hazards we are creating. In the rush after profits found in the manufacture and distribution of so many dangerous and damaging products, we have neglected to question the effect of these chemicals on the human body as well as on the earth. Industry, government, and the public have all failed to ask if we and our planet are capable of adapting to the changes that these chemicals introduce. The clear answer from our experience with EI and CFS is no.

For every person who suffers acute health problems related to the environment, there are many more who unknowingly receive insults to immune function. While many have hidden allergies, others suffer from a series of undiagnosed viral or parasitic infections. There is evidence that low-level exposure to chemicals inhibits our ability to respond to stress and to protect against bacterial and viral invasion. It is widely appreciated that the damage done to our bodies may not be evident until years after the initial exposure. If you consider those suffering from low energy, alienation, and depression, the ranks of those injured by our increasingly toxic world are seen to be enormous.

Rachel Carson, author of *Silent Spring*, wrote, "The contamination of our world is not alone a matter of mass spraying. Indeed, for most of us this is of less importance than the innumerable small-scale exposures to which we are subjected day-by-day, year-after-year." Her work in the 1930s addressed the notion that the human race could no longer upset the balance of nature or exploit the environment without damaging ourselves in the process. As the comic character Pogo Possum so aptly said, "We have met the enemy and the enemy is us." The earth has become allergic to us.

Each person is called on to change his or her habits as a matter of survival. But the average person is not concerned with environmental pollution until he or she is personally affected. Since most of the population are superficially able to adapt to the huge load of environmental chemicals, they aren't concerned with the global threat. Until there is a direct personal threat that is fully felt, few will take self-protective steps. It may be that cases of immune-related illnesses have to become much more widespread before something is done.

Change won't occur until greater numbers experience devastating events striking closer to home. The Bhopal disaster in India was the first enormous, visible display of chemical contamination. Next was the Exxon Valdez oil spill followed by the train wreck in Dunsmuir, California, which caused a toxic spill into the American River. Love Canal, Chernobyl, and many similar incidents have helped amplify public concern, but not enough to send up an outcry demanding change. Spills of this type happen with greater frequency, yet these incidents continue to be met with apathy. Even the difficulties of Gulf War veterans—exposed to pesticides, chemicals, and vaccinations and now exhibiting CFS and EI symptoms—have been minimized.

The Precautionary Principle

Current policies with regard to environmental decision making require strict proof of causal relations between a specific pollutant and one or more illnesses before a particular chemical is restricted in its production and use. Measuring the adverse impact of toxic exposures is difficult. To produce statistically significant results, scientists must dismiss evidence that does not include strict, irrefutable proof of harm. Prevention only occurs after irreversible harm has been documented, and attributed to a specific disease entity.

A 1993 report by Greenpeace on the relationship between breast cancer and chlorine notes, "There is no scientific or ethical reason to presume chemicals harmless until they are proven otherwise. Such an approach allows action only after there has been irreversible harm to health and the environment. We need a new standard of proof. In public health and environmental policy, the precautionary principle should be the framework for evaluating scientific information and for taking action."[2]

The Precautionary Principle requires that industry err on the side of caution, that it is not necessary to wait for scientific proof that a substance causes harm in order to restrict use. The mere possibility that chemicals may cause harm should be enough. This means that a particular chemical should be considered to be guilty until proven innocent, with the burden of proof regarding its safety placed on the shoulders of the manufacturer. It's that simple: chemicals that may cause harm should not be released into the environment. Such a policy would prevent impairment before it happens and does not require that even an indirect demonstration of toxic damage be made.

The Precautionary Principle is currently being used as a basis for some international agreements. Though the validity of the principle is widely accepted, it is not used in most government and industrial policy-making so that regulation of toxins continues to be based on a reactionary approach. Common sense alone should support the use of this principle in an effort to prevent further contamination and harm.

The Politics of Change

Still, there is no unified, loud voice of concern being raised. The United States, by far the greatest technological polluter, doesn't spend sufficient funds on environmental protection and tends to minimize the harm in favor of profits. Government and big business, hand in hand with the public relations (PR) industry, continue to support their own short sighted self-interests.

Let's reconsider the issue of toxic sludge. John Stauber and Sheldon Rampton, authors of the book *Toxic Sludge Is Good for You*, investigated the PR campaign that promoted the "beneficial use" of sewage sludge. In their research, they found "a murky tangle of corporate and government bureaucracies, conflicts of interest, and a cover-up of massive hazards to the environment and human health."[3] In the end, the issue was blown open in the 1980s by Hugh Kaufman, a courageous whistleblower in the hazardous site control division of the EPA. Kaufman refused to keep silent regarding the collaboration between EPA officials and the very industries they were mandated to regulate. In this process his testimony exposed the EPA's failure to deal with mounting chemical wastes.

Then there is the growing, very real concern about global warming. In September of 1995, 2500 scientists serving on the Intergovernmental Panel on Climate Change (IPC) issued an announcement stating that our planet has moved into a period of climatic instability that will likely cause "widespread economic, social and environmental dislocation over the next century."[4] In response to these very real, scientifically substantiated threats, the energy industry has spent millions of dollars using disinformation PR tactics to sell the public the idea that this scientific information is a matter of uncertainty and to downplay the threat of climate change.[5]

Waiting for governments to take responsibility is no longer an option. Our own government fails to accept responsibility that should theoretically reflect having the world's largest consumptive economy. It is not realistic to assume that politicians, protection agencies, or industry will look after our best interest.

In the face of this enormous challenge, it is natural to protect yourself, both emotionally and physically, from the grief and pain of what is happening. You may wish to avoid critical thinking and discernment, and avoid feeling deeply about political and personal issues. But since you are being harmed, you cannot ignore these problems. Both EI and CFS are a wake-up call, a call to action to stop the damage that is being done to the earth.

Since it is not realistic to expect government and industry to do the right thing, it is up to all of us to take personal responsibility for the health of the planet. Since you have made a practical shift in your awareness, it's up to you to use your recovery as an example, as part of the solution. By sharing your personal experiences relating to environmental damage and an excessively stressed life-style, you can aid the causes of prevention and healing.

Those afflicted with environmentally related illnesses are the proverbial canaries in the coal mine. If you have EI, you have already been forced by illness to intervene on your own behalf. People with EI and, to a less overt, but equally significant extent, those with CFS are living testimony of the declining health of the earth.

It is promising that physical and emotional difficulties are beginning to be linked to environmental damage rather than merely being attributed to emotional problems or the deficiency of the human condition. The experience of illness has already forced you to redefine your personal understanding of success and power, while releasing material attachments in the process. Your illness will have deepened your understanding of the challenges that must be faced if we are to save the earth.

By becoming caught up in the values of this culture you may have forgotten your own value. If the human race continues to make choices that express this disconnection, we will not survive. We must find another way. This is a time of unusual opportunity for you—your personal knowledge of the physical damage that is being perpetrated will bridge your inner journey of healing with the healing of our planet. Being alive at this time is an opportunity to participate in a powerful and challenging redirection of the values of the human race.

Activism

Your experiences are the best advertisement for why we must save the earth. Illness has enabled you to focus on what is important; you had no extra energy to spend continuing to grasp and strive in ways you used to. Your geared-down life offers you the chance to observe past neediness and to break free from being dominated by your attachments. In this way, EI and CFS are good for the environment, i.e., in terms of the very simple, uncomplicated, low-impact life-style that they impose.

In your effort to heal yourself, you've become less enslaved by a hunger for possessions and can then come to terms with the deeper purpose of your life. When confronting empty, unfulfilled feelings, you no longer need to buy more stuff; instead you are called on to examine what's preventing you from living fully. As you learn to treasure and care about every aspect of your life, what happens to this earth may emerge as a deep concern. As you take responsibility for your life, you take responsibility for this earth. Inextricably bound together with the earth, we are compelled into action on its behalf.

For those who are acutely sick, it is difficult to undertake any interventions other than those directed at personal survival, let alone any that will benefit the earth. Being able to impact or alter the course of world-damaging events is an overwhelming notion, even for the most robust. But as you find the healing within, you are inevitably making a contribution to the healing of the earth. Developing a spiritual context from which to live your life may evoke an activist stance. From a place of spiritual activism you may be able to move forward, past material achievements, to see the larger picture and act with greater selflessness.

In order to help the world, you must first achieve your own inner balance. This balance, the result of finding compassion for yourself, will make it possible for you to go out into the world to share what you have learned. You cannot manifest balance in the world if you are unable to gain it from within. By nurturing your own growing sense of personal worth and goodness, the next natural step is to cultivate and find goodness in others. Seeing yourself with loving compassion makes it possible for everything else to unfold in a state of pure grace.

You must be as well as possible, at least achieving greater internal balance, before you can move out into the world to become involved; otherwise you will likely become ill again. Frantic efforts to solve the earth's problems before solving your own only obscure the work you need to do on yourself and tend to create more problems. It is easy to become lost in external activities secretly performed for personal acclaim rather than for the greater good.

Think of others you know who use activism in order to develop an impressive set of credentials signifying goodness. Their work is invaluable, but often it serves merely to dispel a lack of self-worth and distracts from living out one's true purpose. If you choose to get involved, be careful not to use these acts exclusively for self-gratification or to create a smoke screen to avoid other issues. It is possible to become so frenetically busy with this work as to obscure your own needs.

Your personal recovery is intertwined with holding the vision of the highest good for yourself first and then the greater society. Surprisingly, the best hope for survival of the planet rests with the work you do to achieve balance within yourself. Once you find balance, it will be easy to express loving-kindness toward yourself. It will then be impossible to prevent spreading this loving-kindness to others. When you truly, deeply love yourself, how you view your relationship to the earth will then change.

Use the time of your recovery wisely, as a unique opportunity to fall in love with every aspect of yourself. The time spent resting can be an opportunity to fill yourself with increased understanding, information, and awareness. Educate yourself as to environmentally safe products and strive to grasp the issues. Most of all, keep your inner life in harmony with the outer world.

Engaging in political activism and self-sacrifice before your personal awareness has fully developed will make you ill again. You will need to admonish yourself to keep a firm reign on your self-sacrificing nature. These self-sacrificing tendencies may partly explain why the illness first appeared in you. Don't be an activist who sacrifices her own needs and whose own development stagnates.

It is hard not to be overwhelmed wondering where to begin in this enormous undertaking to save the earth. Being stuck in overwhelm may prevent you from ever taking up a cause. So how do you start? What can you, as one puny, earnest person, do to help? Identify an area that sparks your interest; choose something you care about, that sets your heart on fire.

Even if you aren't a joiner, or if you are uncomfortable operating within the confines of volunteerism or activist groups, you can carve a unique place that suits you. Anything you do, no matter how small, will make a difference. And try not to get anxious about the myriad of other issues that you are not actively involved in. There will be others who will step in to take up those causes. It isn't up to you to cover all of the bases.

Keep in mind that your involvement may not achieve results today or even next year. Pace yourself and strive for a balance between taking care of your physical welfare and trying to make a difference. You are no good to anyone else if you become depleted. Steel yourself for the long haul and don't get discouraged when inevitable setbacks occur. The ailments of the earth have taken many years to develop and will take time to correct and heal. Keep at it, even if there are no tangible results.

Educate yourself by learning all you can about the subject you have chosen. It will also be necessary to educate yourself about the big picture, not just about the subject you choose to specialize in. Explore issues that make you feel uncomfortable. How about studying the destruction of the ozone layer or the rain forest? By moving through your resistance, the more you come to know, the more you must be held accountable for your actions. Coming from a place of all-inclusive integrity, you also have the right to ask others to be accountable for their actions.

The everyday choices you make have consequences for the future of the earth. Every action you take leaves a permanent imprint, making an impact long after you have moved on to something new. The more you understand and take responsibility for the consequences of your simple choices, the more you will assist in the healing of the earth.

In order to save the planet, your own values must be reshaped. You will no longer be able to have a life-style or career that is essentially a short-term means to a detrimental end. You will have to give up possessions and comforts that have made your life so easy. But you've had a head start: illness has short-circuited acquisitiveness, forcing you to find your essence in the process.

It is imperative to start scaling back on a personal level to reduce your own impact on the earth. You can do this by becoming aware of your own abusive acts as well as how much waste you personally generate. What will be asked of you is to have the courage to examine and restrict your own life and curtail your own acquisitive tendencies.

What You Can Do

Once you are in recovery, feeling more in control and awake regarding your own life, you may feel compelled to express your concern about the environment. The more you have awakened to your own life through the impact of illness, the more difficult it is to shut down a sense of responsibility for what is going on in the world. Bring your insights down to earth, applying them in practical ways.

So what can you do? The most effective thing you can do is change your own awareness and act in concert with this awareness. You may have already started to do this in your own life by making sensible purchases, minimizing the harm you cause the earth, exercising healthy discernment, and letting go of attachment to material trappings. Perhaps your low-impact life-style can model for others a better way to live. Your capacity to take responsibility for your own life can help point the way for others. And your honesty and congruence will make it safe for others to be direct about their needs.

The tools you have accumulated to survive illness can serve as a model for those who touch your life. In the process of awakening to become responsible for yourself, you have begun to awaken to the larger need. Seeking to reenter this damaged earth, you are called on to assist others, including the earth itself, to heal. By helping to seed this idea, you can awaken in others their responsibility toward all of life.

However, it will be difficult getting the political machine to acknowledge that polluting the environment will inevitably disable us and the planet; this subject has little interest for those who are not aware of being made ill by their environment or by their life-style. Predictions that the ranks of the ill will increase with many more individuals diagnosed with CFS and with EI hold little sway with government. But this doesn't mean giving up. It means that you should be alert to every opportunity to assist others to wake up and take notice.

Prevention in the form of a multidimensional approach to change could turn back the tide of environmental damage. First, people will have to awaken to the incredible potential existing within everyone. While no one intervention will solve the environmental crisis, each of us, by embracing a simpler, balanced life-style, could help prevent a worldwide epidemic of toxin-related illness, and prevent the destruction of the earth.

Increased public education can help awaken and activate the consumer voice, leading to the demand for greater governmental regulation and safeguards to personal welfare. The louder and more unified that voice, the more likely that it will be heard. On an individual and group level, you can help guide and bring attention to the human capacity for change, as well as giving witness to the destructive actions perpetrated against the earth.

Get excited. Become creative. Act in ways that constantly keep the larger context in mind. Pay attention to your own responsibility in generating and perpetuating the problem. Ask yourself how you personally are willing to change.

Your purchases have a direct correlation with the health of the earth. Electing to eat organic foods is one very large step toward helping to restore the earth's balance. In so doing, your dietary choices have a powerful impact on the sustaining capabilities of the earth. Supporting organic farmers supports the planet.

The purchases you make are very important. Send a message by selecting clothing and products that are as natural as possible, without the usual infusion of chemicals. Switch to nontoxic cleaning products. Take note of what you throw away. You will help save the trees if you carry a cup, bowl, and utensils when you buy take-out foods. Compost your food and garden scraps. Wear extra sweaters instead of turning up the heat. Challenging yourself to consume less and less will generate less waste.

Ask questions about products before purchasing them. Contact the manufacturer with feedback after you've tried a product. When you consider making a purchase, ask yourself how it will affect the environment of your grandchildren. Support companies that make active efforts to reduce waste. Vote for officials who have the courage to speak out against environmental destruction, in favor of positive change.

If you cannot leave the house, write letters to Congress and to others to express your concerns. Make your letters as personal as possible. Be clear and specific, rather than hostile and demanding. Use recycled paper and specify that you would like a response.

Laura has successfully worked to secure a smoke-free campus at her community college. Because of her efforts, the housekeeping staff now uses less harmful cleaning supplies and has removed deodorizers from the restrooms. You too can be a representative, for example, helping educate the public as to the need for safe access to public buildings.

Josh writes about environmental concerns for such magazines as *Eco-Traveler* and *Lifetimes Magazine*. Gloria has become the director of a Center for Attitudinal Healing, offering support and information for those struggling with illness. And Jamie gives public talks on ways to reduce environmental hazards in the home and workplace.

It can be difficult to generate ongoing enthusiasm if you are working alone day after day, without external support and reinforcement. When people band together to do this work, they can become very powerful. The collective empowerment generated by group work will greatly magnify your own achievements. Find a team you want to join or create a community of those who share your beliefs.

To do this you don't need to invent the wheel; there are a growing number of organizations that are taking a long-term approach to environmental concerns. These groups are working to increase public knowledge of environmental and economic hazards. Activism can start in quiet ways, such as involvement with EI and CFS self-help, support groups. You may wish to investigate local, state, and national EI and CFS organizations, and some of these groups have their own political organizations. There are national and statewide EI and CFS groups aiming their efforts at social and legislative reform. Some of these groups work to enlighten educators and legislators, while others raise funds to help finance research. This is an encouraging upsurge of organized effort.

The Big Picture

Many acts seem like no more than putting a Band-Aid on an elephant. Palliative interventions—planting a tree, adopting a highway, energy-efficient buildings, and an emphasis on public transportation—are important interventions, but they are not enough. Even if the United States were to cut its carbon dioxide emissions, those from other countries would still cause great damage. No intervention can work if it doesn't impact the entire globe.

Not to be discouraged, writer Ross Gelbspan offers interesting thoughts on this matter. "What if the world mobilized around a ten year project to phase out all fossil fuels, to develop renewable energy technologies to extend those technologies to every corner of the world? What if, to minimize the conflict of so massive a dislocation, the world's energy companies were put in charge of the transition...."[5] Most of the technology is already in place to implement such a plan. By guaranteeing the same profits for solar electricity and hydrogen fuel, the energy industries might be assured of maintaining the same position they now enjoy in the world's economy.

The exciting news is that these efforts are already happening. In Sweden, Dr. Karl-Henrick Robert, a cancer researcher and founder of The Natural Step, has established a countrywide consensus-building program based on systems thinking and ongoing dialogue. He has worked with Swedish scientists in an effort to come to a consensus on the cause of and the solution to our environmental problems.

Working in collaboration with Sweden's media and the Department of Education, they now have 20 major corporations that are phasing out all petroleum products, unrecycled minerals, and nonbiodegradable compounds. These corporations are also working to develop ecologically sustainable farming and forestry methods and are lobbying the Swedish Parliament to tax pollution and overuse of energy. If this happens, their government would switch from taxation based on income and investment to taxation based on activities that harm the environment. Similar programs are being developed in Denmark, Holland, Spain, Britain, Switzerland, Norway, Poland, and the United States.[6]

Changing our economy requires that we come to terms with the limitations of our planet. There are many reasons to have hope in this regard. Who could have foreseen the demise of communism throughtout the world? Who would have thought that the world's governments would join together to regulate CFCs? Who could have dreamed that there might someday be peace in the Middle East?

Summary

A culture that has high regard for the human body will also have high regard for earth. Historically, Western civilization has not been nourishing to the planet, and likewise has little regard for the body. Similarly, you may have forgotten your own value. For you to become well, you need to understand and integrate your relationship to your body and to the earth with respect for your well-being. Can you live in a culture that you are a part of, yet not be bound by it? Do you have to remove yourself from your culture in order to survive? How will you find a different way? When you ask these questions, healing and change can result.

Endnotes

[1]Richard Leviton, "Environmental Illness: A Special Report," *Yoga Journal* Nov.–Dec. 1991: 44.

[2]Joe Thornton, *Chlorine, Human Health, and the Environment* (Chicago: Greenpeace, 1993) 50.

[3]John Stauber and Sheldon Ramptom, *Toxic Sludge is Good for You* (Monroe: Common Courage, 1995) 101.

[4]Ross Gelbspan, "The Heat is On," *San Jose Mercury* 17 Dec. 1995: 1P, 4P.

[5]Gelbspan, 4P.

[6]For information regarding the efforts of The Natural Step in the United States, contact http://www.cs.tufts,edu/tns-us/ or contact them for their website in other countries.

Conclusion

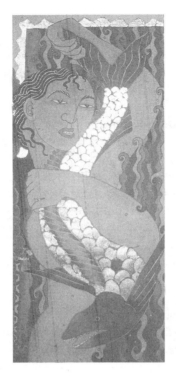

*Sprouting a
Rudder*

*i*llness offers a point of departure from being asleep. It permits you to awaken and unfold to life as you are ready to receive it. At some point in your life prior to becoming ill, everything probably seemed okay on the surface. However, once you begin to wake up, you may realize that all is not quite as it seems. Some part of you may recognize that the things that were promised, the material gains, the great expectations for your life, didn't happen as planned.

Illness often jolts you awake, and is a time in your life in which you may come to question everything. This questioning process can take you far beyond what you know and recognize to be true, stripping away layers that have hidden your true self. Illness strips you of things that you might otherwise have hidden behind; exposed and naked, you can then find clarity as to who you are and your true purpose.

Illness requires that you question everything that is familiar and comfortable. Illness questions your self-worth, along with all ideas of who you are and who you should be. You will find yourself asking important questions. "Can I love myself in spite of being unwell?" "Can I love myself in spite of not being able to make myself well?" "Is it possible for me to love myself in the absence of any sort of traditional guidelines for self-definition?" "Can I love myself in spite of all those others who don't love themselves?" "Can I be my own person in spite of social expectations and learned behaviors that try to shape and influence me?"

Illness drives you to deeper levels, extracting you from your upbringing. When you are ready to heal, you are hollow and naked. The process of recovery involves busting out of old patterns and breaking your own heart over and over again until you are spent. Then, after all the failed hopes and expectations, you are forced to set your own pace for internal healing that allows your heart to grow back together.

In order to heal, you must fearlessly examine the things that are not working, using this information to build and move on without beating yourself up in any way with the information that is revealed. Many of the habitual procedures by which you evaluated yourself in the past have to do with systems that interfere with allowing you to fully love and accept who you are. These systems tend to obscure your fullness.

When you discover that true healing comes when you learn how to love yourself, you will be able to set your own standards for self-evaluation. In this process you will need to scan inward to find your real set of priorities and standards rather than looking to the outside world for confirmation. Looking inward offers the only clear information; everything else is illusion. It can be difficult to get to this clear information because to do so you must go against the grain, against conditioning, against training and social trends.

This process of getting well is about finding your real, whole self amid all of the false versions of who you think you are. To get the most out of this, you must look at yourself, lumps, foibles, and all, and still decide that you are worthy, that you deserve self-love, and deserve to be well. Certainly, nowhere in your being deserves self-punishment.

By now you may have found the general territory in which your real path to healing exists, yet you may often stumble onto the trail only briefly and then lose sight of your way. It is easy to become lost and confused by the excessive options and opinions that pressure you into conformity. Over and over, you will find yourself going back to the trailhead to try again, only to repeatedly lose the path. Yet, each time you get closer, traveling a greater distance on the path of your longing. Each time you cross over the trail or pass by your target, the area will be a little more familiar, allowing you to focus a bit more.

This is a process of sprouting a rudder. In the process of healing, you begin, bit by bit, to take over as the helmsman, readjusting your ship's path in order to get to your destination. When a storm blows up, the waves may seem to overwhelm you; don't fight against them, just flow with them. As the winds, tides, and currents of life interfere with your plans, you must hold fast to the tiller, changing course over and over in order to remain safe. You will eventually reach your destination by adjusting your path. At other times you may really become stuck. By continuing to pay attention and affirming your choice you can reach your end point. The strength of your determination and the efforts you expend to achieve desired results will help you achieve your goal.

As with life, having a rudder is essential to finding and keeping your life on course. This rudder helps steer you through the deep and shallow waters of existence, helping give life direction and meaning. In the process of recovery, it is your job to remain as awake as possible to change your actions and evaluate your behavior in order to steer your life in the direction you choose.

As a result of your upbringing, the rudder may have broken off or you may have suffered damage to the extent that it never had a chance to grow. This damage may have caused your illness. You may have had to suppress your true nature in order to get along, in order to survive. Inevitably, you will no longer be able to suppress your true path. This is when the fire of healing starts to burn. The fire that may have started in the form of illness also triggers growth and a budding strength that causes the rudder to sprout. It is the sprouting and subsequent growth of the rudder that enables you to find your own path.

Like learning to walk, you will take a few steps, then fall and get up again. Each time, you'll travel a little farther. The process of getting well means moving through life's obstacles without a schedule, taking the next thing that comes and doing your best.

Along the way your rudder will grow more firm and solid so it can help steer you with greater accuracy. If you become overwhelmed, you can always pull it up and take a rest. Eventually, the steering process will become second nature as you recognize your innate ability to move through inner territory with greater alignment. It will become easier and quicker to take in the information and practice healthy discernment; catching it with a catcher's mitt, grabbing and examining whatever comes. Examine the information to decide what parts are true for you; if something doesn't fit, toss away what you don't need.

When you are aligned with your own schedule of how things need to be dealt with, it will be easier to use your energy in ways that you choose and you will accomplish more. Rather than struggling against the external forces, you will learn to allow the wind and the currents to work in your favor. While this may not mean moving faster, life will flow with greater efficiency and ease. Charting the path that is your life is an experience that can be filled with delicious curiosity, joy, and engagement.

Sprouting a rudder enables you to reclaim and steer yourself in any direction you choose. Life is about experiencing and creating this journey. And your task in this journey is to uncover the hidden gifts of your illness. Perhaps the greatest gift of all is to find yourself.

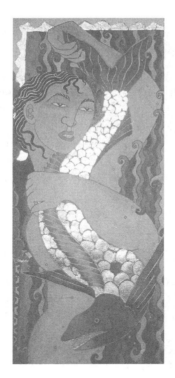

Appendix One

Possible Excitants

*t*he following substances could be making you sick:

acrylics

air and furnace filters

air fresheners

air pollution

alcohol found in vanilla extract,
   cleaning fluids, paint thinner,
   hand lotions, drugs

animal hair

antihistamines

antiperspirants

automotive exhaust

barber and beauty shops

bed sheets

brake drums

carpet and upholstery latex backing

carpeting

chlorine in tap water

cigarettes and cigarette smoke

cleaning supplies

coal- and wood-burning heat

computers

concrete or plaster

construction materials, including insulation and particleboard

cosmetics

counter- and tabletops

dairy products

dental fillings

deodorants
deodorizers
detergents
disinfectants
drapery and upholstery fabric
dried fruits
dust mites
dyes
electrical insulation parts
electronic equipment, including clocks
embalming agents
fabric softener
fabric stores, grocery stores, tire and bike shops, print shops
facial tissues and napkins
feathers
fiberboard
fiberglass
flame retardant in clothes
flavoring agents
flea bombs
fluoride
foam insulation
food additives, including MSG and dyes
foods such as milk, wheat, corn, yeast, and eggs
formaldehyde from furniture and building materials and permanent pressed clothing
Formica
fumes from stoves and heaters
furniture adhesives
furniture finish
gasoline
glues
hair spray
hardware
heating pads and electric blankets
hormones
household cleaning supplies and detergents
lawn and garden equipment

leather goods
lighter fluid
mattresses
medications
mildew preventatives
milk
mothballs
nail polish and polish remover
natural inhalants such as pollen, dust, animal dander, and mold
new cars
new furniture
new homes
newsprint
nylon fibers
office machines
oil and gas-heated stoves and furnaces
paint and wood finishes
paper towels and toilet paper
paper, napkins, cardboard, butcher paper
particleboard
perfume
pesticides
phenol; found in nasal sprays, over-the-counter drugs, ointments, hair products, shampoo, Scotch tape, newsprint, wallpaper, canned foods.
plastics, particularly soft plastic
plumbing fixtures
polyesters and permanent press clothing
preservatives
pressed wood furniture
printers
public places
rayon
resins and oil-based paints
rubber
shampoo
solvents
sprayed fruits and vegetables
stove and refrigerator hardware

synthetic fabrics
synthetic lubricants
tap water
tea bags
toothpaste
treated cotton
TVs

utensil handles
water
waterproofing
water-softening chemicals
wheat grains and agricultural seeds
wool

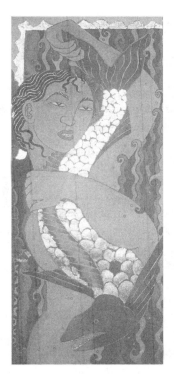

Appendix Two

Resources

*t*he process of researching this book revealed information about organizations and businesses that can help people with EI and CFS to cope and thrive. You may want to contact some of these organizations and companies to see if they have anything to offer you.

Education and Support

Action Against Allergy
Box 278
Twickenham, Middlesex, TW1 422, England

This organization works with people with all kinds of allergic sensitivities, including ME and EI. They offer information and resources, including physicians who specialize in allergy care.

Candida Research and Dysbiosis Foundation (CRDF)
P.O. Box JF
College Station, TX 77841, at (409) 694-8687
   CRDF emphasizes information about candida and other immune-related illnesses. They have a newsletter as well as educational packets.

The Chronic Fatigue Immune Dysfunction (CFIDS) Association
P.O. Box 220398
Charlotte, NC 28222-0398, at (800) 442-3437
   The CFIDS Association is the largest nonprofit CFS organization in existence. They believe research offers the key and consequently seek funds to support research and advocacy activities. Their magazine, *The CFIDS Chronicle*, has the latest information about CFS and related matters.

CFIDS Information Line
(800) 44 CFIDS or 442-3437
(900) 988-CFID or (900) 988-2343
   Offered by the CFIDS Association, this service disseminates up-to-date information about CFS, providing a toll-free number for general information and an information line which charges a fee, allowing you to access the most timely CFS information.

Environmental Health Network (EHN)
P.O. Box 1155
Larkspur, CA 94977, at (415) 541-5075
   EHN is a politically oriented group offering information, referrals, and advocacy for people who have experienced chemical and environmental exposures with the goal of developing responsible public health policies regarding toxins. They have a newsletter, *The New Reactor*, peer counseling, a guest lecture series, and information and referrals regarding safe housing and disability issues.

Human Ecology Action League (HEAL)
P.O. Box 29629
Atlanta, GA 30359, at (404) 248-1898
   HEAL is an organization concerned with environmental health hazards which offers telephone support and a national information and referral service. HEAL has chapters throughout the country and publishes a magazine, as well as resource information about EI-related problems.

The M.E. Association of Canada
246 Queen Street, Suite 400
Ottawa, Ontario, K1P 5E4, Canada, at (613) 563-1565
   This organization assists sufferers of ME, also known as CFS, providing medical and legal counseling by phone, as well as information and referral services, support group linkages, and a newsletter.

The M.E. Association of England
Stanhope House, High Street
Stanford-le-Hope, Essex, England SS17 8EX, at 01375 642466

This association offers information regarding CFS or ME, and has a listening line that is staffed with persons who provide support and counseling.

The Nightingale Research Foundation
383 Danforth Avenue
Ottawa, Ontario, K2A OE1, Canada, at (613) 728-9643

This internationally oriented group conducts research and educational programs for people with ME or CFS, or professionals. They sponsor a self-help network and publish a newsletter.

Share Care and Prayer
P.O. Box 2080
Frazier Park, CA 93225

This group has a free lending library containing educational and inspirational tapes and videos and publishes a newsletter. With an emphasis on EI and CFS, they also focus on emotional and spiritual supports. Postage for borrowed materials is paid for by the organization; amazingly enough, they supply return stamps.

The World Research Foundation
20501 Ventura Boulevard, Suite 100
Woodland Hills, CA 91364, at (818) 999-LIVE

The WRF is a health and environmental network with information regarding all types of health-related treatments. They charge a fee for their information searches: their computer search contains current health-related information, emphasizing allopathic practices and the library search focuses on alternative interventions.

Supplements

CFIDS Buyers Club
(800) 366-6056

This group sells vitamins and supplements at a discount, emphasizing products proven to be beneficial to CFS patients. When you buy a larger quantity they reduce the price. They distribute an informative newsletter of product information, testimonials, and research activities.

National Ecological and Environmental Delivery System (NEEDS)
527 Charles Avenue
Syracuse, NY 13209, at (800) 634-1380

NEEDS provides supplements, vitamins, as well as air, water, and shower filtration products at substantially reduced prices.

Apex Energetics
700 N. Central Avenue, Suite 420
Glendale, CA 91203, at (800) 736-4381

This scientifically based organization has a comprehensive series of homeopathic remedies that address the underlying causes of physical disturbance. Their Antitox Program gradually reduces the total load of toxins with the initial phases preparing the immune system for removal of toxic residue and subsequent steps removing increasingly deeper levels of toxins.

General Information

Center for Science in the Public Interest
1875 Connecticut Avenue NW, Suite 300
Washington, DC 20009-5728, at (202) 332-9110

This organization lobbies to reform government policies on health, food quality, and dietary practices.

The United States Environmental Protection Agency
401 M Street, SW
Washington, DC 20460

The EPA is mandated to do just what its name says: protect the environment. They have several phone numbers; some of these include: the Public Information Center (202) 426-7751; Indoor Air Quality (800) 438-4318; the Drinking Water Hot Line (800) 426-4791: and Right to Know Hot Line (800) 535-0202.

Healing and Health Centers

Bio-Magnetic Educational Foundation
440 Pastoral Place
Sedona, AZ 86336, at (520) 282-2054.

Nancy Lee offers training in Bio-Magnetic healing work, Bio-Magnetic healing treatments, and a list of certified Bio-Magnetic practitioners in your area.

Cancer Support and Education Center (formerly The Creighton Health Institute)
1035 Pine Street
Menlo Park, CA 94025, at (415) 327-6166

This organization offers a unique program of empowerment and healing to people with cancer as well as EI, CFS, and other illnesses. Participants engage in their own healing through counseling, massage therapy, nutritional education and therapy, and group work.

The Cheney Clinic
10620 Park Road, Suite 234
Charlotte, NC 28210, at (704) 542-7444

This clinic specializes in the diagnosis and management of CFS. Dr. Paul Cheney, an internist and widely known expert on CFS, is available for conference calls as well as private consultation.

Environmental Health Center–Dallas
8345 Walnut Hill Lane, Suite 220
Dallas, TX 75231, at (214) 368-4132

Dr. William Rea founded this clinic which specializes in treating EI. It provides comprehensive assessment of all factors influencing health in a highly controlled, toxin-free environment while testing for sensitivities. Interventions include stress management, dietary changes, environmental controls, immunotherapy, and client education.

Light Harmonics
Rt. 19 Box 123
Old Santa Fe Trail
Santa Fe, NM 87505, at (505) 989-4610

Linda Lancaster provides individualized data regarding the effects of environmental pollutants on the subtle energies of the body. These prephysical energies can be detected prior to becoming manifest as clinically measurable illness.

The School for Enlightenment and Healing (SEH)
1742 Garnet Avenue #266
San Diego, CA 92129, at (619) 495-2435

Michael Mamas' three-year program offers intensive training regarding remote and hands-on healing skills, plus it can be a catalyst for spiritual unfoldment. Contact them for graduates' names if you wish a hands-on or long-distance healing.

Miscellaneous

Unity Prayer Line
(800) 669-7729

Any time you wish, you may request that these people pray for you or a loved one. They will do this for free for 30 consecutive days.

The World Wide Web
Since computer web-sites are like mushrooms that come and go after the rains, it is wisest to tell you how to access them, rather than give you specific sites which may disappear before you can get to them. First, you must be a member of an on-line service or have access to the World Wide Web on the Internet. Next, go to

one of the Internet search sites such as Yahoo at http://www.yahoo.com, Web Crawler at http://webcrawler.com, or Lycos at http://www.lycos,com. Once you are there, search for EI, MCS, CFS, CFIDS, or any other topic you might think of. There is a vast array of useful information on-line which can be of great help.

The World Wide Web is the most interesting part of the Internet and the easiest to use, but there are also Usenet newsgroups on the Internet which might be of help. Examples of some of these sites include: alt.med.cfs; alt.med.allergy; alt.med.fibromyalgia; ncf.ss.cfs, in Ottawa Canada; and misc.health.alternative.

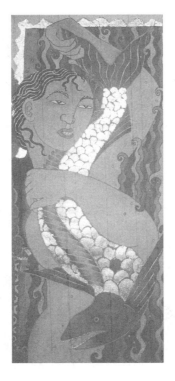

Recommended Reading

Adolph, Jonathan, and Peggy Taylor. "What's so Good About Feeling Bad?" *New Age Journal* Feb. (1991): 32–37, 91–95.

Almass, A. H. *Diamond Heart Book Three* (Berkeley: Diamond, 1990).

Anand, Margo. *The Art of Sexual Ecstasy* (Los Angeles: J. P. Tarcher, 1989).

Baginski, B., and S. Sharmon. *Reiki: Universal Life Energy* (Mendocino: Life Rhythm, 1985).

Bailey, A. A. *Healing in the New Age,* excerpts *Esoteric Healing: A Treatise on the Seven Rays* Vol. IV (New York: Lucis Publishing, 1978).

Barsky, Arthur. *The Worried Sick: Our Troubled Quest for Wellness* (Boston: Little, Brown, 1988).

Baxter, Richard. "Some Public Attitudes About Health and the Environment," *Environmental Health Perspectives* Vol. 88 (Washington, DC: U.S. Department of Health and Human Services, 1990): 261–269.

Beadsley, Joseph, and Jerry Swift. "The Impact of Nutrition, Environment and Lifestyle on the Health of Americans," *The Kellog Report* (New York: Institute of Health Policy and Practice, 1989).

Beck, Charlotte Joko. *Everyday Zen, Love and Work* (New York: Harper & Row, 1989).

Bell, David. *The Disease of a Thousand Names* (Lyndonville: Pollard, 1991).

Bell, Iris. *Clinical Ecology* (Bolinas: Common Knowledge, 1982).

Benzaia, Diana. "New Ways to Fight Allergies," *Consumer Digest* May–June 1989: 56.

Bliznakov, Emile, and Gerald Hunt. *The Miracle Nutrient Co Enzyme Q10* (New York: Bantam, 1987).

Borysenko, Joan. *Minding the Body, Mending the Mind* (Reading: Addison–Wesley, 1987).

Bower, John. *The Healthy House* (New York: Carol, 1989).

Bower, John. *Healthy House Building* (Bloomington, IN: The Healthy House Institute, 1993).

Bower, John. "Pollution Free Housing," *Mother Earth News* Mar.–Apr. 1989: 98.

Bower, John. *Understanding Ventilation* (Bloomington, IN: The Healthy House Institute, 1995).

Bower, Lynn Marie. *The Healthy Household* (Bloomington, IN: The Healthy House Institute, 1995).

Brennan, Barbara Ann. *Hands of Light: A Guide to Healing Through the Human Energy Field* (New York: Bantam, 1988).

Brennan, Barbara Ann. *Light Emerging* (New York: Bantam, 1993).

Brewer, John. "Are You Chemically Sensitive?" *East West Journal* Mar. 1991: 22.

Brodeur, Paul. "Danger in the Schoolyard," *Family Circle* Sept. 1990: 61–66.

Brooke, Connors, and Stern, eds. *With the Power of Each Breath: A Disabled Women's Anthology* (San Francisco: Clesis, 1985).

Cameron, Julia, with Mark Bryan. *The Artists Way* (Los Angeles: J. P. Tarcher, 1992).

Carry, John, *et al.* "Beware 'Sick Building Syndrome,'" *Newsweek* 7 Jan. 1985: 58–60.

Chopra, Deepak. *Quantum Healing* (New York: Bantam, 1989).

Chopra, Deepak. *Creating Health* (Boston: Houghton Mifflin, 1987).

Clark, Hulda. *The Cure for All Cancers* (San Diego: Promotion, 1993).

Colburn, Theo, John P. Myers, and Dianne Dumanowski. *Our Stolen Future* (New York: Dutton, 1996).

Collinge, William. *Recovering from Chronic Fatigue Syndrome* (New York: Perigee, 1993).

Conant, Susan. *Living with Chronic Fatigue* (Dallas, TX, 1990).

Cowley, Geoffrey. "Chronic Fatigue Syndrome," *Newsweek* 12 Nov. 1990: 62–70.

Cowley, Geoffrey, and Mary Hager. "A Clue to Chronic Fatigue," *Newsweek* 30 Sept. 1991: 66.

Crook, William. *The Yeast Connection* (Jackson, MS: Professional, 1986).

Crook, William. *The Yeast Connection and the Woman* (Jackson, MS: Professional: 1995).

Cunningham, Lydia. "30 Easy Ways to Safeguard Your Family from Deadly Toxins," *Women's Day* Sept. 1988: 94.

Dadd, Debra Lynn. *Non Toxic, Natural, and Earthwise* (Los Angeles: J.P. Tarcher, 1990).

Deaver, Korra. *Psychic Power and Soul Consciousness* (Alameda: Hunter House, 1991).

Easwaran, Eknath. *Meditation: An Eight Point Program* (Petaluma: Nilgiri, 1978).

Ellsworth, Barry. *Living in Love with Yourself* (Salt Lake City: Breakthrough, 1988).

English, Thomas. "Skeptical of Skeptics," *JAMA* 265.8 (Feb. 27, 1991): 964.

"Environmental Illness Gains Public Attention and Medical Concern," *Utne Reader* 44 (Mar.–Apr. 1991): 40.

"Environmentally Induced Diseases," *EPA Journal*, Office of Community and Public Affairs, Mar.–Apr. 1990.

Feiden, Karyn. *Hope and Help for Chronic Fatigue Syndrome* (Englewood Cliffs: Prentice–Hall, 1990).

Ferrucci, Piero. *What We May Be: Techniques for Psychological and Spiritual Growth Through Psychosynthesis* (Boston: Houghton Mifflin, 1982).

Fisher, Gregg, Stephan Strauss, Paul Cheney, and James Oleske. *Chronic Fatigue Syndrome: A Victim's Guide to Understanding, Treating and Coping with this Debilitating Illness* (New York: Warner, 1989).

Fuerst, Mark. "Free Yourself from Chronic Fatigue," *Prevention* Jan. 1990: 58–64.

Goldberg, Natalie. *Writing Down the Bones* (Boulder: Shambhala, 1986).

Goldhawk, Tessa. *A Rose to a Sick Friend* (New York: Gateway, 1989).

Golos, Natalie, and Frances Golos-Globitz. *Coping with Your Allergies* (New York: Simon & Schuster, 1986).

Griffin, Susan. *The Eros of Everyday Life* (New York: Doubleday, 1995).

Grof, Christina. *Spiritual Emergency: When Personal Transformation Becomes a Crisis* (Los Angeles: J. P. Tarcher, 1989).

Hanh, Thich Nhat. *The Miracle of Mindfulness: A Manual on Meditation* (Boston: Beacon, 1987).

Harvey, Andrew. *Hidden Journey* (New York: Henry Holt, 1991).

Hay, Louise. *Heal Your Body* (Santa Monica: Hay House, 1988).

Hay, Louise. *You Can Heal Your Life* (Santa Monica: Hay House, 1987).

Hendler, Sheldon Saul. *The Oxygen Breakthrough: 30 Days to an Illness Free Life* (New York: Simon & Schuster, 1989).

Hillesum, Etty. *An Interrupted Life: The Diaries of Etty Hillesum 1941–1943* (New York: Washington Square, 1985).

"Information Sheet: Natural Gas," *Human Ecology Action League* (Atlanta, Sept. 1990).

Jaffe, Dennis. *Healing from Within* (New York: Simon & Schuster, 1988).

Jamplosky, Gerald. *Love is Letting Go of Fear* (New York: Bantam, 1981).

Johnson, Hillary. *Osler's Web* (New York: Crown, 1995).

Justice, Blair. *Who Gets Sick?* (Los Angeles: J. P. Tarcher, 1988).

Kaptchuk, Ted. *The Web that has No Weaver—Understanding Chinese Medicine* (New York: Congdon Weed, 1983).

Kjellstrom, Tord. "Health Hazards of the Environment: Measuring the Harm," *World Health* (Switzerland: World Health Organization, June 1988).

Knaster, Mirka. "Alternative Health's Answer People," *East West Journal* Mar. 1991: 48.

Krieger, D. *The Therapeutic Touch* (Englewood Cliffs: Prentice–Hall, 1979).

Lefferts, Lisa, and Stephen Schmidt. "Nutritional Action," Center for Science in the Public Interest, Human Ecology Action League, 17 Apr. 1990.

Leonard, Jim, and Phil Laut. *Rebirthing: The Science of Enjoying All of Your Life* (Cincinnati, 1983).

Levy, Emily, and Nancy Magidson. "Two Women Speak Out on E.I.," *Matrix* Feb. 1991: 7.

Lind-Kyle, Patt. *When Sleeping Beauty Wakes Up* (Portland: Swan-Raven, 1992).

McNamara, Rita. *Toward Balance: Psycho Physical Integration and Vibrational Therapy* (New York: Samuel Weiser, 1989).

Mamas, Michael. *Consciousness Unfolding* (San Diego: School of Enlightenment and Healing, 1996).

Mitchell, Stephen. *Tao Te Ching* (New York: Harper & Row, 1943).

Palmer, Harry. *Creativism: The Art of Living Deliberately* (Longwood: Star's Edge International, 1990).

Peck, M. Scott. *A World Waiting to Be Born* (New York: Bantam, 1993).

Pennington, M. Basil. *Thomas Merton Brother Monk: The Quest for True Freedom* (New York: Harper & Row, 1987).

Penzer, Victor. "Amalgam Toxicity: The Grand Deception," *International Journal of Orthodontics* 24 (Spring 1986): 21–24.

Potts, Eve, and Marion Morra. *Understanding Your Immune System* (New York: Avon, 1986).

Randolph, Theron. *Human Ecology and Susceptibility to the Chemical Environment* (Springfield: Charles C. Thomas, 1962).

Randolph, Theron, and R. M. Wisner. *Detoxification: Personal Survival in a Chemical World* (New York: HealthMed Inc., 1988).

Randolph, Theron, and R. M. Wisner. *Alternative Approaches to Allergies: The New Field of Clinical Ecology Unravels Environmental Causes of Mental and Physical Ills* (New York: Harper & Row, 1988).

Rea, W. J., R. R. Johnson, E. Fenyves, and J. Butler. "The Environmental Aspects of the Post Polio Syndrome," *The Journal: Birth Defects Original Article Series* 23 (1987): 173–181.

Register, Cheri. *Living with Chronic Illness* (New York: Macmillan Co., 1987).

Remington, Dennis, and Barbara Higa. *Back to Health: A Comprehensive Medical and Nutritional Yeast Control Program* (Salt Lake City: Vitality House International, 1989).

Rinpoche, Sogyal. *The Tibetan Book of Living and Dying* (San Francisco: HarperCollins, 1992).

Rose, Barbara. *Cleanliness is Godliness* (Birmingham: Purity, 1991).

Rosenbaum, Michael, and Murray Susser. *Solving the Puzzle of Chronic Fatigue Syndrome* (Tacoma: Life Sciences Press, 1992).

Rossman, Martin. *Healing Yourself* (New York: Pocket Books, 1987).

Rotz, Francine. "50 Ways to Better Women's Health," *East West: The Journal of Natural Health* Nov. 1990: 46–50.

Rousseau, David, W. J. Rea, and Jean Enwright. *Your Home, Your Health and Well Being* (Ann Arbor: Ten Speed, 1988).

Saplonsky, Robert. *Why Zebras Don't Get Ulcers* (San Francisco: Freeman, 1994).

Selby, John. *Immune System Activation: Practical Programs for Maximizing Your Recovery Potential* (New York: E. P. Dutton, 1989).

Siegel, Bernie. *Peace Love and Healing: Body Mind Communication and the Path to Self Healing: An Exploration* (New York: Harper & Row, 1989).

Skrabanek, Peter, and James McCormick. *Follies and Fallacies in Medicine* (Buffalo: Prometheus, 1990).

Slomski, Anita. "Is Your Home Poisoning You?" *Consumer Digest* Sept.–Oct. 1989: 65.

Solomon, Neil. *Sick and Tired of Being Sick and Tired* (New York: Wynwood, 1989).

South, James. "The Liver, Master Organ for Optimal Nutrition," *Optimal Nutritional Health Review* 1.31 (July 1989).

Stoff, Jesse, and Charles Pellegrino. *Chronic Fatigue Syndrome: The Hidden Epidemic* (New York: Random House, 1988).

Trungpa, Chogyam. *Shambala: The Sacred Path of the Warrior* (New York: Bantam, 1986).

Tulku, Tarthang. *Gesture of Balance* (Berkeley: Dharma Publishers, 1982).

Vanauken, Sheldon. *A Severe Mercy* (New York: Harper & Row, 1977).

Weil, Andrew. *Health and Healing: Understanding Conventional and Alternative Medicine* (Boston: Houghton Mifflin, 1983).

Weiner, Michael. *Maximum Immunity* (Boston: Houghton Mifflin, 1986).

Wilkinson, Steve. *Chronic Fatigue Syndrome: A Natural Guide to Healing* (New York: Sterling, 1990).

Williams, Linda. "Stalking a Shadowy Assailant," *Newsweek* 14 May 1990: 66.

Winslow, Ron. "Virus May Have a Role in Causing Chronic Fatigue," *The New York Times* Sept. 1991: B1, B2.

Zamm, Alfred, and Alfred Gannon. *Why Your House May Endanger Your Health* (New York: Simon & Schuster, 1980).

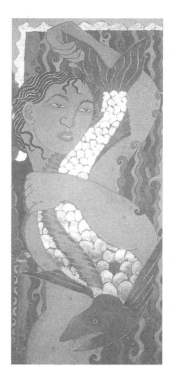

Glossary

Acid   A substance that yields hydrogen ions in a solution. A decrease in pH from a neutral reading indicates an acid state.

Acupressure   A practice similar to acupuncture that involves the application of manual pressure to parts of the body to treat imbalance and disease.

Acupuncture   The Chinese practice of puncturing the body with special needles to treat disease.

Adrenal   Either of a pair of endocrine glands lying immediately above the kidneys, consisting of an inner medulla, which produces epinephrine and norepinephrine, and an outer cortex, which produces a variety of steroid hormones.

Alkaline   An increase in bicarbonate, pH, and carbon dioxide combining power resulting in an increase in pH from a neutral reading.

Allergy   Hypersensitivity to a specific substance, such as a food, pollen, dust, or others. A condition that in similar amounts is harmless to most people, but in some manifests as a physical disorder.

Antibodies   Specialized protein molecules produced by certain lymphocytes capable of recognizing and neutralizing antigens.

Antigen   A protein, toxin, or other substance to which the body reacts by producing antibodies.

Antioxidant   A substance that opposes oxidation or inhibits reactions promoted by oxygen or peroxides. Some antioxidants are enzymes that donate electrons to free radicals, preventing further tissue damage.

Autoimmunity   Overactive immune response against the body's own tissues, which can damage normal, healthy parts of the body. Examples include EI, Hashimoto's thyroiditis, and rheumatoid arthritis.

B cells   Any of the lymphocytes that have immunoglobulin molecules on the surface and comprise the antibody-secreting plasma cells.

Basal body temperature   Body temperature that is measured when the body is in the lowest possible resting state. A measurement used to determine thyroid function, in which a lower than normal temperature is suggestive of hypothyroidism.

Bio-accumulation   The process whereby fat-soluble toxic chemicals become localized in fatty tissue.

Biofeedback   A therapeutically used form of meditation that teaches how to interrupt emotional or body conditions by consciously learning to modify autonomic body functions such as blood pressure or heart rate.

Bio-Magnetics   A simple, hands-on healing method that uses light touch directed to specific points to stimulate the body's ability to heal itself.

Brain-fogging   State marked by moodiness, confused thinking, inability to concentrate, and acute loss of memory.

Candida   Any of a genus of parasitic yeastlike imperfect fungi. Overgrowth of *Candida albicans* can lead to serious internal and chronic conditions.

Carbon monoxide   A colorless, odorless, highly poisonous gas that is produced by the incomplete combustion of carbonaceous materials.

Cell-mediated immunity   The portion of the immune system that is mediated by the T cells and is important in the defense against malignant cells, viral infection, fungal infection and some bacteria.

CFS   See Chronic fatigue syndrome.

Chronic fatigue syndrome   Illness whose hallmark is chronic debilitating fatigue that interferes with the ability to perform normal, everyday activities.

Clinical ecology   Study of the environmental causes of illness.

Cocoa Pulse Test   A pulse test used to determine which foods are prompting allergic reactivity.

Coenzyme Q10   Enzyme that is essential to the production of cellular energy.

Cranial–Sacral Therapy   A form of healing in which gentle pressure is applied to release energy trapped in the bones, membranes, and fluids.

Cytokines   Hormones produced by the immune cells intended to regulate the immune response. Symptoms of EI and CFS may result from overproduction of cytokines.

Dehydroepiandrosterone   Also known as DHEA, one of the steroid hormones produced by the adrenal gland that converts to other hormones.

Detoxification   Activities involved in assisting the body in the mobilization and excretion of toxins, with the net effect of reducing the burden to the immune system, thereby allowing greater health.

Digestive enzymes   Enzymes of the digestive system that break down proteins, carbohydrates, fats, and sugars in order to provide nourishment and energy for the body. These include lipase, protease, cellulase, lactose, and amylase.

Digestive system   The part of the body including the mouth, teeth, pharynx, esophagus, stomach, and intestines that converts food by the action of gastric and intestinal juices, enzymes, and bacteria into a form that can be absorbed by the body.

EI   See Environmental illness.

Electromagnetic radiation   The complete range of frequencies of electromagnetic waves, including radio, infrared, visible light, ultraviolet, X-ray, and gamma ray waves. These forms of radiation can influence human cellular activity and can be immunosuppressive.

Elimination diet   After restricting dietary intake for 7 days, foods are reintroduced one at a time to determine which ones cause allergic reactions.

Endocrine system   The glands that regulate body activity by producing hormones, including the pituitary, thyroid, thymus, adrenals, pineal, pancreas, and sex glands; the testes; and the ovaries.

Environmental illness   An illness in which individuals are intolerant of foods, chemicals, and other natural or synthetic agents in the environment, being reactive to substances that are generally tolerated by the majority of the population. This multisystem disorder can cause mild discomfort or total disability.

Eosinophil   A white blood cell that increases in number under certain allergic and parasitic conditions.

Fibromyalgia   A syndrome characterized by widespread pain (lasting over 3 months, on both sides of the body, and pain on manual palpation in 11 of 18 tender point sites) and aching muscles. Some believe this illness to be a variation of CFS.

Formaldehyde   A colorless gas; the most common indoor air contaminant.

Free radicals   An atom or molecule that has at least one unpaired electron, causing it to be unstable and therefore causing damage to human cells and impairing the body's ability to fight illness.

Gallbladder   A sac connected by various ducts to the liver, in which excess gall or bile is stored and concentrated.

Grief   A natural, healthy reaction to loss that sometimes manifests as intense emotional suffering.

Hashimoto's thyroiditis   An autoimmune disorder characterized by autoantibodies to thyroglobulin, the microbes of thyroid epithelial cells.

"Healing crisis"   The exacerbation of symptoms while the body is ridding itself of accumulated toxic substances. In this temporary state, the individual can feel worse in the process of becoming well.

Heavy metals   Substances such as cadmium, lead, mercury, and aluminum that can be absorbed by the body and reduce immune capability.

Homeopathy Therapeutic system of medicine, developed by Samuel Hahnemann, based on the "law of similars," that a causative substance administered in minute doses will stimulate the body's natural defenses in order to return the person to health.

Humoral immunity The portion of the immune system that is mediated by antibodies produced by B cells.

Immune system A complex system that protects the body from infection and abnormal growth and acts to neutralize poisons, thereby aiding in the body's defense against disease.

Leukocyte See White blood cell.

Light therapy The use of full-spectrum light to produce healing on both mental and physical levels. It has been demonstrated to have a positive impact on people with immune illnesses such as CFS, AIDS, Gulf War syndrome, cancer, and leukemia.

Liver The major organ of detoxification; works to break down toxins into metabolites and harmless waste chemicals.

Lymphocytes Leukocytes that are found in lymphatic tissue and the whole blood circulatory pool; important in the synthesis of antibodies.

Macrophage A large phagocytic cell found in connective tissue, lymphatic tissue, bone marrow, etc.

MCS See Multiple chemical sensitivities.

ME See Myalgic encephalomyelitis.

Meditation The act of deep reflection, of clearing the mind in order to create stillness or relaxation; often a part of spiritual practice.

Mercury A toxic heavy metal commonly found in dental amalgam fillings that can cause mutagenic effects and suppression of immune response. Capable of causing allergic reactivity when present in the body in small amounts.

Mindfulness The act of being fully present and aware in each moment.

Mold Any fungus that produces a growth on the surface of organic matter; common in the presence of dampness and decay.

Monocytes A large white blood cell.

Multiple chemical sensitivities (MCS) Synonym for environmental illness.

Myalgic encephalomyelitis (ME) Synonym for chronic fatigue syndrome.

Natural gas A mixture of gaseous hydrocarbons, mainly methane, occurring naturally in the earth and used as a fuel. A major source of allergic reactivity for the chemically sensitive.

Natural killer cells Autonomous cells of the immune system that are able to detect cancerous and virus-infected cells and destroy them.

Negative ions An electrically charged atom or group of atoms that have excess electrons. The oceans and forests have an abundance of negative ions.

Neurally mediated hypotention   A state that results when the autonomic nervous system misinterprets the body's needs, causing a reduction in heart rate and blood pressure when the opposite is what is actually needed.

Neutrophil   A phagocytic white blood cell.

NK cells   See Natural killer cells.

Outgas   Release of gases from a solid material.

Ozone   An unstable gas with an acrid odor that is formed by electrical discharge in air and used as an oxidizing, deodorizing, and bleaching agent.

Pancreas   An elongated gland located behind the stomach that secretes a digestive juice, pancreatic juice, into the small intestine and that contains groups of cells that produce the hormone insulin.

Parasite   Any one of a number of organisms that lives on or in a host from which it derives sustenance or protection without benefit to, and usually with harmful effects on, the host. Viruses are sometimes considered to be parasites.

Pesticides   Any chemical used to kill weeds and insects; often highly toxic to the human body.

Phagocytes   Any cell, but particularly leukocytes that ingest and destroy other cells.

Phobia   An excessive, persistent fear of a particular thing or situation. The purpose of the fear may be to warn and protect against danger.

Pineal   A gland located in the brain that produces the hormone melatonin.

Pituitary   The master gland of the endocrine system, which secretes hormones influencing growth and metabolism and controls the hormone production of other glands.

Positive ions   An electrically charged atom or group of atoms that are missing an electron, making them unstable. Positive ions are abundant in closed ventilation buildings and auto exhaust and in the presence of synthetic materials.

Psychoneuroimmunology   A science that holds that everything is linked and that emotions and emotional states impact physical health.

Radionics   A branch of esoteric science that works to psychically diagnose human energy imbalances using instrumentation in the form of a "black box."

Reflexology   A combination of massage and acupressure that holds that specific places on the hands and feet correspond to certain body parts; when those areas are stimulated, there is a beneficial impact on the corresponding part of the body.

Reiki   A form of hands-on energetic healing that can be useful in healing and energizing the body.

Secondary gains   The hidden benefits of a situation that on the surface seems to have only detrimental effects.

Sound healing   Use of sound to heal the body.

Stress   A force, external or internal, that causes mental or physical strain.

T cells   Any of the lymphocytes that are affected by the thymus and are engaged in the rejection of foreign tissue, regulation of cellular immunity, and controlling production of antibodies in the presence of an antigen. Types include T helper, T killer, and T memory cells.

Thymus   A two-lobed, ductless gland situated behind the upper part of the sternum and extending into the neck, involved in the production of lymphocytes.

Thyroid   A ductless gland lying in front and on either side of the trachea that secretes hormones that regulate body growth and metabolism. It also serves as a storehouse for iodine.

Thyroiditis   Inflammation of the thyroid gland.

Toxins   Poisonous manmade compounds, or those occurring in nature or found in the body in the form of microorganisms that have an adverse impact on immune function.

Twelve-Point Recovery Plan   Twelve interventions that can support EI and CFS sufferers in their return to health.

"Universal reactors"   Individuals who react to everything, including substances considered benign; they display the phenomenon of intense allergic reactivity.

Visualization   The use of specific mental images in a directed manner in order to heal the body, mind, or spirit.

White blood cell   A blood cell that is important in the body's defenses against infection. Types include lymphocytes, monocytes, macrophages, neutrophils, basophils, and eosinophils.

Whole live foods   Raw, organic, unprocessed foods including vegetables, fruits, germinated seeds and nuts, grains, sea vegetables, and freshly made juices. Such sources are enzyme rich, offering greater life energy.

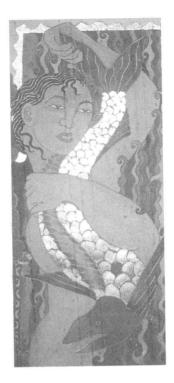

Index

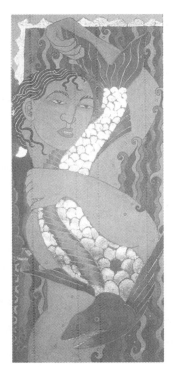

About the Author

*t*he author is a writer, healer, and registered nurse who became ill with EI and CFS in 1983. For years illness was the hallmark of her existence. Her life began for the second time in 1989 when she nearly died as a result of surgical complications, an experience that, surprisingly enough, enabled her to create a totally new relationship with life. Until then, her premise about healing had to do with fixing her body, thinking that once she became well her life would start anew.

Nearly dying woke her up to see that she could choose to live life fully, despite the experience of ongoing illness. Today she is mostly well, but still works day to day, continuing to make gains on all levels of mind, body, and spirit. For her, illness has been a catalyst for change which has prompted her to develop an intense hunger to deepen the process of her own healing. Working as a mental health crisis specialist, writer, and in private practice, she lives in Santa Cruz, California, with her husband John and three hilarious cats. For information regarding her work, send a self-addressed stamped envelope to: Janice Strubbe Wittenberg, P.O. Box 272, Capitola, CA 95010, contact her on the Internet at wittnbrg@cruzio.com, or visit the Web-site http://members.cruzio.com./~ johnw.